Case Studies in Urologic Disorders

Case Studies in Urologic Disorders

Editor: Adrian Price

AMERICAN
MEDICAL PUBLISHERS
www.americanmedicalpublishers.com

AMERICAN
MEDICAL PUBLISHERS
www.americanmedicalpublishers.com

Cataloging-in-Publication Data

Case studies in urologic disorders / edited by Adrian Price.
p. cm.
Includes bibliographical references and index.
ISBN 979-8-88740-617-6
1. Urinary organs--Diseases. 2. Urinary organs--Diseases--Treatment.
3. Urinary organs--Diseases--Diagnosis. 4. Urology. I. Price, Adrian
RC900 .C55 2023
616.6--dc23

American Medical Publishers,
41 Flatbush Avenue,
1st Floor, New York,
NY 11217, USA

ISBN 979-8-88740-617-6 (Hardback)

Contents

Preface

I am honored to present to you this unique book which encompasses the most up-to-date data in the field. I was extremely pleased to get this opportunity of editing the work of experts from across the globe. I have also written papers in this field and researched the various aspects revolving around the progress of the discipline. I have tried to unify my knowledge along with that of stalwarts from every corner of the world, to produce a text which not only benefits the readers but also facilitates the growth of the field.

Urologic disorders encompass a wide range of conditions that affect the urinary system and the male reproductive organs. The urinary system consists of the kidneys, ureters, bladder and urethra, while the male reproductive organs include the testes, prostate gland and penis. A few of the common urologic disorders are kidney stones, urinary tract infections (UTIs), urinary incontinence, urinary retention, bladder and kidney cancers, prostate enlargement (benign prostatic hyperplasia), infertility, and sexually transmitted infections. Kidney stones are hard deposits that form in the kidneys and can cause severe pain when they pass through the urinary tract. UTIs occur when bacteria enter the urinary tract and cause infection. Its prominent symptoms are frequent urination, pain or burning during urination, and cloudy or bloody urine. This book brings forth some of the recent studies on the diagnosis and treatment of urological disorders. It will provide comprehensive knowledge to the readers.

Finally, I would like to thank all the contributing authors for their valuable time and contributions. This book would not have been possible without their efforts. I would also like to thank my friends and family for their constant support.

Editor

1

Case Report: Prolapsed Ureterocele—A Differential Diagnosis of Urethral Cists

Francisco Renan Doth Sales, Georgia Alexsandra Colantonio Dourado, Ana Carolina Montes Ribeiro, Humberto de Holanda Madeira Barros, David Sucupira Cristino, Antonio Augusto Guterres Castro, and Francisco José Cabral Mesquita

Department of Urology, Doctor Cesár Cals General Hospital, Fortaleza, Ceará, Brazil

Correspondence should be addressed to Francisco Renan Doth Sales; renandoth.rd@gmail.com

Academic Editor: Tun-Chieh Chen

Ureterocele is a cystic dilatation of submucosal distal ureter. It presents a higher incidence in infants and young children but is rare in adults. The urethral prolapse of ureterocele is extremely rare, and its clinical presentation includes vulvar mass, hematuria, and urinary tract dysfunction. We present a case of ureterocele prolapse in a 45-year-old woman who has a 3-day-evolution vulvar mass and intense urethral bleeding. The patient underwent armed cystoscopy and ureteroscopy, ureterocele resection, and biopsy. She evolved with good postoperative condition and was then discharged.

1. Introduction

Ureterocele is a cystic dilatation of submucosal distal ureter. This condition presents an incidence about 1/5000 to 1/12000 [1] and is higher in infants and young children and rare in adults and adolescents [2]. It is more frequent in women [1], and the presentation as urethral prolapse is extremely rare, appearing in only 5% of cases. [3] There are few cases in the literature presenting ureterocele prolapsed through the urethra, most of them in adult Caucasian women [3]. The diagnosis should be considered in young children presenting urinary tract infection in the first months after birth, Caucasian women with vulvar mass, urinary obstruction, and other urinary tract dysfunction associated [3].

2. Case Report

A 45-year-old patient, a menopausal woman, sought medical attention complaining of a "mass" in the genital region (Figure 1). She reported long-standing dyspareunia and a 3-day evolution of heaviness in the pelvis and the exteriorization of a "mass" in the vulvar region, associated with episodes of intense urethral bleeding. She noticed progressive change in the mucosal coloration, presented fever, and reduced urinary frequency and volume. She denied associated dysuria. Her previous pathological history includes dyslipidemia and an obstetric history of three vaginal deliveries and one miscarriage. The physical examination showed tachycardia, pallor, and a necrotic/hemorrhagic aspect of the cyst originating in the urethra, not showing correlation with the vagina. A transvaginal ultrasound was performed, showing a heterogeneous oval image, located in the vulvar region, visible on physical examination, with debris and septations in the center, measuring $4.7 \times 4.0 \times 3.1$ cm. She underwent armed cystoscopy and ureteroscopy in which there were no injuries in the urethra and no evidence of stenosis or diverticula. It was observed an ureterocele with necrotic area and dilated right ureteral ostium and ureter. There were no anomalies in the left ureteral ostium. The exam also showed bladder with sparse trabeculations. Therefore, it was decided to perform transurethral resection of ureterocele, bleeding point hemostasis, and biopsy of the mass. The procedure occurred without complications. Patient remained on a bladder catheter for 3 days after the procedure and evolved

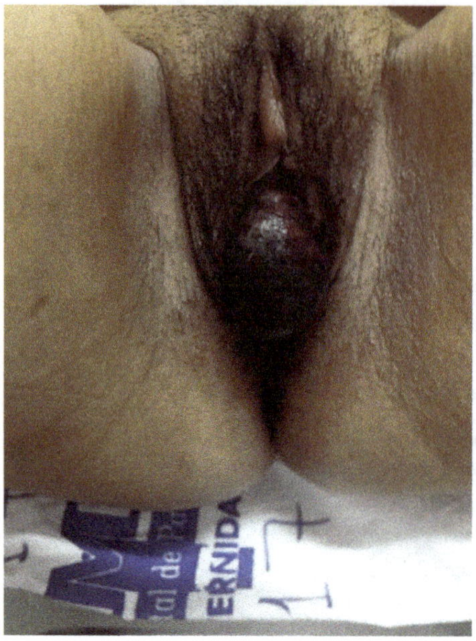

FIGURE 1: Necrotic mass in the vulvar region, requiring careful observation and examination to confirm urethral origin.

without hematuria. The histopathological report of the surgical specimen was compatible with urothelial mucosa fragments without atypia, granulation tissue in the lamina propria, and absence of signs of neoplasia or dysplasia. The patient evolved with good postoperative condition and was then was discharged on the fifth postoperative day, after antibiotic therapy with ceftriaxone and clindamycin. After the procedure, estrogen cream was oriented.

3. Discussion

The first ever reported case of prolapsed ureterocele was first described in 1982 in a 45-year-old female patient with a 2-month evolution of hesitancy, nocturia, and suprapubic discomfort, in addition to a swelling in her vulvar region. [4] That report leads other medical services to consider prolapsed ureterocele as a differential diagnosis to patients who present the same findings as this first one.

The most accepted theory of the origin of ureterocele is an embryogenesis failure in the canalization of the ureteral bud [5], which would explain the predominance of the disease in infants and even more in girls than in boys (7:1) [6]. There are few reported cases of ureterocele in adults, and the presentation of the disease prolapsing through the urethra is even more rare [3]. Therefore, once presenting urinary complaints, a female middle-aged patient should exclude other differential diagnosis before confirming prolapsed ureterocele.

As many reports showed, including ours, the symptoms have a quick evolution, from days to months [1–4, 7–9], and are summed up on urinary symptoms (poor urinary stream, dysuria, infection, and bleeding) and the feeling or the appearance of a mass through the urethra [8]. Considering that, one of the first pathologies to discard is urethral diverticulum. Its incidence varies to 0,6%-5% [10] and is most common in middle-aged females whom had previous obstetric trauma or frequent urethral infection [6]. Its symptoms include lower urinary tract disorder, dyspareunia, post-micturition dribbling and purulent urethral discharge (this last one being pathognomonic of urethral diverticulum, which can help us to distinguish the pathologies) [6, 11]. The diagnosis is basically considering the history and performing cystourethroscopy and urethrography [11].

Another differential diagnosis is pelvic organ prolapses (POP), which is a "herniated vagina" containing one pelvic organ (bladder, rectum, or uterus) [12]. Although the urinary symptoms in the POPs are similar to the prolapsed ureterocele, such as sensation of heaviness in the pelvis, urinary urgency or frequency, voiding dysfunction, and others [13], we can distinguish from prolapsed ureterocele observing the prolapse from the vagina, not from the urethra, through pelvic examination with a Sims' speculum or a bivalve speculum [13].

References

[1] W. L. M. Robson, M. A. Thomason, R. W. Newell, R. S. Abrams, and M. W. L. Gauderer, "Picture of the month," *Archives of Pediatrics & Adolescent Medicine*, vol. 151, no. 1, pp. 95-96, 1997.

[2] S. C. Pike, M. P. Cain, and R. C. Rink, "Ureterocele prolapse—rare presentation in an adolescent girl," *Urology*, vol. 57, no. 3, p. 554, 2001.

[3] M. L. Fernández, J. U. Fernández, and F. M. Madrid, "Ureterocele prolapsado: un diagnóstico para tener en cuenta ante una masa vulvar en una lactante. A propósito de un caso," *Archivos Argentinos de Pediatría*, vol. 115, no. 1, pp. e43–e46, 2017.

[4] T. Moore, "Orthotopic ureterocele presenting as swelling at the external urinary meatus," *British Journal of Urology*, vol. 54, no. 2, pp. 197–197, 1982.

[5] E. A. Tanagho, "Embryologic basis for lower ureteral anomalies: a hypothesis," *Urology*, vol. 7, no. 5, pp. 451–464, 1976.

[6] SMITH, *Urologia Geral*, Tanagho & Mcaninch, 17th edition, 2010.

[7] L. K. Sahu and R. Mohanty, "Prolapsed ureterocele presenting as a vulval mass in a woman," *The Journal of Urology*, vol. 138, no. 1, p. 136, 1987.

[8] L. Anveden-Hertzberg, M. W. L. Gauderer, and J. S. Elder, "Urethral prolapse: an often misdiagnosed cause of urogenital bleeding in girls," *Pediatric Emergency Care*, vol. 11, no. 4, pp. 212–214, 1995.

[9] M. A. W. Miller, A. J. Cornaby, M. S. Nathan, A. Pope, and R. J. Morgan, "Prolapsed ureterocele: a rare vulval mass," *British Journal of Urology*, vol. 73, no. 1, pp. 109-110, 1994.

[10] M. J. F. Andersen, "The incidence of diverticula in the female urethra," *The Journal of Urology*, vol. 98, no. 1, pp. 96–98, 1967.

[11] B. L. Davis and D. G. Robinson, "Diverticula of the female urethra: assay of 120 cases," *The Journal of Urology*, vol. 104, no. 6, pp. 850–853, 1970.

[12] W. Horst, J. B. do Valle, J. C. Silva, and C. L. L. Gascho, "Pelvic organ prolapse: prevalence and risk factors in a Brazilian population," *International Urogynecology Journal*, vol. 28, no. 8, pp. 1165–1170, 2017.

[13] J. E. Jelovsek, C. Maher, and M. D. Barber, "Pelvic organ prolapse," *The Lancet*, vol. 369, no. 9566, pp. 1027–1038, 2007.

2

Persistent Müllerian Duct Syndrome: Understanding the Challenges

Irene Chua[1] **and Naeem Samnakay**[1,2]

[1]Department of Paediatric Surgery, Perth Children's Hospital, Western Australia, Australia
[2]Division of Surgery, Medical School, The University of Western Australia, Western Australia, Australia

Correspondence should be addressed to Naeem Samnakay; naeem_samnakay@hotmail.com

Academic Editor: Walid Farhat

Persistent Müllerian duct syndrome (PMDS) is a rare autosomal recessive condition defined by the presence of Müllerian duct-derived structures in an otherwise normally masculinized phenotypical and genotypical (46,XY) male. We describe the case of an infant diagnosed with PMDS, managed and followed up for 7 years. The diagnosis of PMDS was made at laparoscopy at 6 months of age for investigation and management of bilateral impalpable testes. A Müllerian structure resembling a uterus with bilateral fallopian tube-like structures was seen in the pelvis, along with bilateral intra-abdominal testes. Gonadal biopsy confirmed normal testicular tissue. The child underwent successful bilateral two-stage Fowler-Stephens orchidopexies. The Müllerian remnant was preserved to maintain testicular vascularity. At the most recent follow-up, the testes are intrascrotal and normal on palpation. There have been no clinical symptoms or concerns with the Müllerian remnant during surveillance with ultrasound and MRI. To date, there are less than 300 cases described in the medical literature, with limited consensus on management. We reflect on challenges the condition poses, including fertility preservation in PMDS, testicular and Müllerian malignancy risk in PMDS, and optimal management and surveillance of PMDS.

1. Introduction

Persistent Müllerian duct syndrome (PMDS) is a rare genetic condition defined by the presence of Müllerian duct-derived structures (fallopian tubes, uterus, and upper vagina) in an otherwise normally masculinized phenotypical and genotypical (46,XY) male. Accurate incidence remains largely unknown. There are less than 300 cases described in the medical literature, with various management options for the condition described [1–3]. In this paper, we present a case of PMDS diagnosed and managed in infancy, with follow-up over a 7-year period. We review the current up-to-date evidence for the management of PMDS and reflect on challenges the condition poses.

2. Case Presentation

A healthy, first-born 6-month-old male infant was referred by a pediatrician for the management of bilateral impalpable testes. The infant was born at term, with no significant family history or consanguinity between parents. On examination, he was noted to have a normal penis with complete prepuce and glanular urethral meatus. The scrotum was well formed but empty. The testes were impalpable bilaterally. Initial ultrasound scan of the scrotum and pelvis did not identify the testes and did not detect any pelvic abnormality.

Diagnostic laparoscopy for impalpable testes at age 6 months revealed bilateral intra-abdominal testes, with normal and expected testicular structure and appearance. However, a Müllerian structure resembling the uterus, with bilateral fallopian tubes and round ligaments, was also noted. Vasa deferentia were clearly identified in close association with the fallopian-tube like structures (Figures 1(a) and 1(b)). A pole-to-pole gonadal biopsy was performed to assess gonadal histological structure. Cystourethroscopy did not reveal an obvious channel between the Müllerian structure and the urethra. Although PMDS was clinically suspected,

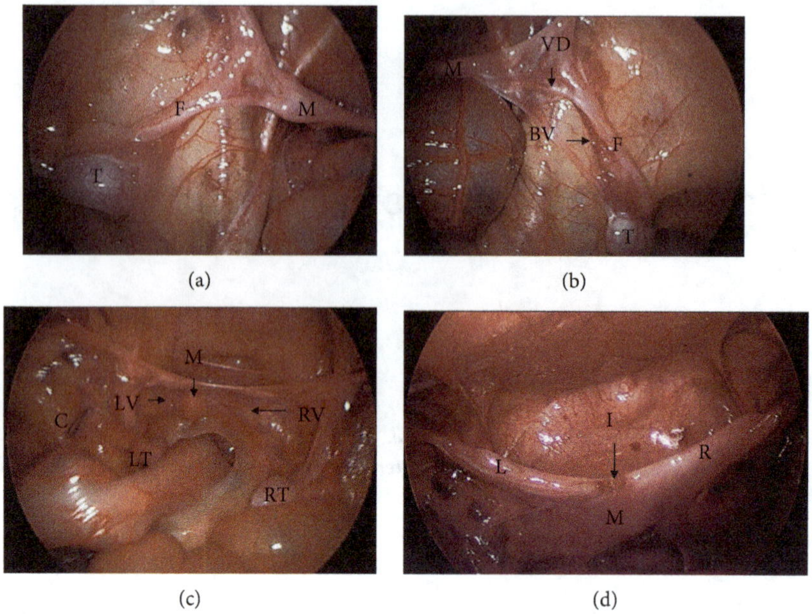

FIGURE 1: (a) Diagnostic laparoscopy showing the left testicle and fallopian tube-like structure. Key: M: persistent Müllerian duct structure; F: fallopian tube-like structure; T: left testicle. (b) The right testicle and fallopian tube-like structure. Key: M: persistent Müllerian duct structure; F: fallopian tube-like structure; T: right testicle; VD: right vas deferens closely associated with fallopian tube-like structure; BV: blood vessels along vas and fallopian tube-like structure. (c) Laparoscopic view showing completed first-stage FSO bilaterally. Key: M: persistent Müllerian duct structure; RV: right vas deferens; RT: right testis; LV: left vas deferens; LT: left testis; C: clips on the distal end of left gonadal vessels. (d) Laparoscopic view illustrating completed second-stage bilateral FSO. Small midline incision at the dome of persistent Müllerian duct structure was made to allow tension-free orchidopexy. Key: M: persistent Müllerian duct structure; I: midline incision in the Müllerian duct structure; R: right fallopian tube-like structure with associated vas and blood vessels exiting the abdominal wall; L: left fallopian tube-like structure with associated vas and blood vessels exiting the abdominal wall.

no further surgery was performed at this stage. Parents were counselled about the operative findings; results of gonadal biopsy, endocrine work-up, and karyotype were awaited.

Histology of bilateral gonadal biopsy showed normal testicular tissue. Sex-determining region (SRY) on the Y chromosome was present on fluorescence in situ hybridisation. 46,XY karyotype was confirmed. Hormonal studies revealed age-appropriate levels of luteinising hormone (LH), follicle stimulating hormone (FSH), and testosterone. Serum anti-Mullerian hormone (AMH) was normal for age (serum AMH level 526 pmol/L; normal range for <1 year old: 454-944 pmol/L). HCG stimulation test showed robust stimulation of testosterone production (baseline level was <1 nmol/L, and stimulated level 72 hours later was 18 nmol/L).

The child underwent a planned bilateral laparoscopic two-stage Fowler-Stephens orchidopexy (FSO). In order for sufficient mobility for the testes to be brought down, the limiting length of the gonadal vessels was divided (Figure 1(c)). The vasa and associated vasal vasculature ran in close association with the fallopian tube-like arms of the Müllerian structure (Figure 1(b)). The Müllerian structure was therefore left intact to limit any damage to the vas or vessels. A small midline longitudinal apical incision was made in the Mullerian structure to allow greater splay of the fallopian tube-like arms and facilitate tension free orchidopexy (Figure 1(d)). Both intra-abdominal testes were successfully moved to an intrascrotal position with the vasa and vasal blood supply intact.

The child has had annual follow-up with pelvic and scrotal surveillance ultrasound for seven years, plus a pelvic baseline MRI at age six. The Müllerian structure has remained small and stable on ultrasound follow-up (Figure 2). The testes are both intrascrotal and normal in structure and volume for age. On MRI of the pelvis, the Müllerian remnant was well visualised and small (Figure 3). Further periodic surveillance, MRI would be a useful adjunct to annual USS surveillance. The child has not had any urological symptoms relating to the Müllerian structure, such as epididymitis, urinary tract infection, or urinary incontinence.

3. Discussion

First described in the literature in 1939 by Nilson [4], PMDS is a rare disorder of internal male sex development, with persistence of Müllerian duct-derived structures in addition to Wolffian duct-derived structures. PMDS is transmitted as an autosomal recessive condition [3]. It may also occur as a sporadic *de novo* mutation.

Sexual dimorphism, although determined genetically at the time of fertilisation, does not occur until the seventh week of embryological development. Initially, the embryo possesses two pairs of genetic ducts, the Wolffian and Müllerian ducts. The presence of SRY on the Y chromosome leads to differentiation of the primordial gonad into testis. The process of male sex development depends on

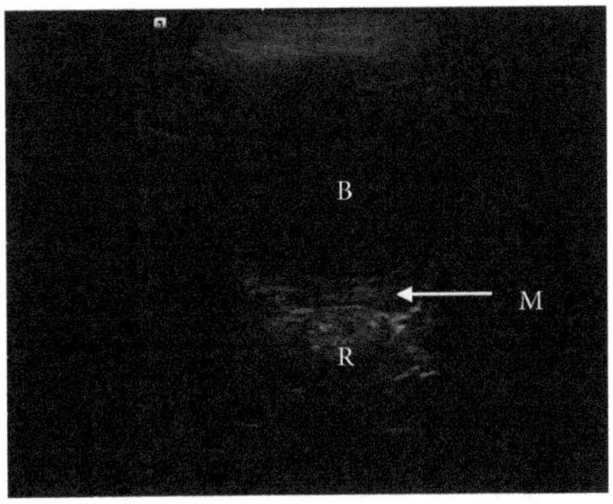

FIGURE 2: Müllerian remnant viewed on surveillance pelvic ultrasound scan. Key: M: Müllerian remnant; B: bladder; R: rectum.

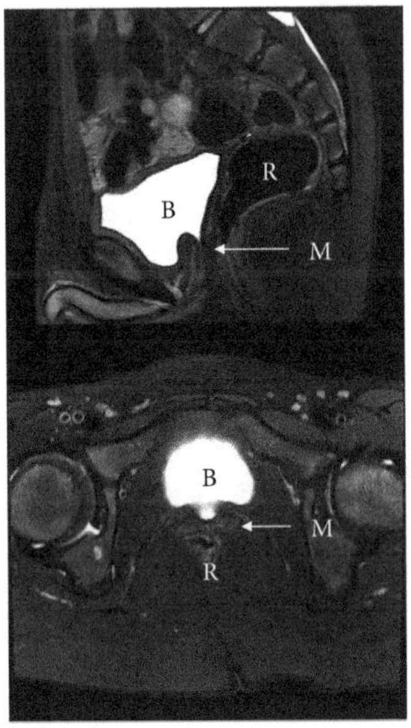

FIGURE 3: Magnetic resonance imaging (MRI) sagittal and axial views showing Müllerian remnant. Key: M: Müllerian remnant; B: bladder; R: rectum.

testosterone, dihydrotestosterone, and anti-Müllerian hormone (AMH) [5]. At the end of the seventh gestational week, AMH is produced by fetal Sertoli cells. This leads to the regression of the Müllerian duct and its derivatives. Failure to do so leads the Müllerian duct to differentiate into uterus, fallopian tubes, and upper vagina. In addition, the presence of Leydig cells results in the secretion of testosterone, which directs localised differentiation of Wolffian duct structures including the epididymis, vas deferens, seminal vesicles, and ejaculatory ducts.

It is a defect in AMH or AMH receptors which results in the manifestation of PMDS. It is estimated that 85% of cases of PMDS occur because of a mutation in either the AMH synthesis gene on chromosome 19 (type I PMDS, 45%) or a defect in the AMH receptor (AMHR) gene on chromosome 12 (type II PMDS, 40%) [6, 7]. In the remaining, the cause for PMDS is unknown (idiopathic PMDS). In our described case, serum AMH levels were normal, suggesting a likely AMHR mutation as the underlying aetiology. Genetic testing to clarify the likely molecular aetiology has not been performed as yet but is an important consideration.

The defect results in the coexistence of both Wolffian and Müllerian duct structures in a phenotypic male, as external virilisation is complete due to the presence of testosterone.

PMDS usually presents incidentally in a male presenting with cryptorchid testes or inguinal hernia in childhood or sometimes in adulthood or testicular tumor or abdominal mass in adulthood [3, 8, 9].

PMDS is classified based on the location of testes and Müllerian structures. There are three clinical anatomical variants described in the literature (Figure 4).

PMDS-female type (FT). This is the most common type reported in the literature (Figure 4(a)). In FT PMDS, both testes are intra-abdominal, in the ovarian position, with the vasa and associated vasculature closely applied to the fallopian tube-like structures. Gonadal biopsy usually demonstrates normal testicular structure on histology. Our described case had FT PMDS.

In children, preservation of fertility potential and hormonal function should be an overriding aim. Gonadal malignancy risk reduction should be maximised by early orchidopexy, as for any child with intra-abdominal testes.

PMDS-hernia uteri inguinale (HUI). This is the next most commonly reported variant (Figure 4(b)). It is also known as male-type PMDS. HUI usually presents with an ipsilateral hernia with ipsilateral descended testis and Müllerian structures within the hernia. The contralateral testis is usually undescended or intraabdominal.

PMDS-transverse testicular ectopia (TTE). This is considered the rarest type of PMDS (Figure 4(c)). Both testes and the Müllerian structures are herniated into one hemiscrotum [10, 11]. Not all cases of TTE are associated with PMDS. Type 1 TTE comprises up to 50% of cases, associated with inguinal hernia only. Type 2 TTE comprises up to 30% cases, associated with persistent Müllerian structures. Type 3 TTE is associated with other anomalies such as scrotal anomalies, hypospadias, fused vas deferens, and horseshoe kidney [12].

4. Clinical Management of PMDS in Children: Evidence and Challenges

The surgical management and subsequent follow-up of PMDS may not have conformity, but some important guiding principles are highlighted by reviewing the literature.

4.1. Principle 1: Recognition and Diagnosis of PMDS. With investigative laparoscopy for impalpable testes now commonplace, the recognition of FT PMDS in infancy has increased [3]. When both Müllerian and Wolffian structures are present together at laparoscopy, it is generally considered prudent to make a careful assessment for other possible variants or differences of sex development, such as gonadal dysgenesis. Mixed gonadal dysgenesis is unlikely in the presence of a normally formed penis. If there is any doubt, it is recommended to initially perform gonadal biopsies to confirm that they comprise testicular tissue. Gonadal biopsy

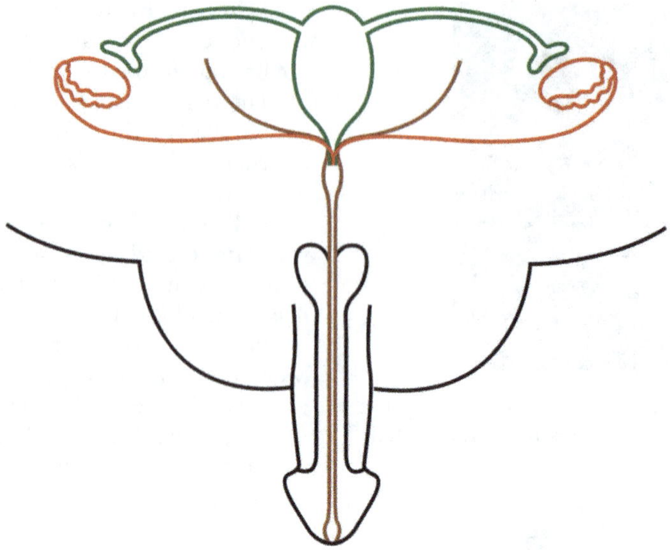

(a) Female type—bilateral intraabdominal testes in "ovarian" position

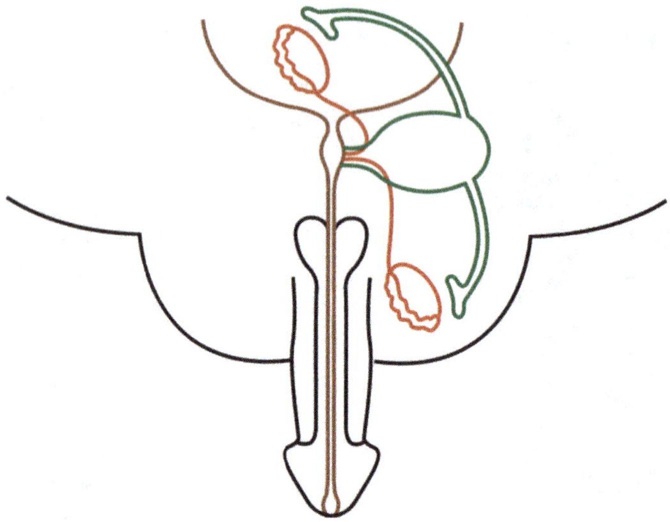

(b) Male type or "hernia uteri inguinale" type—one testis along with Müllerian remnant and Fallopian tube-like structure in the hernia sac

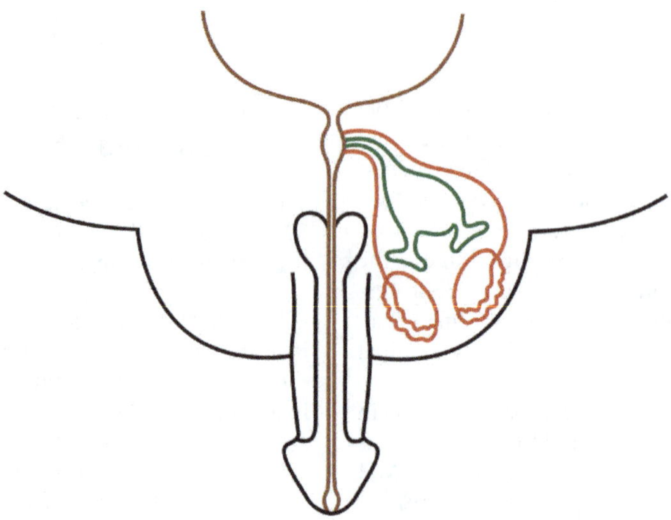

(c) Transverse testicular ectopia—both testes with Müllerian structures in one hemiscrotum

Figure 4: Three described anatomical variants of PMDS. Key: red: Wolffian structures plus testes; green: persistent Müllerian structures; brown: bladder and urethra.

and karyotype before proceeding to orchidopexy will help to give the family time to understand the condition, to get reassurance about the karyotype, and to get objective reassurance about the presence of normal testicular tissue.

HUI and TTE both commonly present with inguinal hernia. During hernia repair, the Müllerian structures are noted. In some cases, the Müllerian structures are left in situ to preserve testicular vascularity and ductal structures [13]; in other reports, the Mullerian structures are excised, especially in adults [12, 14]. In children with HUI, it is recommended that the cryptorchid contralateral testis undergo orchidopexy. In adults presenting with HUI, the undescended or intraabdominal testis is often excised due to concerns about malignancy risk.

In children with TTE, the testes can be placed in separate hemiscrota by transseptal orchidopexy [15].

4.2. Principle 2: Preserving Gonadal Function and Fertility Potential. The literature documents fertility impairment in adults with PMDS [3]; however, there are reports of fertility and paternity in men with PMDS, including in FT PMDS [3, 16–18].

It is not clear what contributes, and to what degree, to the reported fertility impairment—it may be due to uncorrected cryptorchidism, or due to coexisting congenital gonadal and Wolffian duct anomalies, or due to ischemic and structural damage to the vas and testis secondary to excision of Müllerian remnants.

In children with PMDS, the gonads show normal testicular tissue on biopsy but are undescended [2]. The benefit of early orchidopexy in potentiating fertility is well established in the literature for cryptorchidism in general [19]. Thus, for children with PMDS, early orchidopexy to place the testes into the scrotum is indicated. Care should be taken to maximise preservation of gonadal vascularity and limit any damage to Wolffian ductal structures during hernia repair, orchidopexy, and, if deemed necessary, excision of Müllerian structures. Priority should be given to gonadal preservation and successful orchidopexy. For example, in FT PMDS, if excision of the Müllerian remnant is considered likely to damage the vasal vessels supplying the testes or the vas and ductal structures, then it should preferably be left in situ and surveilled [13]. If despite sacrificing gonadal vessels, the descent of the testes is limited by the short length of the fallopian tubes, the literature describes dividing the main body of the Mullerian structure sagittally to allow lateral splitting of each half, thus giving extra length for testicular descent without compromising the vasa or testicular vasculature (Figure 1(d)) [20].

4.3. Principle 3: Reducing Future Gonadal Malignancy Risk. The reported incidence of malignant change in the testes in PMDS generally ranges from 5 to 18%, a rate which is similar to abdominal undescended testes in men without PMDS. However, some reviews suggest gonadal malignancy risk in PMDS is as high as 33% [3]. Seminomas are most commonly recorded, but other Germ cell neoplasia in situ-(GCNIS-) derived testicular tumours are also reported [3].

Orchidopexy early in childhood has been shown to reduce malignancy risk in cryptorchidism [19]. Early orchidopexy should be offered to children with PMDS.

4.4. Principle 4: Being Aware of the Risk of Malignancy in Müllerian Remnants. The rate of Müllerian malignancy in the literature ranges from 3.1% to 8.4% [3]. In one paper describing malignancies in Müllerian remnants, 3 of the 11 described malignancy cases qualified as having PMDS [1]. Described Müllerian malignancies in PMDS include adenocarcinomas and adenosarcoma [8].

The risk of Müllerian malignancy is generally considered lower than the risk of malignancy in the associated undescended testes. The age of documented Müllerian malignancy in PMDS ranges from as young as 4 years old to 68 years old [1]. How to manage this risk of malignancy remains unclear.

If the Müllerian remnant is left in situ, the literature advocates regular ultrasound surveillance, such as annually, to assess for change in size or new mass lesions [21]. Soft tissue MRI is also a useful modality to follow up with and assess for changes in the Müllerian remnant. At present, there is no data to suggest whether one modality is superior for surveillance purposes, and there is no data to guide the frequency of surveillance should it be undertaken. If a change is detected on surveillance, then appropriate intervention will need to be undertaken.

5. Conclusion

PMDS is a rare disorder of internal male sexual development. The main surgical considerations are repairing associated inguinal hernias; preserving gonadal function and fertility and minimising the risk of malignant change by early orchidopexy and careful preservation of gonadal vasculature and vasal and ductal structures; and long-term surveillance for potential malignancy in pexed testes and retained Müllerian structures.

Disclosure

An early version of this abstract was presented at the conjoined Asia Pacific Association of Paediatric Urology (APAPU) and Society of Pediatric Urology of New Zealand and Australia (SPUNZA) meeting in December 2019.

References

[1] J. Farikullah, S. Ehtisham, S. Nappo, L. Patel, and S. Hennayake, "Persistent Müllerian duct syndrome: lessons learned from managing a series of eight patients over a 10-year period and review of literature regarding malignant risk from the Müllerian remnants," *BJU international*, vol. 110, no. 11c, pp. E1084–E1089, 2012.

[2] M. M. Shalaby, A. Kurkar, M. A. Zarzour, A. A. Faddan, M. Khalil, and M. F. Abdelhafez, "The management of the persistent Müllerian duct syndrome," *Arab Journal of Urology*, vol. 12, no. 3, pp. 239–244, 2014.

[3] J. Y. Picard, R. L. Cate, C. Racine, and N. Josso, "The persistent Müllerian duct syndrome: an update based upon a personal experience of 157 cases," *Sexual Development*, vol. 11, no. 3, pp. 109–125, 2017.

[4] O. Nilson, "Hernia Uteri inguinalis bein Manne," *Acta Chir Scand*, vol. 83, pp. 231–249, 1939.

[5] A. Jost, "Problems of fetal endocrinology: the adrenal glands," *Recent Progress in Hormone Research*, vol. 22, pp. 541–574, 1966.

[6] O. Cohen-Haguenauer, J. Y. Picard, M. G. Mattei et al., "Mapping of the gene for anti-Müllerian hormone to the short arm of human chromosome 19," *Cytogenetics and Cell Genetics*, vol. 44, no. 1, pp. 2–6, 2004.

[7] S. Imbeaud, E. Faure, I. Lamarre et al., "Insensitivity to anti-Mullerian hormone due to a mutation in the human anti-Mullerian hormone receptor," *Nature Genetics*, vol. 11, no. 4, pp. 382–388, 1995.

[8] M. Saleem, U. Ather, B. Mirza et al., "Persistent mullerian duct syndrome: a 24-year experience," *Journal of Pediatric Surgery*, vol. 51, no. 10, pp. 1721–1724, 2016.

[9] A. Al-Asmar, A. Abu-Qamar, N. Al-Saidah, A. Al-Kaabneh, A. Al-Qaralleh, and A. Al-Hiari, "Persistant Mullerian duct syndrome with intra-abdominal seminoma," *Urology Case Reports*, vol. 33, p. 101342, 2020.

[10] M. Wuerstle, T. Lesser, R. Hurwitz, H. Applebaum, and S. L. Lee, "Persistent mullerian duct syndrome and transverse testicular ectopia: embryology, presentation, and management," *Journal of Pediatric Surgery*, vol. 42, no. 12, pp. 2116–2119, 2007.

[11] K. A. Deepika and A. Kumar, "Persistent mullerian duct syndrome with transverse testicular ectopia: rare entity," *Journal of Clinical and Diagnostic Research*, vol. 8, no. 3, pp. 162-163, 2014.

[12] G. Zhou, J. Yin, M. Jiang, Z. Yang, and S. Li, "Clinical characteristics, ultrasonographic findings, and treatment of pediatric transverse testicular ectopia: a 10-year retrospective review," *Urology*, vol. 154, pp. 249–254, 2021.

[13] D. R. Vandersteen, A. K. Chaumeton, K. Ireland, and E. S. Tank, "Surgical management of persistent mullerian duct syndrome," *Urology*, vol. 49, no. 6, pp. 941–945, 1997.

[14] M. U. Mukhtar, S. A. K. Niazi, M. Z. Sarwar, and S. A. Naqi, "Transverse testicular ectopia with persistent Mullerian duct syndrome: an operative eureka," *International Journal of Surgery Case Reports*, vol. 71, pp. 338–340, 2020.

[15] M. Arora, J. Kaur, and R. Kulshreshtha, "A rare case of transverse testicular ectopia," *Journal of Indian Association of Pediatric Surgeons*, vol. 24, no. 2, pp. 150-151, 2019.

[16] T. I. Farag, "Familial persistent Müllerian duct syndrome in Kuwait and neighboring populations," *American Journal of Medical Genetics*, vol. 47, no. 3, pp. 432–434, 1993.

[17] A. S. Agrawal and R. Kataria, "Persistent Müllerian duct syndrome (PMDS): a rare anomaly the general surgeon must know about," *The Indian Journal of Surgery*, vol. 77, no. 3, pp. 217–221, 2015.

[18] J. Modi, D. Modi, and L. Bachani, "Acute urinary retention caused by seminoma in a case of persistent Mullerian duct syndrome," *Indian Journal of Pathology & Microbiology*, vol. 58, no. 1, pp. 83–85, 2015.

[19] F. J. Schneuer, E. Milne, S. E. Jamieson et al., Association between male genital anomalies and adult male reproductive disorders: a population-based data linkage study spanning more than 40 years," *The Lancet Child & Adolescent Health*, vol. 2, no. 10, pp. 736–743, 2018.

[20] D. W. Brandli, C. Akbal, E. Eugsster, N. Hadad, R. J. Havlik, and M. Kaefer, "Persistent Mullerian duct syndrome with bilateral abdominal testis: surgical approach and review of the literature," *Journal of Pediatric Urology*, vol. 1, no. 6, pp. 423–427, 2005.

[21] S. Sancar, E. Ozcakir, and M. Kaya, "Management of the patients with persistent Müllerian duct syndrome: is the ultimate goal testicular descent?," *Turkish Journal of Urology*, vol. 44, no. 2, pp. 166–171, 2018.

3

Right Transverse Testicular Ectopia: A Nonclassified Variant Confirmed on Laparoscopy

Landry Mbouché,[1,2] E. Njuma Tamufor,[1] K. G. Fossi,[1] A. S. Salihou,[1] D. E. C. Dikongue,[1] Salihou Fadi,[1] Bienvenu Binwe,[1] and F. F. Mouafo Tambo[1,2]

[1]*Faculty of Medicine and Biomedical Sciences, University of Yaounde I, Cameroon*
[2]*Yaounde Gynaeco-Obstetric and Paediatric Hospital, Cameroon*

Correspondence should be addressed to Landry Mbouché; landrymbouche@gmail.com

Academic Editor: Walid Farhat

Transverse testicular ectopia is a rare anomaly characterized by testicular descent into the scrotum through the same inguinal canal. Here, we report the case of a 15-year-old boy diagnosed with transverse testicular ectopia wherein both testes descended through separate inguinal canals. He underwent a diagnostic laparoscopy which helped to identify both spermatic cords entering both inguinal canals separately. During scrotal exploration, both testes were found in the same side. Transseptal orchidopexy was performed. The short-term follow-up is uneventful.

1. Introduction

Ectopic testis is the migration of the testis away from its normal route of descent. The common sites for ectopic testes include the superficial inguinal pouch, femoral canal, perineum, pubopenile region, and opposite scrotum and is also called transverse testicular ectopia (TTE). The latter is a rare form of testicular ectopia wherein both testes descend along the same inguinal route and are found in the same hemiscrotum [1]. Following the first description by Von Lenhossek in 1886 [2], it has been reported in the literature in over a hundred cases as crossed testicular ectopia, pseudoduplication, unilateral double testes, transverse aberrant testicular maldescent, or transverse testicular ectopia [3] with patients' ages ranging from 3 days to 77 years [4]. These cases have been reported with various associated malformations. We present here the case of a 15-year-old boy with a transverse testicular ectopia. Laparoscopy and scrotal operation showed both spermatic cords entering their independent inguinal canals while the testes are located on the same side.

2. Case Presentation

We received a 15-year-old male at our outpatient consultation with complaints of an abnormal looking scrotum and a left scrotal swelling. He denied testicular pain. His past history was notable for the presence of this scrotal anomaly from birth with several consultations done in infancy and no definitive diagnosis nor management proposed. On examination, there was a vacant, hypoplastic right hemiscrotum with no palpable right testis along its normal course; a normal looking left hemiscrotum containing a testis; an ovoid shaped mass at the left suprascrotal area which was firm, nontender and not fixed to the deep or superficial plane (Figures 1 and 2). There was no hypogastric mass, no palpable kidney mass, and no disorder of sex development. The penis was uncircumcised.

An abdominal ultrasound found no renal anomalies, and description of the left suprapubic mass was inconclusive. A diagnostic laparoscopy was planned to explore the right testis and any anomaly. On laparoscopic evaluation under general anesthesia, the right spermatic vessels and vas were seen

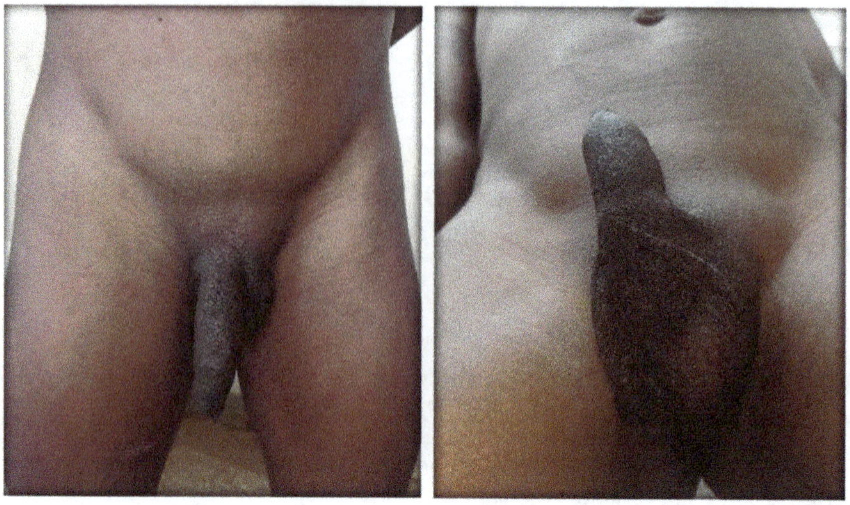

Figure 1: Patient in standing and lying positions showing hypoplasia of right hemiscrotum and left suprascrotal bulge.

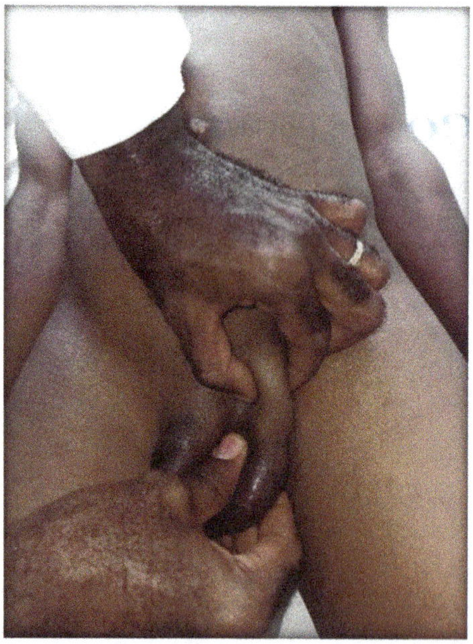

Figure 2: Examiner isolating two separate masses on the left path of testicular descent.

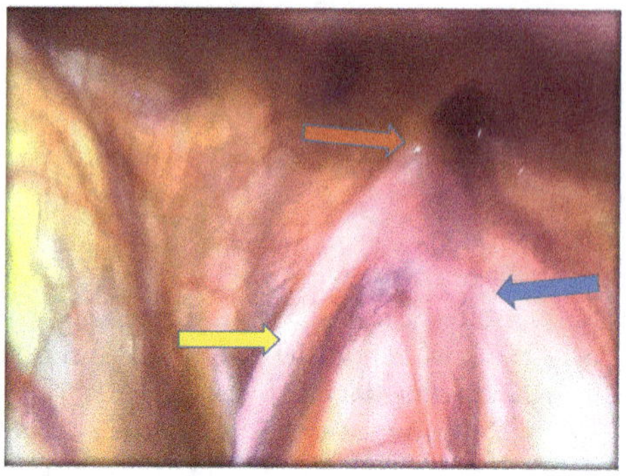

Figure 3: Laparoscopic view of the spermatic vessels (blue arrow) and vas deferens (yellow arrow) exiting the right "open" deep inguinal ring (red arrow).

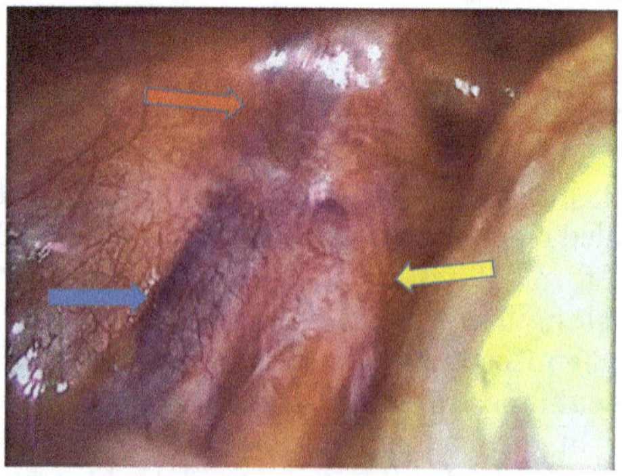

Figure 4: Laparoscopic view of the spermatic vessels (blue arrow) and vas deferens (yellow arrow) exiting the left "closed" deep inguinal ring (red arrow).

going through an open right deep inguinal ring (Figure 3). The spermatic vessels and vas on the left were seen traversing their corresponding closed deep inguinal ring (Figure 4). There were no Müllerian remnants. To identify the origin of the two left-sided scrotal masses during laparoscopy, the lowermost intrascrotal mass was tugged and the effect was seen at the right deep inguinal ring. Meanwhile, tugging of the higher-placed suprascrotal mass resulted in denting of the left deep inguinal ring structures with no effect on the right deep inguinal ring.

A scrototomy through a median raphe incision was made. The lowermost testis was easily dissected and its cord traced to the right side passing front of the root of the penis. The higher placed testis' dissection was more laborious with adhesions and an inflammatory tunica. Both testis appeared macroscopically normal with no epididymotesticular fusion anomaly and unfused vasa deferentia (Figure 5). A right inguinal exploration found a patent processus vaginalis which was transected and closed at the deep ring. Transseptal orchidopexy was undertaken for the right testis with its longer cord length (Figure 6), and an ipsilateral orchidopexy was done for the nondescended suprascrotal left testis

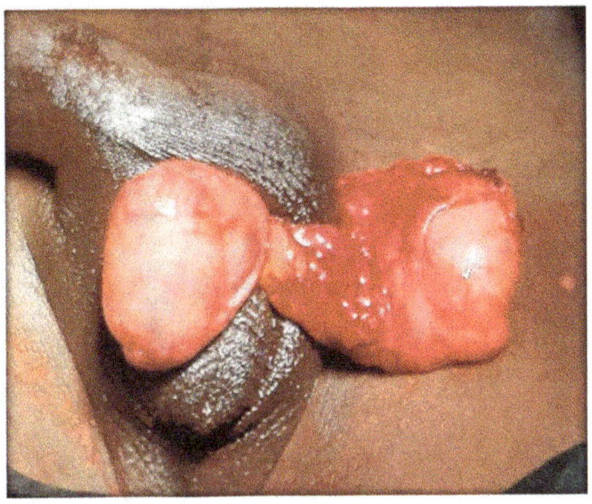

(a)

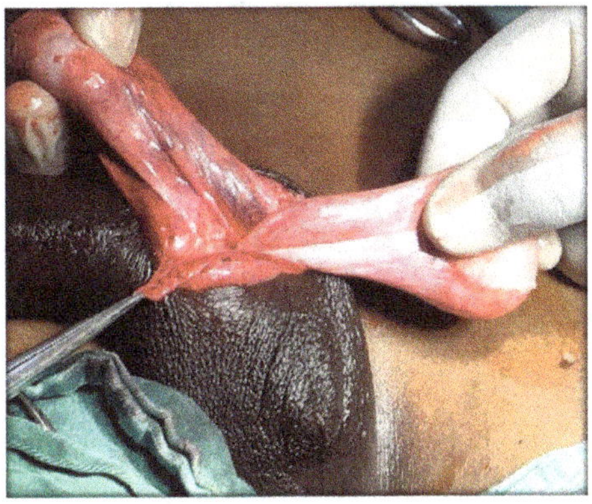

(b)

FIGURE 5: (a) Left and right testes shown through a median raphe scrototomy looking macroscopically normal. (b) No fusion of vessels nor vasa, nor epididymotesticular separation.

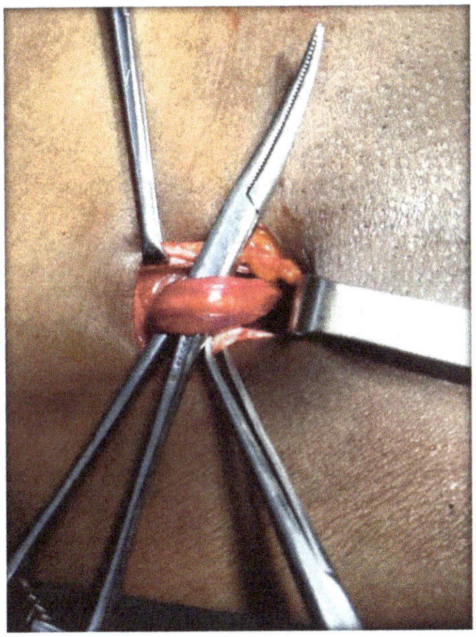

(a)

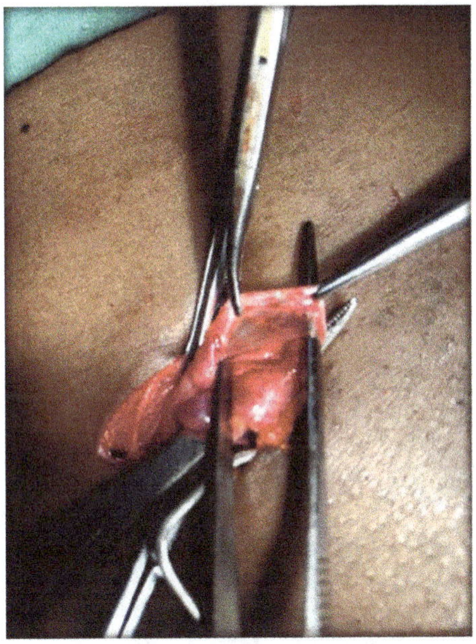

(b)

FIGURE 6: (a) Right inguinal dissection. (b) Closure of a right patent processus vaginalis.

(Figure 7). Circumcision was done. The early postoperative period was uneventful with mild tenderness on palpation and a full-looking scrotum (Figures 8 and 9).

3. Discussion

Some theories have been postulated to explain this singular anomaly of testicular descent which vary depending on the presentation and associated anomalies. A faulty development of both testes on the same side was proposed by Lenhossek and later Berg [5]. Kimura [6] concluded that if both vasa deferentia arose from one side, there had been unilateral origin but if there was bilateral origin, one testis had crossed over due to some compression force. Gupta and Das [7] postulated that adherence and fusion of the developing Wolffian ducts took place early and that descent of one testis caused the second one to follow. This has been referred to as mechanical hindrance by Chacko and colleagues [8]. Defective implantation of the gubernaculum or an obstruction of the inguinal canal preventing testicular descent on the ipsilateral side was confirmed on rat models [9]. The presence of Müllerian structures in persistent Müllerian duct syndrome (PMDS) may bind to vasa and affect their descent [10, 11].

The spectrum of associated clinical findings most commonly includes ipsilateral inguinal hernia, hypospadias, PMDS, disorder of sex differentiation (DSD), fusion of vas deferens, seminal vesicle cysts, renal agenesis, and scrotal abnormalities [12, 13]. The classification proposed by Gauderer et al. [14] is based on the presence of associated abnormalities: Type 1, the most common type (40-50%) is associated with ipsilateral inguinal hernia alone; Type 2 (30%) is associated with persistent Müllerian duct structures; and Type 3 (20%) is associated with other genitourinary

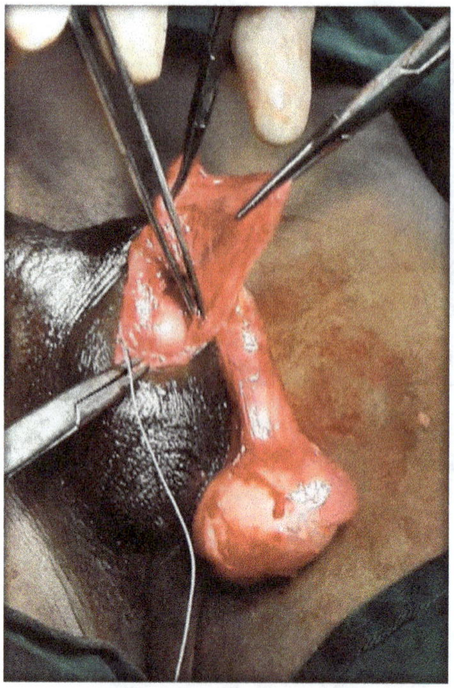

FIGURE 7: Transseptal orchidopexy of the right testis and closure of the scrotal septum.

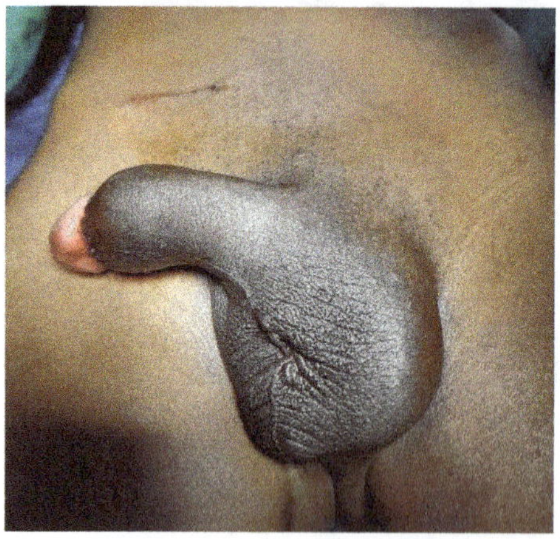

FIGURE 8: Final aspect after bilateral orchidopexy and routine circumcision.

abnormalities without Müllerian remnants. We present a form of TTE wherein the spermatic cords go through their individual inguinal canals to end up in the same hemiscrotum. In our case, the right testis probably reached the contralateral scrotum first and acted as an obstacle to the normal descent of the left testis into its scrotal sac. A similar anatomic configuration has been described previously involving the left testicle [1].

The diagnosis was confirmed by laparoscopic visualization of cord structures passing through their separate deep inguinal rings, respectively. The left internal inguinal ring was closed but the right deep inguinal ring was open. This underscores the importance of laparoscopic exploration as a diagnostic modality to investigate undescended nonpalpable testes in place of other imaging like magnetic resonance imaging, ultrasonography, and computed tomography [15–17] which may describe some of the abnormalities associated with TTE.

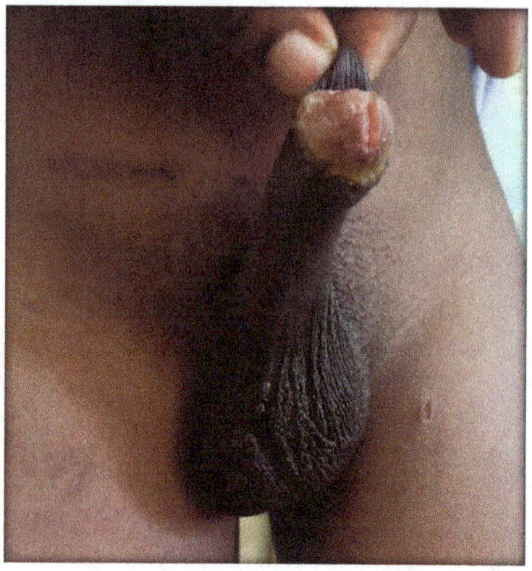

FIGURE 9: Scrotal aspect on day 5 postoperative.

The management goals are fixation of the testes, search for Müllerian duct remnants, and long-term follow-up for malignancy and fertility [18]. The overall incidence of malignant transformation of gonads is 18% [19]. There is no formal consensus on the management due to the rarity of the pathology and its varied presentation [20]. Nonetheless, algorithms based on extensive dissection of the cord [21] or none at all [22] have been proposed to guide management after intraoperative findings. Still, some authors advocate complete dissection to individualize the testes and spermatic cords with transseptal or extraperitoneal orchidopexy through an inguinal or scrotal approach [18]. Laparoscopic surgery with or without inguinal exploration has been described for management of TTE and associated anomalies in staged or single procedures [23, 24]. We used laparoscopy for diagnosis and then a scrotal approach to explore the left hemiscrotum and successfully placed both testes in separate scrotal compartments through a transseptal orchidopexy. There was no need for an ipsilateral inguinal incision because deep inguinal ring was closed on laparoscopic exploration. The follow-up will be ensured by regular examination of the testis through physical examination and ultrasound.

4. Conclusion

Nonpalpable testis in a child associated with contralateral full scrotum should lead to researching all potential sites of testicular ectopy. Laparoscopy should be privileged in the exploration as it can identify the paths of the different cords and avoid additional dissection. A new classification and consensus in the management of transverse testicular ectopy could be considered with regard to the variant form presented. In early or late presentation, a follow-up is warranted in terms of testicular size, functional status, and malignant transformation.

Consent

Informed consent was obtained from the patient's guardian for publication of this case report.

Acknowledgments

We would like to acknowledge Dr He Guo Lin, from the Chinese Medical Team in the Yaounde Gynaeco-Obstetric and Paediatric Hospital, who participated in the laparoscopic exploration.

References

[1] L. Kumar, P. Garg, A. Kumar, and A. S. N. Rao, "Transverse testicular ectopia with bilateral pyocoele: case report and brief review of literature," *Journal of Surgical Technique and Case Report*, vol. 6, no. 2, pp. 55–57, 2014.

[2] M. N. Von Lenhossek, "Ectopia testis transversa," *Anatomischer Anzeiger*, vol. 1, pp. 376–381, 1886.

[3] S. Naouar, K. Maazoun, L. Sahnoun et al., "Transverse testicular ectopia: a three-case report and review of the literature," *Urology*, vol. 71, no. 6, pp. 1070–1073, 2008.

[4] P. Debnath, R. Tripathi, L. Agarwal, E. Malik, and S. Sharma, "Tuberculosis in transverse testicular ectopic testis: a diagnostic dilemma: case report," *The Indian Journal of Tuberculosis*, vol. 53, p. 27, 2006.

[5] A. A. Berg, "Transverse ectopy of the testis," *Annals of Surgery*, vol. 40, pp. 223-224, 1904.

[6] T. Kimura, "Transverse ectopy of the testis with masculine uterus," *Annals of Surgery*, vol. 68, no. 4, pp. 420–425, 1918.

[7] R. L. Gupta and P. Das, "Ectopia testis transversa," *Journal of the Indian Medical Association*, vol. 16, no. 35, pp. 547–549, 1960.

[8] J. K. Chacko, P. D. Furness III, and G. C. Mingin, "Presentation of fused vas deferens," *Urology*, vol. 67, no. 5, pp. 1085.e17–1085.e18, 2006.

[9] H. L. Frey and J. Rajfer, "Role of the gubernaculum and intraabdominal pressure in the process of testicular descent," *The Journal of Urology*, vol. 131, no. 3, pp. 574–579, 1984.

[10] C. G. Thevathasan, "Transverse ectopia of the testis," *The Australian and New Zealand Journal of Surgery*, vol. 37, no. 2, pp. 93–102, 1967.

[11] A. Inugala, "Tranverse testicular ectopia with persistent Müllerian duct syndrome and inginal hernia – a case report," *Asian Journal of Case Reports in Surgery*, vol. 5, no. 3, pp. 10–14, 2020.

[12] S. Barrack, "Crossed testicular ectopia with fused bilateral duplication of the vasa deferential: an unusual finding in crytochidism," *East African Medical Journal*, vol. 71, no. 6, p. 398, 1994.

[13] P. Kajal, K. N. Rattan, N. Bhutani, and V. Sangwan, "Transverse testicular ectopia with scrotal hypospadias but without inguinal hernia - case report of a rare association," *International Journal of Surgery Case Reports*, vol. 31, pp. 167–169, 2017.

[14] M. W. L. Gauderer, E. R. Grisoni, T. A. Stellato, J. L. Ponsky, and R. J. Izant Jr., "Transverse testicular ectopia," *Journal of Pediatric Surgery*, vol. 17, no. 1, pp. 43–47, 1982.

[15] T. F. Kolon, C. D. A. Herndon, L. A. Baker et al., "Evaluation and treatment of cryptorchidism: AUA guideline," *The Journal of Urology*, vol. 192, no. 2, pp. 337–345, 2014.

[16] C. Sommer, E. Stathopoulos, M. C. Antoniou, K. Busiah, M. Hauschild, and O. Sanchez, "An empty hemiscrotum: transverse testicular ectopia," *Journal of Pediatric Surgery Case Reports*, vol. 59, p. 101532, 2020.

[17] W. W. Lam, S. D. Le, L. Chan, F. L. Chan, and P. K. Tam, "Transverse testicular ectopia detected by MR imaging and MR venography," *Pediatric Radiology*, vol. 32, no. 2, pp. 126–129, 2002.

[18] C. Gkekas, E. N. Symeonidis, I. Tsifountoudis et al., "A Rare Variation of Transverse Testicular Ectopia (TTE) in a Young Adult as an Incidental Finding during Investigation for Testicular Pain," *Case Reports in Urology*, vol. 2018, 4 pages.

[19] F. Berkmen, "Persistent Mullerian duct syndrome with or without transverse testicular ectopia and testis tumours," *British Journal of Urology*, vol. 79, no. 1, pp. 122–126, 1997.

[20] B. Erginel, S. Bilici, Ş. Gedik et al., "Crossed testicular ectopia: report of six cases," *African Journal of Paediatric Surgery*, vol. 11, no. 3, pp. 269–272, 2014.

[21] R. Bascuna Jr., J. Y. Ha, Y. S. Lee, H. Y. Lee, Y. J. Im, and S. W. Han, "Transverse testis ectopia: diagnostic and management algorithm," *International Journal of Urology*, vol. 22, no. 3, pp. 330-331, 2015.

[22] V. Raj, R. G. Redkar, S. Krishna, and S. Tewari, "Rare case of transverse testicular ectopia - case report and review of literature," *International Journal of Surgery Case Reports*, vol. 41, pp. 407–410, 2017.

[23] K. Evans and A. Desai, "Total laparoscopic correction of transverse testicular ectopia," *Journal of Pediatric Urology*, vol. 4, no. 3, pp. 245-246, 2008.

[24] R. S. Kamble, R. K. Gupta, A. R. Gupta, P. R. Kothari, K. V. Dikshit, and K. K. Kesan, "Laparoscopic management of transverse testicular ectopia with persistent Müllerian duct syndrome," *Journal of Minimal Access Surgery*, vol. 11, no. 3, pp. 213–215, 2015.

4

Congenital Megaprepuce: Literature Review and Surgical Correction

Zachary Werner, Ali Hajiran, and Osama Al-Omar

Suite 6300, Health Sciences Center, Morgantown, WV 26506, USA

Correspondence should be addressed to Zachary Werner; zwerner@hsc.wvu.edu

Academic Editor: Nicola Zampieri

Congenital megaprepuce (CMP) is a type of buried penis characterized by extensive redundancy and ballooning of the inner prepuce as a result of preputial stenosis and phimosis. The malformation typically presents with difficulty voiding, often requiring manual expression of stagnant urine. Multiple techniques have been reported for the treatment of CMP with varying levels of positive outcomes. The authors provide a review of published literature, in addition to describing the procedure and results of our surgical technique in three children aged eleven months, two years, and twelve years. The literature review was conducted using PubMed with keywords "congenital megaprepuce," "megaprepuce," "buried penis," "CMP," and "correction." Results were then differentiated based on presence or absence of true congenital megaprepuce and the surgical correction thereof. Regarding our cases, all patients completed the procedure with excellent cosmesis and without complication. Our technique is shown to provide consistent, excellent esthetic outcome across a wide range of ages and may be replicated by others.

1. Introduction

Congenital megaprepuce is a subtype of buried penis. Maizels et al. defined buried penis as a penis of normal size hidden by preputial skin [1]. We conducted a literature review of techniques and cases using this definition as a guideline. It differs from various other forms of buried penis including webbed penis, buried penis secondary to circumcision, secondary to large suprapubic fat pad, and secondary to large hernia or hydrocele. Although Summerton et al. theorized that phimosis played little role in the abnormality, multiple modern authors refute this [2–5]. Congenital megaprepuce typically presents with a stenotic preputial ring with inner preputial ballooning as a result of the hydrostatic pressure of accrued urine [4, 6, 7]. Multiple sources have suggested that the etiology of this condition is an abnormal development of the migrational planes of the penis resulting in decreased ventral skin, dysplastic dartos fascia, and improper anchoring of the skin at the base of the penis [7–9].

The condition can present as early as birth but commonly is diagnosed later in infancy, most often due to parental concern regarding the need for manual urine expression and abnormal appearance [3, 6, 7, 10, 11]. While infants often present with benign micturition difficulties without lasting effects, adolescents with CMP may suffer psychological damage both from appearance and difficulty with penetration [4, 10]. Most authors assert that CMP should be treated surgically, often soon after diagnosis [3, 6, 10, 11]. Circumcision is contraindicated in these children as the preputial skin is required for repair.

Various methods have been used for the correction of CMP including the ventral v-plasty, Cuckow's technique, preputial unfurling, and a multitude of other methods; however, there is no "gold-standard" or consensus of the most efficacious technique [2, 3, 5–8, 10, 11]. Here, we describe our surgical strategy, which produced excellent cosmesis and repair.

2. Case Descriptions

Three cases of CMP, aged eleven months, two years, and twelve years, were surgically treated in 2017-2018 at our institution via excision of excess preputial skin, penile reconstruction, and scrotoplasty.

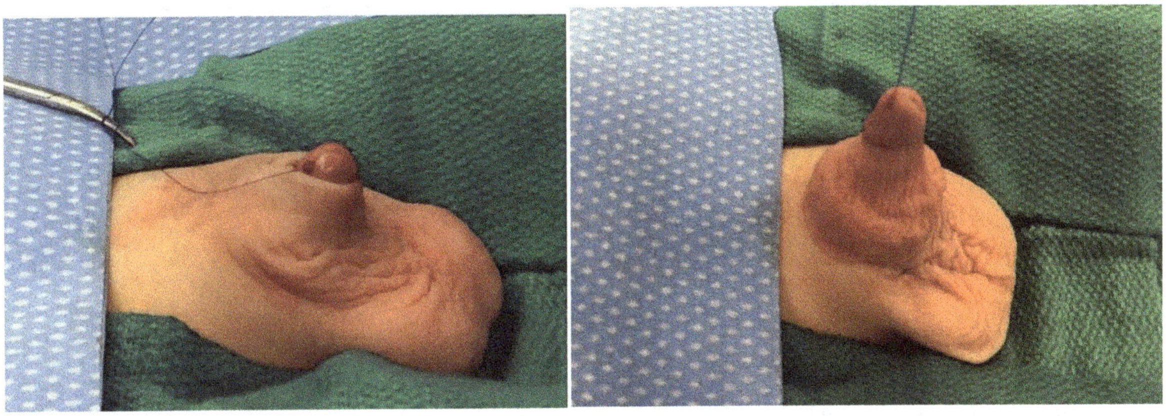

FIGURE 1: (a) shows the buried penis in normal position. (b) further details the extent of the excess inner prepuce.

The eleven-month-old had a history of preterm birth at 24 weeks. He underwent unsuccessful circumcision at an outside facility and was sent to us for difficulty with micturition with ballooning and manual expression, in addition to requirement of circumcision revision. Upon examination, he was noted to have a phimotic ring and right-sided cryptorchidism.

The two-year-old presented to the Urology clinic with difficulty of micturition and ballooning, sometimes requiring parental manual expression of foul urine. Upon examination, he was noted to have severe phimosis and buried penis with a large amount of trapped urine (Figures 1(a) and 1(b)).

The twelve-year-old presented to the Urology clinic primarily for circumcision. He also described the need for postvoiding manual expression of urine.

2.1. Surgical Technique. All surgeries were performed under general anesthesia. Using a hemostat, the glans of the penis was exposed by ventrally or dorsally opening the phimotic ring. A 5.0 PDS stitch was placed in the glans for intraoperative control of the penile shaft, as shown in Figure 1(b). The key steps in the surgery are as follows:

(1) Radical degloving of the penis: a circumferential incision 10 mm from the coronal sulcus was made. The penile shaft skin then incised ventrally and longitudinally down to the penoscrotal junction in order to radically deglove the penis to Buck's fascia until reaching the penile base deep in the scrotum.

(2) Radical excision of the dysplastic and thick dartos muscle down to the base of the penis (Figure 2).

(3) Excision of the redundant inner prepuce and preparing the penile shaft Byer skin flaps, which were rotated ventrally in order to have sufficient penile shaft skin coverage.

(4) Recreation of the penopubic and penoscrotal angles by using two PDS anchoring stitches dorsally and ventrally, retrospectively, between the dermis and Buck's fascia at the dorsal and ventral base of the penis. The scrotum was reapproximated in two layers at the midline using 4.0 Monocryl sutures and the ventral penile skin was similarly reapproximated at the ventral midline and circumferentially as shown in Figures 3 and 4.

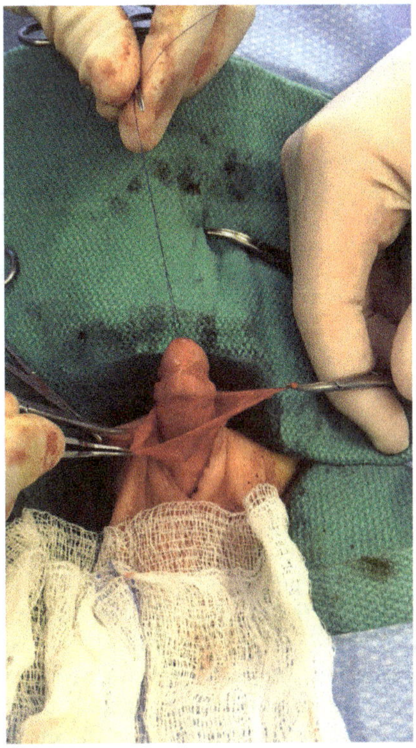

FIGURE 2: Isolated dysplastic dartos muscle prior to excision.

All patients completed the procedure with excellent cosmesis. No immediate postoperative complications such as infection, bleeding, or urinary retention were observed.

The two-year-old boy showed excellent cosmesis and parental satisfaction at eleven-month follow-up visit (Figure 5).

Unfortunately, the twelve-year-old and eleven-month-old failed to appear for follow-up and cannot be reached for short-term results.

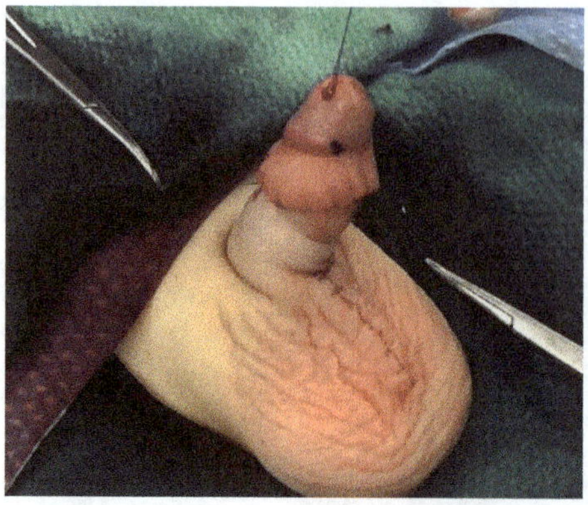

FIGURE 3: Good recreation of the penoscrotal and penopubic angle is shown, in addition to scrotal reapproximation at the midline.

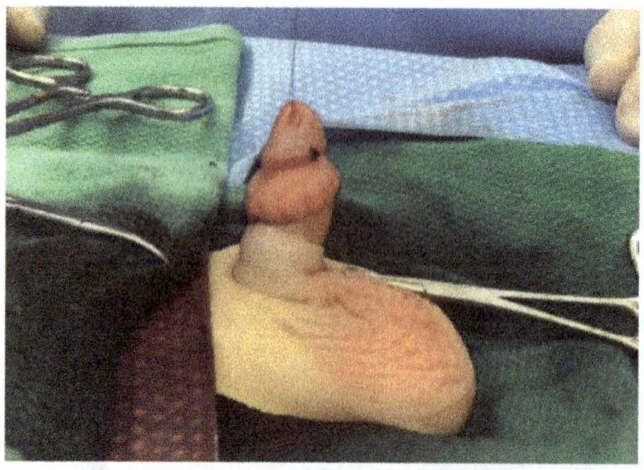

FIGURE 4: Redemonstration of the penopubic and penoscrotal angles in the two-year-old patient.

3. Discussion

Discussion regarding the condition of congenital megaprepuce can be especially confusing given the ill-defined nomenclature surrounding the disease. The first case of congenital megaprepuce was described in 1994 [12]. Various terms such as buried penis, trapped penis, webbed, concealed, or entrapped were all seemingly used interchangeably in the past. We use the definitions defined by Maizels et al. which defines buried penis as a subtype of concealed penis [1]. Further, we consider congenital megaprepuce to be describing a childhood disease characterized by phimosis and ballooning of the inner prepuce [5, 6]. Congenital megaprepuce is a condition best treated by surgical correction, often at the time of diagnosis. There is an abundance of literature and techniques for describing and treating general buried penis [13–25]. However, upon a review of the literature, we found there is significantly less literature regarding specific surgical correction of CMP. Table 1 lists the various articles found upon review that are specific to CMP, many of which contain techniques for general buried penis that have been repurposed for the treatment of CMP [2, 3, 5–8, 11, 26–33]. The majority of the papers describe incision of the stenotic ring, unfurling of the prepuce with subsequent inner preputial resection, followed by a variety of resurfacing techniques [2, 3, 5–8, 11, 26–33].

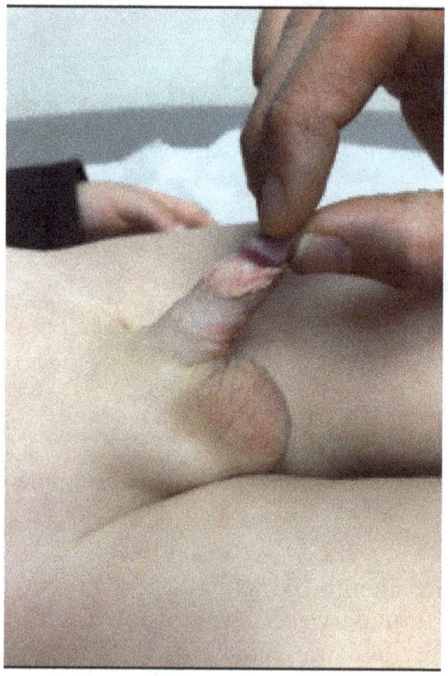

FIGURE 5: Demonstration of excellent cosmesis at eleven-month follow-up.

Our method of correction provided similar levels of cosmetic repair in patients of very different ages and is thus applicable across a wide spectrum of patients. The technique reaffirms some of the most important aspects of repair including removal of the stenotic ring, excision of redundant inner preputial skin, and anchoring of the skin to Buck's fascia to recreate the penopubic and penoscrotal angles. However, we believe that the most important step in correcting CMP is excising the dysplastic dartos muscle which helps achieve excellent penile skin reconstruction, penoscrotal angle, penopubic angle, and penile shaft skin approximation, based on our limited case series. Leaving the dartos muscle results in downward retraction of the penile skin with thick and poor cosmesis of the penile skin reapproximation. This critical step is described in the majority of papers reviewed.

Although the ventral v-plasty technique described by Alexander et al. has shown good results, we believe a dorsal skin flap provides excellent cosmetic repair [7, 11]. This sentiment was echoed by other authors who have similarly used dorsal skin to achieve a normal circumcised appearance [6, 11]. Additionally, we are proponents of penile coverage with the outer preputial skin with excision of the redundant inner prepuce, as replacement of the inner prepuce has been shown to cause postoperative edema and poor esthetics [2, 6, 7, 26]. It should be noted though that of the 134 patients treated by Chin et al. most of their patients' postoperative edema resolved by one month, although one patient did require a second surgery due to persistent swelling [27]. We did not induce artificial erection as penile degloving in our cases did not indicate any concern regarding penile chordee, although Liu et al. have made it part of their standard procedure [26].

TABLE 1: Results of congenital megaprepuce literature review.

First author	Title	Cases	Minimum age	Maximum age	Average age
Ruiz	Simplified surgical approach to Congenital Megaprepuce. Fixing, Unfurling, and Tailoring Revisited	26	2 months	19 months	6 months
Alexander	The Ventral V-plasty: a simple procedure for the reconstruction of a congenital megaprepuce	10	8 months	3 years	20 months
Lin	An Arc Incision Surgical Approach in Congenital Megaprepuce	32	10 months	3 years	Unknown
Summerton	Congenital megaprepuce: an emerging condition. How to recognize and treat it	20	6 months	3.6 years	16 months
Rod	Congenital megaprepuce: a 12-year experience (52 cases) of this specific form of buried penis	52	4 months	2.3 years	13 months
Liu	Congenital completely buried penis in boys: anatomical basis and surgical technique	22	2.5 years	5.8 years	4.2 years
Chin	Modified prepuce unfurling for buried penis: a report of 12 years of experience	134	2 months	33 years	5.5 years
Shenoy	Surgical correction of congenital megaprepuce	3	3 months	6 months	5 months
Buluggiu	Congenital Megaprepuce: surgical approach	5	6 months	7 years	2.5 years
Murakami	A single surgeon's experience of 65 cases of penoplasty for congenital megaprepuce, with special reference to mid- to long-term follow-up	65	4.8 months	13.9 years	5.9 years
Leao	Congenital megaprepuce: a new alternative technique for surgical correction	5	2 years	5 years	Unknown
Delgado	Congenital megaprepuce: diagnosis and therapeutic management	4	Unknown	Unknown	Unknown
Callewaert	Double longitudinal megapreputium Incision Technique: the Dolomite	6	7 months	2.1 years	13.3 months
Podesta	Megaprepuce Reconstruction: A Single Center Experience	15	3 months	20 months	9 months
Serrano-Durba	Secondary congenital megaprepuce	1	Unknown	Unknown	3 months

One of the most important aspects of CMP is early recognition and proper age of surgical correction. Murakami et al. reported a common misbelief among parents that the patients would eventually grow out of the appearance of their penis [11]. Liu et al. recommended waiting until completion of toilet training to initiate surgical treatment [26]. Multiple sources dispute this recommendation, citing significant psychological damage with delayed surgical correction as an unneeded side effect [3, 6, 9, 10]. De Jesus et al. recommend surgery for buried penis between ages one and three to prevent psychological damage [10]. Despite CMP presenting in infancy, the average age at repair for our review was 24.5 months, although one can assume that age at initial presentation plays a large role in age at repair. We believe surgical correction is best conducted at time of initial diagnosis.

Given the rarity of this disease, it is difficult to have a sample size large enough for strong recommendations on technique. In addition to having a larger sample size to draw conclusions from, longer follow-up is needed to confirm parental and patient satisfaction, lack of recurrent buried penis, and general results of cosmesis and repair. In our humble series, the lack of follow-up with the twelve-year-old is especially disappointing, as he is one of the oldest presenting patients we found during our review of the literature.

References

[1] M. Maizels, M. Zaontz, J. Donovan, P. N. Bushnick, and C. F. Firlit, "Surgical correction of the buried penis: Description of a classification system and a technique to correct the disorder," *The Journal of Urology*, vol. 136, no. 1, pp. 268–271, 1986.

[2] D. Summerton, J. Mcnally, A. Denny, and P. Malone, "Congenital megaprepuce: an emerging condition - how to recognize and treat it," *BJU International*, vol. 86, no. 4, pp. 519–522, 2000.

[3] J. Rod, A. Desmonts, T. Petit, and P. Ravasse, "Congenital megaprepuce: A 12-year experience (52 cases) of this specific form of buried penis," *Journal of Pediatric Urology*, vol. 9, no. 6, pp. 784–788, 2013.

[4] M. Cimador, P. Catalano, R. Ortolano, and M. Giuffrè, "The inconspicuous penis in children," *Nature Reviews Urology*, vol. 12, no. 4, pp. 205–215, 2015.

[5] E. Ruiz, R. Vagni, C. Apostolo et al., "Simplified surgical approach to congenital megaprepuce: Fixing, unfurling and tailoring revisited," *The Journal of Urology*, vol. 185, no. 6, pp. 2487–2490, 2011.

[6] A. Buluggiu, N. Panait, R. Anastasescu, T. Merrot, and P. Alessandrini, "Congenital megaprepuce: surgical approach," *Urology*, vol. 81, no. 3, pp. 649–652, 2013.

[7] A. Alexander, A. J. Lorenzo, J. L. P. Salle, and H. Rode, "The ventral v-plasty: a simple procedure for the reconstruction of a congenital megaprepuce," *Journal of Pediatric Surgery*, vol. 45, no. 8, pp. 1741–1747, 2010.

[8] H.-W. Lin, L. Zhang, H.-Q. Geng et al., "An arc incision surgical approach in congenital megaprepuce," *Chinese Medical Journal*, vol. 128, no. 4, pp. 555–557, 2015.

[9] I. C. C. King, A. Tahir, C. Ramanathan, and H. Siddiqui, "Buried penis: evaluation of outcomes in children and adults, modification of a unified treatment algorithm, and review of the literature," *ISRN Urology*, vol. 2013, Article ID 109349, 7 pages, 2013.

[10] L. E. De Jesus, S. Dekermacher, and K. M. Anderson, "Severe forms of concealed penis without hypospadias: Surgical strategies," *Indian Journal of Urology*, vol. 31, no. 4, pp. 344–348, 2015.

[11] H. Murakami, Y. Yazaki, S. Seo et al., "A single surgeon's experience of 65 cases of penoplasty for congenital megaprepuce, with special reference to mid- to long-term follow-up," *Pediatric Surgery International*, vol. 31, no. 1, pp. 89–92, 2015.

[12] A. O'brien, A. M. J. Shapiro, and J. D. Frank, "Phimosis or congenital megaprepuce?" *British Journal of Urology*, vol. 73, no. 6, pp. 719-720, 1994.

[13] M. Abbas, A. Liard, F. Elbaz, and B. Bachy, "Outcome of surgical management of concealed penis," *Journal of Pediatric Urology*, vol. 3, no. 6, pp. 490–494, 2007.

[14] P. Brisson, H. Patel, M. Chan, and N. Feins, "Penoplasty for buried penis in children: Report of 50 cases," *Journal of Pediatric Surgery*, vol. 36, no. 3, pp. 421–425, 2001.

[15] J.-H. Chuang, L.-Y. Chen, C.-S. Shieh, and S.-Y. Lee, "Surgical correction of buried penis: A review of 60 cases," *Journal of Pediatric Surgery*, vol. 36, no. 3, pp. 426–429, 2001.

[16] M. Wollin, P. G. Duffy, P. S. Malone, and P. G. Ransley, "Buried penis. a novel approach," *British Journal of Urology*, vol. 65, no. 1, pp. 97–100, 1990.

[17] C.-C. Chu, Y.-H. Chen, G.-Y. Diau, I.-W. Loh, and K.-C. Chen, "Preputial flaps to correct buried penis," *Pediatric Surgery International*, vol. 23, no. 11, pp. 1119–1121, 2007.

[18] G. J. Alter and R. M. Ehrlich, "A new technique for correction of the hidden penis in children and adults," *The Journal of Urology*, vol. 161, no. 2, pp. 455–459, 1999.

[19] P. K. Donahoe and M. A. Keating, "Preputial unfurling to correct the buried penis," *Journal of Pediatric Surgery*, vol. 21, no. 12, pp. 1055–1057, 1986.

[20] C. D. A. Herndon, A. J. Casale, M. P. Cain, R. C. Rink, and J. Pope, "Long-term outcome of the surgical treatment of concealed penis," *The Journal of Urology*, vol. 170, no. 4, pp. 1695–1697, 2003.

[21] S. R. Shapiro, "Surgical treatment of the "buried" penis," *Urology*, vol. 30, no. 6, pp. 554–559, 1987.

[22] P. S. Bergeson, R. J. Hopkin, R. B. Bailey Jr., L. C. McGill, and J. P. Piatt, "The inconspicuous penis," *Pediatrics*, vol. 92, no. 6, pp. 794–799, 1993.

[23] N. Smeulders, D. T. Wilcox, and P. M. Cuckow, "The buried penis - An anatomical approach," *BJU International*, vol. 86, no. 4, pp. 523–526, 2000.

[24] L. Perger, R. S. Hanley, and N. R. Feins, "Penoplasty for buried penis in infants and children: Report of 100 cases," *Pediatric Surgery International*, vol. 25, no. 2, pp. 175–180, 2009.

[25] A. Borsellino, A. Spagnoli, S. Vallasciani, L. Martini, and F. Ferro, "Surgical approach to concealed penis: technical refinements and outcome," *Urology*, vol. 69, no. 6, pp. 1195–1198, 2007.

[26] X. Liu, D.-W. He, Y. Hua, D.-Y. Zhang, and G.-H. Wei, "Congenital completely buried penis in boys: Anatomical basis and surgical technique," *BJU International*, vol. 112, no. 2, pp. 271–275, 2013.

[27] T.-W. Chin, H.-L. Tsai, and C.-S. Liu, "Modified prepuce unfurling for buried penis: A report of 12 years of experience," *Asian Journal of Surgery*, vol. 38, no. 2, pp. 74–78, 2015.

[28] M. U. Shenoy and C. H. Rance, "Surgical correction of congenital megaprepuce," *Pediatric Surgery International*, vol. 15, no. 8, pp. 593-594, 1999.

[29] J. Q. Leao, L. G. F. Filho, A. L. Gomes, A. C. Heinsich, and J. Carnevale, "Congenital megaprepuce: A new alternative technique for surgical correction," *International Brazilian Journal of Urology*, vol. 34, no. 3, pp. 313–318, 2008.

[30] F. J. Delgado Oliva, C. Domínguez Hinarejos, S. Serrano Durbá, F. Estornell Moragues, M. Martínez Verduch, and F. García Ibarra, "Congenital megaprepuce: Diagnosis and terapeutic management," *Actas Urológicas Españolas*, vol. 30, no. 10, pp. 1038–1042, 2006.

[31] P. R. H. Callewaert, M. S. Rahnama'I, M. N. C. Guimarães, D. M. J. Vrijens, and P. E. V. A. Van Kerrebroeck, "DOuble longitudinal megapreputium incision technique: the dolomite," *Urology*, vol. 83, no. 5, pp. 1149–1154, 2014.

[32] M. L. Podestá and M. Podestá, "Megaprepuce reconstruction: A single center experience," *Frontiers in Pediatrics*, vol. 6, 2018.

[33] A. Serrano-Durbá, C. Dominguez-Hinarejos, C. Reig-Ruiz, and F. Garcia-Ibarra, "Secondary congenital megaprepuce," *Scandinavian Journal of Urology*, vol. 32, no. 5, pp. 360-361, 1998.

5

Unusual Presentation of Priapism Associated with Acute and Chronic Myeloid Leukemia in Two Patients: Emergency Management

Oumar Gaye,[1] Ngor Mack Thiam,[1] Ayun Cassell,[2] Serigne Mourtalla Gueye,[3] Yaya Sow,[1] Boubacar Fall,[1] and Alain Khassim Ndoye[1]

[1]*Urology-Andrology Department, Hôpital Aristide Le Dantec, Senegal*
[2]*Urology-Andrology Department, Hôpital Général Idrissa Pouye, Senegal*
[3]*Centre National de Transfusion Sanguine, Dakar, Senegal*

Correspondence should be addressed to Oumar Gaye; oumargaye-uro@outlook.fr

Academic Editor: Francesco M. Solivetti

Priapism is a rare urological emergency. It is rarely a telltale sign of myeloid leukemia. We report two cases of acute myeloid leukemia in a child and chronic myeloid leukemia in a young adult presenting with priapism. Puncture irrigation of the corpora cavernosa followed by systemic treatment to lower the hyperviscosity of the blood due to leukemia provided optimal outcome. Prompt emergency management is required to lower the complication of erectile dysfunction.

1. Introduction

Priapism is defined as the persistence of a complete or partial erection beyond four hours, after orgasm/cessation or without any sexual stimulation.

There are three different types of priapism: high-flow priapism, ischemic priapism, and recurrent priapism [1]. Ischemic priapism is the most frequent and serious type requiring emergency management to avoid complications such as erectile dysfunction. [1]. In the United States, ischemic priapism presents more commonly with an incidence of up to 5.34 per 100,000 men per year [2].

The hematological disorder is responsible to 20% of priapism [3]. Priapism resulting from acute or chronic myeloid leukemia is unusual [4]. In adult patients with leukemia, the incidence of priapism is estimated to be approximately 5% [5] and 15% in the pediatric population [6].

Emergency management requires combined systemic treatment along with local treatment of the corpora cavernosa [7]. We report two clinical cases of priapism occurring with of myeloid leukemia received in the urological emergency department.

2. Case 1

A case of a 46-year-old male patient was consulted for a painful erection for 48 hours without any previous sexual stimulation, trauma, or medication intake.

Physical assessment revealed a male with good general condition, grade 1 splenomegaly, hepatomegaly with hepatic notch at 14 cm, rigidity of the corpora cavernosa, and a flaccid glans penis.

The emergency laboratory workup showed Hemoglobin: 9.7 g/dl, Reds cells: 2920000/mm^3, White Blood Cell: 526000/mm^3, Platelets: 412000/mm^3, Lactate Dehydrogenase: 1491 U/I, Urea: 0.23 g/L, and Creatinine level: 7.8 mg/L.

Blood smear (Figure 1) showed Myeloblast: 12%, Promyelocytes: 85%, Myelocytes: 11%, and Eosinophil: 4%.

The emergency management consisted of rehydration, an infusion of sodium bicarbonate, a puncture of the corpora

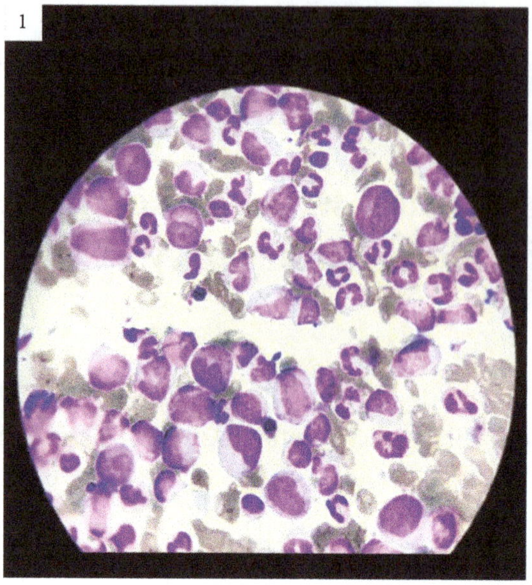

Figure 1: Blood smear showing myeloblast, promyelocytes, myelocytes, and eosinophil.

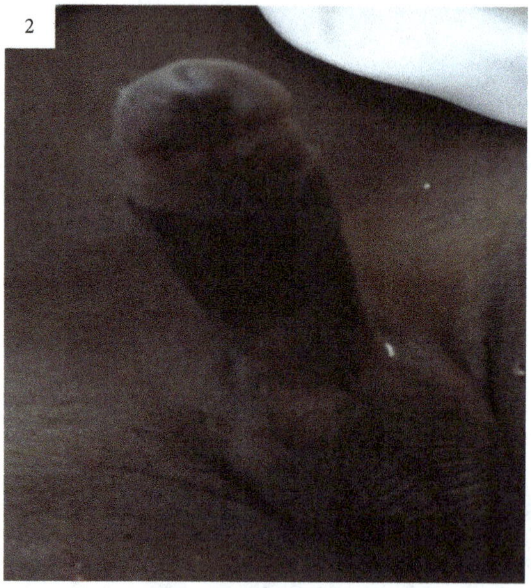

Figure 2: Rigidity of the corpora cavernosa and a flaccid glans penis.

cavernosa, injection of phenylephrine along with administration of hydroxycarbamide. Detumescence was achieved after 36 hours.

Subsequently, a myelogram showed bone marrow hyperplasia and a karyotype revealed a translocation between chromosomes 9 and 22 confirming the diagnosis of chronic myeloid leukemia. The patient was continued with doses of imatinib.

3. Case 2

A case of a 9-year-old child was seen in the emergency department for a sudden onset of a painful erection evolving for about 36 hours without any previous sexual stimulation, trauma, or medication intake.

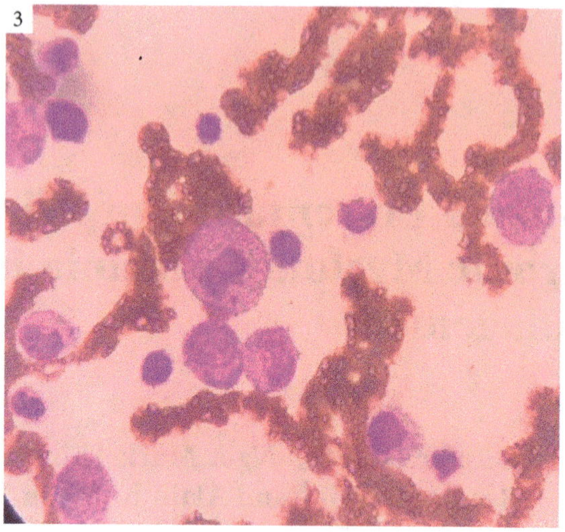

Figure 3: Bone marrow biopsy showing blast cell infiltration, leukemic infiltrate, mitoses, and presence of inflammatory cells.

The examination showed Pallor of the conjunctival mucosa, grade 1 splenomegaly, gingival enlargement, rigidity of the corpora cavernosa, and a flaccid glans penis (Figure 2).

The emergency laboratory workup: Hemoglobin: 3.4 g/dl, Reds cells: $1090000/mm^3$, White Blood Cell: $82000/mm^3$, Platelets: $81000/mm^3$, Neutrophils: 1% or $824/mm^3$, Eosinophils: 4% or $3296/mm^3$, Lymphocytes-h: 3% or $2472/mm^3$, Hematocrit: 11%, Urea: 0.21 g/L Creatinine level: 06 mg/L, and Blood smear: Blasts: 92%.

The emergency management consisted of penile skin refrigeration, rehydration, puncture of the corpora cavernosa with injection of phenylephrine, and induction of chemotherapy with vincristine and prednisolone, which achieved detumescence in 12 hours.

The bone marrow biopsy performed later confirmed an acute myeloid leukemia (Figure 3). Hemoglobin electrophoresis was performed and ruled out sickle cell disease.

4. Discussion

Priapism is a rare urological emergency. Ischemic priapism results from an obstruction of the venous blood and is manifested by a painful erection with rigidity of the corpora cavernosa and a flaccid glans penis [7]. It is the most urgent and frequent type requiring emergency care to prevent complications such as erectile dysfunction.

To date, less than 20 cases of priapism and chronic myeloid leukemia [2, 3, 5, 8–15] have been reported and 2 cases of priapism and acute lymphoblastic leukemia [16, 17] (Table 1).

In Senegal, sickle cell disease is responsible for the majority of priapism cases [18]. Leukemia is rarely complicated by priapism. When it occurs, it is most often caused by chronic myeloid leukemia and more rarely by acute lymphoid leukemia or acute myeloid leukemia [9].

Hyperleukocytosis is considered the underlying pathology of priapism in these instances. The main mechanism is

Table 1: Literature review of priapism and leukemia from 2003 to 2020 using the PubMed database.

Series	Age	Diagnosis	Presenting symptoms	WBC cell/mm^3	Platelet count cell/mm^3	Treatment of priapism and leukemia	Outcome
Becerra-Pedraza et al. [2]	52 yrs	Chronic myeloid leukemia	Priapism for 144 hrs, fatigue, pallor	282 000		Corpora cavernosa drainage-irrigation penile shunts. Dasatinib	No ED on follow-up
Hazra et al. [3]	14 yrs	Chronic myeloid leukemia	Priapism for 24 hrs	226 900	310 000	Cavernosal aspiration and phenylephrine irrigation	No recurrence at 2-month follow-up
Khan et al. [5]	16 yrs	Chronic myeloid leukemia	Priapism for 264 hrs	614 800	7 090 000	Glans-cavernosal shunt hydroxyurea and allopurinol	Achieved detumescence. No info on ED
Nerli et al. [8]	19 yrs	Chronic myeloid leukemia	Priapism for 24 hrs	296 800	936 000	Corporal aspiration and phenylephrine irrigation hydroxyurea and imatinib	Achieved detumescence. No info on ED
Minckler et al. [9]	18 yrs	Chronic myeloid leukemia	Recurrent priapism	5 880 000	1 090 000	Hydroxyurea and imatinib	No info on follow-up
Chang et al. [10]	21 yrs	Chronic myeloid leukemia	Priapism for 19 hrs	216 800	1 746 000	Cavernosa aspiration and epinephrine irrigation hydroxyurea and interferon	No ED on follow-up
Qu et al. [11]	18 yrs	Chronic myeloid leukemia	Priapism for 72 hrs	257 000	5 450 000	Cavernosa-corpus spongiosum shunt, imatinib	No ED at 3-month follow-up
Yoshida et al. [12]	29 yrs	Chronic myeloid leukemia	Priapism for 48 hrs	263 000		Glans-cavernosal shunt hydroxyurea and imatinib	No ED at 5-month follow-up
Tazi [13]	33 yrs	Chronic myeloid leukemia	Priapism for 22 hrs	400 000	1 200 000	Cavernosa aspiration and epinephrine irrigation	No recurrence on follow-up
Ponniah et al. [14]	19 yrs	Chronic myeloid leukemia	Priapism for 18 hrs	513 000		Failed cavernosal aspiration + leukapheresis	No ED on follow-up
Ergenc et al. [15]	18 yrs	Chronic myeloid leukemia	Priapism for 72 hrs	100 000	1 002 000	İmatinib, allopurinol + leukapheresis	No ED at 6-month follow-up
Gupta et al. [16]	10 yrs	Acute lymphoblastic leukemia	Priapism, fever, headache	693 000	40 000	Corporal aspiration followed by phenylephrine irrigation, allopurinol + steroids	Died after 48 hours
Güzelküçük et al. [17]	9 yrs	Acute lymphoblastic leukemia	Priapism for 18 hrs	583 000	51 000	Corporal aspiration followed by hydroxyurea, allopurinol + leukapheresis	Achieved detumescence

ED: erectile dysfunction; Hrs: hours; WBC: White Blood Cell; Yrs: years.

the aggregation of leukemia cells in the corpora cavernosa and the dorsal vein of the penis. Other accessory mechanisms are venous congestion of the corpora cavernosa secondary to mechanical pressure from the abdominal veins draining the spleen or infiltration of the sacral nerves or the central nervous system by leukemia cells [9].

Vadakan and Ortega described a case of priapism, which occurred from an acute lymphoid leukemia without hyperleukocytosis suggesting a disturbance of the central or peripheral nervous system [19]. Chang et al. have described priapism secondary to acute myeloid leukemia due to the direct penetration of the penis by leukemia cells [8]. As in most of the reports described [9–17], hyperleukocytosis was the most likely cause of priapism in the two cases of this report.

The American Urology Association [7] recommended combining systemic treatment of the organic cause with local treatment of the corpora cavernosa in cases of priapism secondary to leukemia. Systemic treatment is indicated for cytoreduction. It combines hydroxyurea with imatinib with or without leukapheresis to reduce hyperviscosity in chronic myeloid leukemia [8, 9, 20, 21] and chemotherapy in acute myeloid leukemia [22].

The local treatment at the level of the cavernous bodies involves a puncture evacuating the blood of the cavernous bodies along the lateral route at the penoscrotal or trans-glandular junction with an injection of alpha sympathomimetic agent. Amongst these agents, the use of etilefrine or phenylephrine has been favored because of their pure alpha-stimulating nature and better cardiac tolerance [21].

Other treatments such as radiotherapy of the penis, spinal anesthesia [23], irradiation of the spine [23, 24], the application of hot compresses [25], or penile refrigeration [19, 23] have been described with less satisfactory results.

The review showed that corporal aspiration/irrigation or a distal shunt was sufficient in achieving at least partial detumescence [2, 5, 8]. These procedures were followed by the treatment of the underlying leukemia with adequate hydration, hydroxyurea, imatinib, and leukapheresis [10–17]. The reports showed disease remission at a maximum 6-month follow-up with adequate erectile function.

5. Conclusion

Priapism is a usual presentation of myeloid leukemia and exceptionally rare association. A blood cell count showing hyperleukocytosis should suggest leukemia.

Emergent combination of systemic treatment with local treatment in the corpora cavernosa provides satisfactory results.

Consent

A written and signed consent was received from the patient for publication of this report.

Acknowledgments

Special thanks are due to the Urology-andrology department, Hôpital Aristide Le Dantec (Sénégal).

References

[1] S. Droupy and F. Giuliano, "Priapismes," *Progrès en Urologie*, vol. 23, no. 9, pp. 638–646, 2013.

[2] L. C. Becerra-Pedraza, L. E. Jiménez-Martínez, I. Peña-Morfin, R. Nava-Esquivel, and J. A. Villegas-Martínez, "Priapism as the initial sign in hematologic disease: case report and literature review," *International Journal of Surgery Case Reports*, vol. 43, pp. 13–17, 2018.

[3] S. P. Hazra, V. Priyadarshi, D. Gogoi, P. K. Sharma, D. K. Pal, and S. C. Chakraborty, "Pediatric priapism: a rare first manifestation of leukemia," *APSP Journal of Case Reports*, vol. 4, no. 3, p. 39, 2013.

[4] R. Rodgers, Z. Latif, and M. Copland, "How I manage priapism in chronic myeloid leukaemia patients," *British Journal of Haematology*, vol. 158, no. 2, pp. 155–164, 2012.

[5] A. Khan, I. Shafiq, M. H. Shah, S. Khan, G. Shahid, and M. Arabdin, "Chronic myeloid leukaemia presenting as priapism: a case report from Khyber Pakhtunkhwa," *The Journal of the Pakistan Medical Association*, vol. 68, no. 6, pp. 942–944, 2018.

[6] N. Paladino, D. Roldán, and M. S. Caram, "Priapismo en pediatría: presentación inicial de una leucemia mieloide crónica," *Archivos Argentinos de Pediatría*, vol. 109, no. 5, pp. e104–e108, 2011.

[7] D. K. Montague, J. Jarow, G. A. Broderick et al., "American Urological Association guideline on the management of priapism," *The Journal of Urology*, vol. 170, 4 Part 1, pp. 1318–1324, 2003.

[8] R. B. Nerli, P. V. Magdum, S. C. Hiremath et al., "Priapism – a rare presentation in chronic myeloid leukemia: case report," *Urology Case Reports*, vol. 4, no. 4, pp. 8–10, 2016.

[9] M. R. Minckler, E. Conser, J. J. Figueroa, A. J. Scott, J. Gaither, and R. Amini, "The semantics of priapism and the first sign of chronic myeloid leukemia," *Case Reports in Emergency Medicine*, vol. 2017, Article ID 2656203, 3 pages, 2017.

[10] M. W. Chang, C. C. Tang, and S. S. Chang, "Priapism a rare presentation in chronic myeloid leukemia: case report and review of the literature," *Chang Gung Medical Journal*, vol. 26, no. 4, pp. 288–292, 2003.

[11] M. Qu, X. Lu, L. Wang, Z. Liu, Y. Sun, and X. Gao, "Priapism secondary to chronic myeloid leukemia treated by a surgical cavernosa-corpus spongiosum shunt: case report," *Asian Journal of Urology*, vol. 6, no. 4, pp. 373–376, 2019.

[12] K. Yoshida, H. Kinoshita, H. Taniguti et al., "Priapism complicated by chronic myelogenous leukemia (CML); a case report," *Acta Urologica Japonica*, vol. 53, no. 5, pp. 323–325, 2007.

[13] I. Tazi, "Priapism as the first manifestation of chronic myeloid leukemia," *Annals of Saudi Medicine*, vol. 29, no. 5, p. 412, 2009.

[14] A. Ponniah, C. T. Brown, and P. Taylor, "Priapism secondary to leukemia: effective management with prompt leukapheresis," *International Journal of Urology*, vol. 11, no. 9, pp. 809-810, 2004.

[15] C. Varım, C. Karacaer, D. Çekdemir, and H. Ergenc, "Chronic myeloid leukemia presented with priapism: effective management with prompt leukapheresis," *Nigerian Journal of Clinical Practice*, vol. 18, no. 6, pp. 828–830, 2015.

[16] G. Gupta, D. Kumar, and M. Trivedi, "Acute lymphoblastic leukemia in a child presenting primarily with priapism," *Journal of Indian Association of Pediatric Surgeons*, vol. 25, no. 1, pp. 52–54, 2020.

[17] Z. Güzelküçük, D. Kaçar, R. Demir, M. Kürtül, H. N. Yaralı, and N. Y. Özbek, "Priapism: a rare presentation of precursor B-cell acute lymphoblastic leukemia," *The Turkish Journal of Pediatrics*, vol. 61, no. 2, pp. 311-312, 2019.

[18] C. Sylla, M. Ba, A. Ndoye et al., "Penile emergencies," *Annales d'Urologie*, vol. 34, no. 3, pp. 203–207, 2000.

[19] V. V. Vadakan and J. ORTEGA, "Priapism in acute lymphoblastic leukemia," *Cancer*, vol. 30, no. 2, pp. 373–375, 1972.

[20] B. D. Adams, R. Baker, J. A. Lopez, and S. Spencer, "Myeloproliferative disorders and the hyperviscosity syndrome," *Emergency Medicine Clinics of North America*, vol. 27, no. 3, pp. 459–476, 2009.

[21] T. Jameel and K. Mehmood, "Priapism—an unusual presentation in chronic myeloid leukaemia: case report and review of the literature," *Biomédica*, vol. 25, pp. 197–199, 2009.

[22] A. L. Burnett and T. J. Bivalacqua, "Priapism: new concepts in medical and surgical management," *The Urologic Clinics of North America*, vol. 38, no. 2, pp. 185–194, 2011.

[23] D. A. Grace and C. C. Winter, "Priapism an appraisal of management of twenty-three patients," *The Journal of Urology*, vol. 99, no. 3, pp. 301–310, 1968.

[24] R. G. Graw Jr., R. T. Skeel, and P. P. Carbone, "Priapism in a child with chronic granulocytic leukemia," *The Journal of Pediatrics*, vol. 74, no. 5, pp. 788–790, 1969.

[25] G. Maciotta, "Priapism as a symptom of leukemic myelosis in a 10 year old boy," *Pediatria (Bucur)*, vol. 42, pp. 1093-1094, 1934.

KRAS Mutation in Serous Borderline Tumor of the Testis: Report of a Case and Review of the Literature

Sarah Bouri,[1,2] **Jean-Christophe Noël**,[1,2] **Xavier Catteau**,[1,2] **Walid Al Hajj Obeid**,[3] **Ilyas Svistakov**,[3] **Thierry Roumeguère**,[3] **Nicky D'Haene**,[1,2] **and Sandrine Rorive**[1,2]

[1]*Department of Pathology, Erasme Hospital, Université Libre de Bruxelles, Brussels, Belgium*
[2]*Department of Pathology, Centre Universitaire Inter Regional d'Expertise en Anatomie Pathologique Hospitalière, Jumet, Belgium*
[3]*Department of Urology, Erasme Hospital, Université Libre de Bruxelles, Brussels, Belgium*

Correspondence should be addressed to Sarah Bouri; sarah.bouri@erasme.ulb.ac.be

Academic Editor: Mehraj Sheikh

Ovarian-like epithelial tumors of the testis, including serous borderline tumors, are rare entities. We report the case of a 60-year-old man with a left intratesticular mass who had a radical orchidectomy. Histologically, the tumor was identical to the ovarian counterpart showing a well-delineated cystic lesion characterized by intraluminal papillae. The papillae are lined by atypical cuboidal or ciliated cells and are associated with psammoma bodies. The tumor cells express cytokeratin 7 (CK7), cytokeratin 5-6 (CK5-6), cancer antigen 125 (CA125), estrogen (ER), progesterone (PR), Wilm's tumor gene (WT1), paired box gene 8 (PAX8), Ber-EP4, and epithelial membrane antigen (EMA). The diagnosis of a serous borderline tumor of the testis was proposed. Mutation testing using next-generation sequencing showed a Q61K KRAS gene mutation. To the best of our knowledge, this is the second case report of a serous borderline tumor of the testis with a Q61K KRAS gene mutation.

1. Introduction

Ovarian Mullerian-like epithelial tumors of the testis are exceedingly rare tumors with about 50 cases described in the literature [1–5]. Like in the ovarian counterpart, serous, mucinous, clear cell, and seromucinous carcinomas have been previously reported [6–8]. The mutational molecular profile of these tumors is poorly understood with only 5 previous cases well documented. In particular, in the serous tumor of the testis, only one previous article had suggested that like in the ovarian neoplasms, KRAS mutation could play a role in the development of these tumors [9]. Here, we report the second case of a serous borderline tumor of the testis in which a mutation of the Q61K KRAS gene is demonstrated. Our data were analysed in the highlight of the literature concerning the molecular profile of this unusual neoplasm.

2. Case Presentation

A 60-year-old man was referred to the urological consultation of Erasme University Hospital for a left intratesticular mass felt by the patient for about six months. At the ultrasound, this tumor of approximately 20×13 mm was heterogenous and hypoechogenic and contained calcifications (Figure 1).

The epididymis and right testis were normal. Testicular cancer tumor markers such as human chorionic gonadotropin (hCG), alpha-foetoprotein (AFP), and lactate dehydrogenase (LDH) were within normal limits. Therefore, a left radical orchidectomy was performed. Macroscopic examination revealed an intratesticular heterogenous cystic lesion measuring 18×13 mm and containing an endoluminal whitish area (Figure 2).

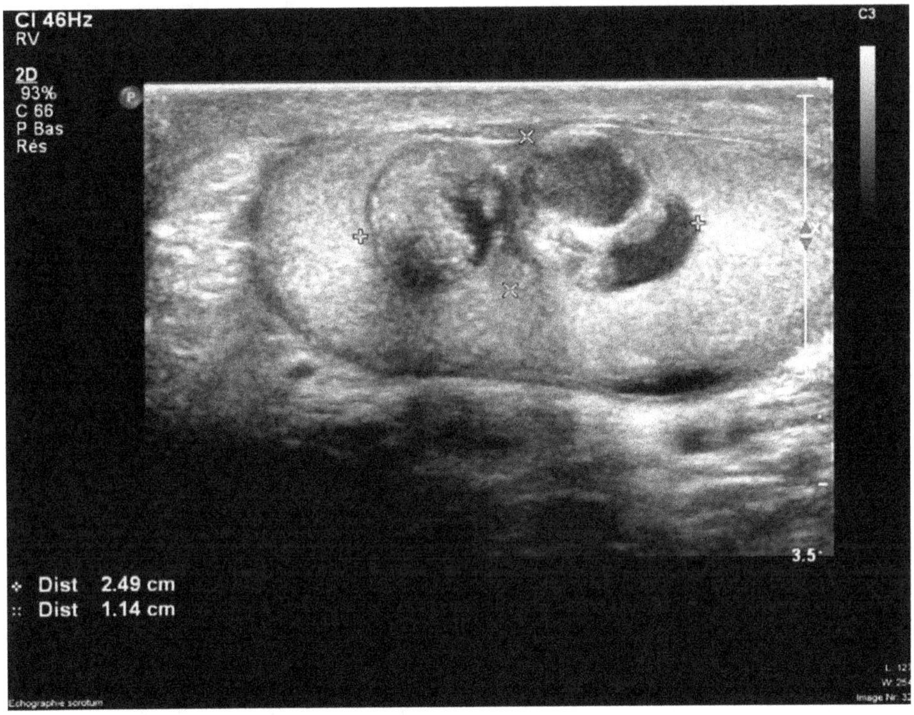

FIGURE 1: Ultrasound features: heterogenous, hypoechogenic, and cystic tumor of 20 mm.

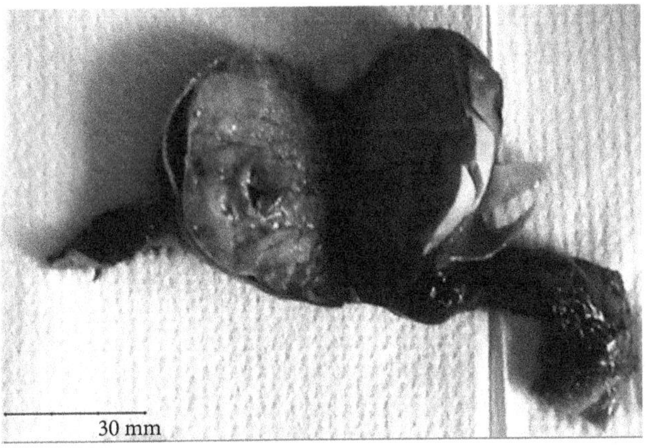

FIGURE 2: Macroscopically, the intratesticular tumor appeared cystic with an endoluminal solid area.

Microscopically, the tumor was well delineated and characterized by intraluminal papillae. The papillae are lined by pseudo- or pluristratified atypical cuboidal and/or ciliated epithelium. The mitotic index is less than 5 mitoses per HPF (×400). Rare psammoma bodies are also observed. No capsular invasion or vascular involvement is noted (Figure 3).

The tumor cells express cytokeratin-7 (CK7 clone *OV/TL12/30*, 1 : 400, Leica Newcastle, United Kingdom), cytokeratin 5-6 (CK 5-6 clone *D 5/6 B4*, 1 : 100, Dako, Glostrup, Denmark), cancer antigen 125 (CA-125 clone *M1*, ready to use, Dako, Glostrup, Denmark), estrogen (ER clone *EP1*, 1 : 50, Dako, Glostrup, Denmark), progesterone (PR clone *16+SAN27*, 1 : 500, Leica Newcastle, United Kingdom), Wilm's tumor gene (WT1 clone *6F-H2*, 1 : 150, Dako, Glostrup, Denmark), paired box gene 8 (PAX8 clone *MRQ-50*, ready to use, Menarini, Firenze, Italy), Ber-EP4 (clone *Ber-EP4*, 1 : 800, Dako, Glostrup, Denmark), and epithelial membrane antigen (EMA clone E29, 1 : 400, Dako, Glostrup Denmark). We do not observe immunopositivity for cytokeratin 20 (CK20 clone *Ks 20.8*, 1 : 100, Dako, Glostrup, Denmark), CDX2 gene (clone *DAK-CDX2*, 1 : 100, Dako, Glostrup, Denmark), Sal-like protein 4 (SALL4, clone *6E3*, 1 : 100, Cell-Marque, California, United States), human chorionic gonadotropin (beta-HCG clone *GA508*, ready to use, Dako, Glostrup, Denmark), alpha-foetoprotein (AFP clone *GA500*, ready to use, Dako, Glostrup, Denmark), podoplanin (clone D2-40, ready to use, Dako, Glostrup, Denmark), and calretinin (clone *DAK Calret 1*, 1 : 300, Dako, Glostrup, Denmark). p53 protein (clone *DO-7*, 1 : 200, Dako, Glostrup, Denmark) expression is weak and patchy. The proliferative index evaluated by Ki-67 antibody (clone *MIB-1*, 1 : 200, Dako, Glostrup, Denmark) is about 10%.

The molecular profile of the lesion was performed using next-generation sequencing (NGS) with a panel of 16 genes, described in Table 1 [10]. Briefly, DNA was isolated from formalin-fixed and paraffin-embedded (FFPE) tumor samples using the QIAamp FFPE tissue kit (Qiagen, Antwerp, Belgium), according to the manufacturer's instructions. First of all, tumor tissue was manually microdissected with a scalpel on a 10 μm paraffin slide using the H&E-stained slide cut from the same block. This H&E-stained slide was previously reviewed by a pathologist to evaluate the tumor cell percentage in the tumor area. DNA was then quantified using the Qubit® fluorometer and Qubit® ds DNA HS assay kit (Life Technologies, Gent, Belgium). Detection of mutations was performed using a next-generation platform (Ion Torrent, Life Technologies) with a panel of 16 genes (Table 1)

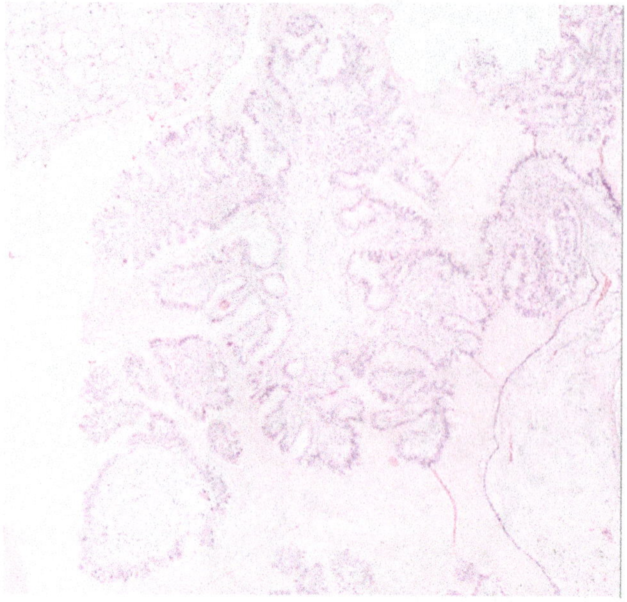

FIGURE 3: Microscopic view: cystic tumor with papillae lined by pseudo- or pluristratified atypical epithelium (hematoxylin and eosin) (×10).

TABLE 1: Cancer hotspot panel used by next-generation sequencing.

AKT1	DICER1	FOXL2	POLE
BRAF	ERBB2	KRAS	PTEN
CDKN2A	FBXW7	PIK3CA	RB1
CTNNB1	FGFR2	PIK3R1	TP53

previously validated at the Department of Pathology at Erasme Hospital (Brussels, Belgium) [10, 11]. The mutational analysis revealed a Q61K KRAS gene mutation in the testicular tumor.

3. Discussion

Ovarian-like epithelial tumors of the testis are extremely rare [1–5]. All types of epithelial tumors, serous, mucinous, seromucinous, and clear cell tumors, have been reported in the testis [6–8]. The most frequently reported types are serous borderline tumors, which share histological and immunohistological similarities with their ovarian counterpart.

These similarities found in such ovarian and testicular serous neoplasms can provide a better comprehension of the pathogenesis of serous borderline testis tumors.

Indeed, several hypotheses are proposed [12]; these tumors may arise from (1) embryological Mullerian remnants in paratesticular tissue, spermatic cord, or epididymis or (2) Mullerian metaplasia of intratesticular inclusions of the tunica vaginalis. This second hypothesis shows a similarity with the origin of the development of the ovarian counterpart, which seems to grow from germinal surface epithelium [13].

TABLE 2: Summary of gene mutations described in the serous borderline tumor of the testis.

	Gwiti et al., 2017 [9]	Burger et al., 2015 [12]	Cundell et al., 2015 [14]
Mutational analysis (number of cases)	7	2	1
No mutation	4	1	0
KRAS gene mutation	1	0	0
BRAF gene mutation	3	1	1

However, the mutational profile of such testicular tumors is poorly understood, probably due to the rarity of these entities [9, 12, 14].

We report here a case of a serous borderline tumor of the testis showing a Q61K KRAS gene mutation. This is the second reported case of a KRAS gene mutation in this type of testis tumor. The other gene mutations in these tumors include BRAF gene mutations (Table 2) [9, 12, 14].

Interestingly, in ovarian serous borderline neoplasms, BRAF and KRAS gene mutations are frequently found and known to be involved in the carcinogenesis of these tumors and support common pathogenesis in serous borderline tumors of both female and male, possibly arising from Mullerian origin/remnants [15–17]. BRAF and KRAS are protooncogenes involved in the mitogen-activated protein kinase (MAPK) pathway. The activation of this pathway involves the cascade of activation of signaling proteins such as RAS, RAF, MEK, and ERK, which leads to increased cell growth and differentiation. Mutations in BRAF or KRAS gene result in the constitutional activation of the MAPK pathway and aberrant cell proliferation [18, 19].

Low-grade serous lesions of the testis and their ovarian counterpart have the potentiality of recurrence and metastasis after surgery [20, 21]. Classically, this kind of tumors has shown a low response rate to cytotoxic chemotherapy [20–22]. Therefore, the RAS/RAF/MEK/ERK pathway could constitute an attractive target for cancer drugs in patients with KRAS and/or BRAF mutations [23].

Naturally, due to the rarity of these tumors in testis, their mutational status should be confirmed in the future in a larger series.

References

[1] A. S. Ibrahim, C. Li, and M. S. al-Jafari, "Borderline serous papillary tumour of the testis: a case report and review of the literature," *Anticancer Research*, vol. 32, no. 11, pp. 5011–5013, 2012.

[2] H. Maruyama, N. Ohyama, Y. Hosokawa et al., "Serous borderline tumor of the paratestis," *Pathology International*, vol. 58, no. 5, pp. 311–316, 2008.

[3] L. S. Abdullah, R. Gupta, and A. Arnst, "Intratesticular borderline serous tumor," *International Journal of Urology*, vol. 13, no. 12, pp. 1536–1538, 2006.

[4] R. F. McClure, G. L. Keeney, T. J. Sebo, and J. C. Cheville, "Serous borderline tumor of the paratestis: a report of seven cases," *The American Journal of Surgical Pathology*, vol. 25, no. 3, pp. 373–378, 2001.

[5] R. Guarch, A. Rivas, A. Puras, and C. Pesce, "Papillary serous carcinoma of ovarian type of the testis with borderline differentiation," *Histopathology*, vol. 46, no. 5, pp. 588–590, 2005.

[6] A. Z. Thomas, T. E. D. McDermott, S. Crowther, and J. A. Thornhill, "Primary clear cell carcinoma of the rete testis: 1st report," *Case Reports*, vol. 2015, 2015.

[7] B. Scholz, M. Beckert, V. Mordstein, N. Hohmann, R. Walther, and T. Papadopoulos, "Seromucinous borderline tumor of the testis—a case report," *Human Pathology*, vol. 60, pp. 188–191, 2017.

[8] S. Menon, S. Desai, and S. Ahmed, "Primary borderline mucinous neoplasm of the testis: a case report and literature review," *Indian Journal of Urology*, vol. 28, no. 2, pp. 224–226, 2012.

[9] P. Gwiti, I. Vereczkey, D. Cundell et al., "The mutational frequency ofBRAFandKRASin low-grade serous testicular neoplasms-a case series," *Histopathology*, vol. 71, no. 5, pp. 686–692, 2017.

[10] L. Bienfait, N. D'Haene, X. Catteau, and J. C. Noël, "PIK3CA and p53 mutations by next generation sequencing in lymphoepithelioma-like carcinoma of the endometrium," *Case Reports in Pathology*, vol. 2018, Article ID 5894589, 5 pages, 2018.

[11] C. Koopmansch, C. Maris, P. Demetter et al., "Differentiated-type intraepithelial neoplasia-like lesion associated with squamous cell carcinoma of the anus: a case report with molecular profile," *Case Reports in Pathology*, vol. 2019, Article ID 2301640, 5 pages, 2019.

[12] T. Bürger, H.-U. Schildhaus, R. Inniger et al., "Ovarian-type epithelial tumours of the testis: immunohistochemical and molecular analysis of two serous borderline tumours of the testis," *Diagnostic Pathology*, vol. 10, no. 1, p. 118, 2015.

[13] M. Michal, D. V. Kazakov, D. Kacerovska et al., "Paratesticular cystadenomas with ovarian stroma, metaplastic serous Müllerian epithelium, and male adnexal tumor of probable Wolffian origin: a series of 5 hitherto poorly recognized testicular tumors," *Annals of Diagnostic Pathology*, vol. 17, no. 2, pp. 151–158, 2013.

[14] D. Cundell, J. Pawade, M. Sohail, and Z. Melegh, "The V600E BRAF mutation in a borderline serous tumour of the testis is genotypic evidence of similarity with its phenotypic ovarian counterpart," *Histopathology*, vol. 67, no. 1, pp. 142–144, 2015.

[15] I. M. Shih and R. J. Kurman, "Ovarian tumorigenesis: a proposed model based on morphological and molecular genetic analysis," *The American Journal of Pathology*, vol. 164, no. 5, pp. 1511–1518, 2004.

[16] D. Mayr, A. Hirschmann, U. Löhrs, and J. Diebold, "KRAS and BRAF mutations in ovarian tumors: a comprehensive study of invasive carcinomas, borderline tumors and extraovarian implants," *Gynecologic Oncology*, vol. 103, no. 3, pp. 883–887, 2006.

[17] G. Singer, R. Oldt, Y. Cohen et al., "Mutations in BRAF and KRAS characterize the development of low-grade ovarian serous carcinoma," *Journal of the National Cancer Institute*, vol. 95, no. 6, pp. 484–486, 2003.

[18] M. Burotto, V. L. Chiou, J. M. Lee, and E. C. Kohn, "The MAPK pathway across different malignancies: a new perspective," *Cancer*, vol. 120, no. 22, pp. 3446–3456, 2014.

[19] P. T. C. Wan, M. J. Garnett, S. M. Roe et al., "Mechanism of activation of the RAF-ERK signaling pathway by oncogenic mutations of B-RAF," *Cell*, vol. 116, no. 6, pp. 855–867, 2004.

[20] M. A. Jones, R. H. Young, J. R. Srigley, and R. E. Scully, "Paratesticular serous papillary carcinoma a report of six cases," *The American Journal of Surgical Pathology*, vol. 19, no. 12, pp. 1359–1365, 1995.

[21] Y. T. Ma, S. Chaudhri, and M. H. Cullen, "Metastatic serous carcinoma of the testis: a case report and review of the literature," *Case Reports in Oncology*, vol. 4, no. 1, pp. 246–249, 2011.

[22] C.-H. Yeh, P.-P. Hsieh, S.-J. Lin et al., "Testicular serous carcinoma of ovarian epithelial type," *Journal of Cancer Research and Practice*, vol. 4, no. 2, pp. 76–79, 2017.

[23] P. J. Roberts and C. J. Der, "Targeting the Raf-MEK-ERK mitogen-activated protein kinase cascade for the treatment of cancer," *Oncogene*, vol. 26, no. 22, pp. 3291–3310, 2007.

7

Malignant Priapism as a Result of Metastatic Thyroid Cancer: A Hard Reality

Ethan Vargo,[1] Bryson Cook,[2] Jason Lane,[3] Eric Speakman,[3] and Neel Parekh[1]

[1]*Cleveland Clinic Akron General Department of Urology, Akron General Avenue, Akron, OH 44307, USA*
[2]*Northeast Ohio Medical University, 4209 St, OH-44, Rootstown, OH 44272, USA*
[3]*Cleveland Clinic Akron General Department of Pathology, Akron General Avenue, Akron, OH 44307, USA*

Correspondence should be addressed to Ethan Vargo; vargoe@ccf.org

Academic Editor: Claudio Simeone

Metastasis to the penis is an extremely rare entity. Malignant priapism is defined as a persistent, nonsexual erection that is refractory to pharmacologic treatment, corporal aspiration, and surgical shunts. Furthermore, it is typically a hallmark of an advanced cancer that has metastasized, most commonly from regional organs like the prostate or bladder. We report an unusual case of malignant priapism in the setting of metastatic follicular thyroid carcinoma. To date, this is the second reported case of penile metastasis due to thyroid carcinoma and the first incidence of priapism secondary to follicular thyroid carcinoma metastasis.

1. Introduction

Primary cancer of the penis is a rare occurrence in North America and Europe, with rates approaching 1 in 100,000 men annually [1]. Metastases to the penis and malignant priapism, however, are exceedingly rare phenomena. Metastatic rectal adenocarcinoma to the penis was the first reported case of penile metastasis, as described by Eberth in 1870 [2]. While the vast majority of cases involving metastasis to the penis involve regional organs, there have been a limited number of cases originating from the head and neck region [3, 4]. Although a very rare occurrence, this report describes the phenomenon of metastasis to the penis resulting in a sustained erection and highlights the importance of considering metastatic disease as a differential diagnosis, especially in a patient with known malignancy presenting with priapism.

2. Case Presentation

The patient is a 73-year-old male with a past medical history of metastatic follicular thyroid carcinoma that was initially diagnosed in 2013. The patient underwent total thyroidectomy with radioactive iodine ablation in 2014. He was then found to have metastasis to the liver and underwent liver ablations in 2016 and 2018. In early 2020, the patient underwent positron emission tomography (PET) which demonstrated several metastatic sites involving the lung and bone and recurrent lesions within the liver. At this time, the patient underwent palliative radiation and was initiated on immunotherapy. Follow-up imaging in mid-2020 demonstrated regression of the previously identified pulmonary nodules.

The patient initially presented in August of 2020 to the urology service in the emergency department with a chief complaint of penile edema and pain for the previous few days. On physical examination, the penile shaft was significantly edematous, tender to palpation, and appeared to be erect. Based on the patient's history and physical exam, a diagnosis of priapism was made. A corporal blood gas was subsequently obtained. The corporal blood gas exhibited a pH of 6.999, consistent with ischemic priapism. Bedside corporal aspiration was then performed yielding a scant amount of thick, dark blood. Given the significant penile edema, it was difficult to ascertain the degree of improvement following corporal aspiration. The patient's pain, however, was well controlled, and he was discharged home with plans for close follow-up.

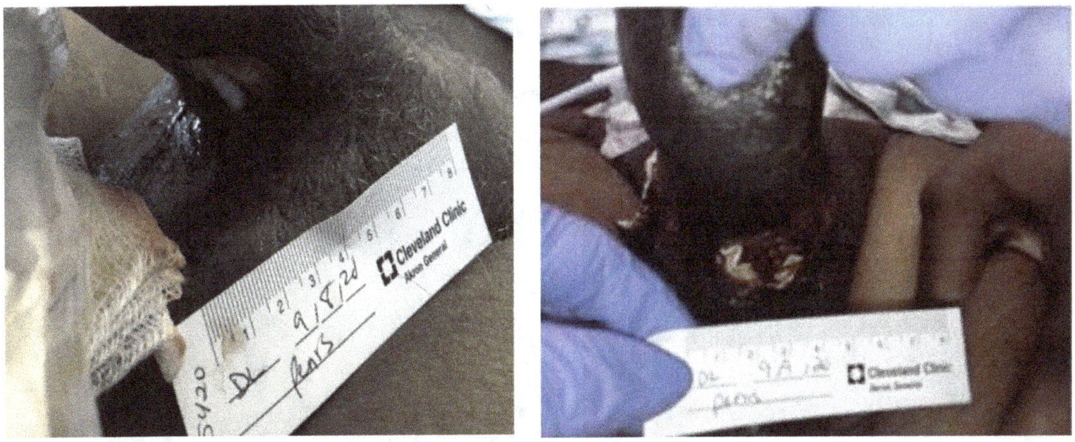

(a) (b)

FIGURE 1: Physical exam findings prior to surgery demonstrated ventral urethral erosion and a visible Foley catheter (a). Postsurgical outcome after debridement and a visible Penrose drain at the base of ventral penile shaft (b).

The patient was admitted to the hospital two days later with shortness of breath, and he was found to have extensive metastatic disease to the lungs. Additionally, the patient also experienced new onset urinary retention and a Foley catheter was placed. Upon evaluation, the patient's physical exam was relatively unchanged from a few days prior. An inpatient pelvic MRI was ordered; however, it was unable to be obtained due to patient-reported claustrophobia. Within 24 hours of the Foley catheter placement, a new two-centimeter ulcerative lesion at the base of the ventral penile shaft was noted. There did appear to be erosion into the ventral bulbar urethra, as the Foley catheter that was previously placed for retention was now visible. Sloughing of the skin was present and the wound was foul smelling (Figure 1(a)). A decision was made to take the patient to the operating room urgently for exploration and debridement.

Initially, cystoscopy was performed to fully evaluate the urethra given the new ulcerative lesion on the ventral aspect of the penis eroding into the urethra. A flexible cystoscope was used as a rigid cystoscope was unable to bypass the area of necrosis. Once the gangrenous area was traversed and the bladder was entered, pan cystoscopy did not demonstrate any additional abnormalities in the urethra or bladder. A suprapubic catheter was placed. With the urine diverted, attention was then turned to the bulbar urethra. The wound was copiously irrigated and debrided. Bilateral penoscrotal decompression and corporal biopsies were performed. A Penrose drain was left, and the wound was packed with wet to dry gauze (Figure 1(b)). Minimal improvement of the patient's penile edema and priapism was noted on postoperative day one. A computed tomography (CT) scan of the abdomen and pelvis with IV contrast was obtained following surgery. This demonstrated several new hepatic lesions, a right adrenal mass, and portacaval adenopathy (Figure 2(a)). There was also enlargement of a right posterior ilium osteolytic lesion (Figure 2(b)). Additionally, enlargement of the penis at the base was noted (Figures 3(a) and 3(b)).

Pathology from the intraoperative biopsies demonstrated poorly differentiated carcinoma with dyscohesive malignant epithelioid cells demonstrating pleomorphism in a background of necrosis (Figure 4(a)). Additionally, the cells stained positive for pan-keratin, paired box gene 8 (PAX-8) (Figure 4(b)), and epithelial membrane antigen (EMA) (Figure 4(c)) confirming a dedifferentiated or anaplastic process related to the patient's known history of metastatic follicular cell carcinoma of the thyroid.

Surgical options were discussed with the patient including penectomy; however, the patient was reluctant. Palliative radiation was deemed to be of minimal benefit by radiation oncology. The patient was ultimately discharged home, admitted to home hospice, and expired shortly after hospice initiation.

3. Discussion

Overall, metastasis to the penis is a rare phenomenon with fewer than 500 reported cases in the literature. Priapism, or a sustained erection for greater than four hours, represents 40% of the cases of metastatic disease to the penis [4]. Other manifestations of penile metastasis include penile masses, pain within the penis or perineum, voiding symptoms, and widespread swelling [5]. The most common sites of carcinoma origin in cases of metastasis to the penis include the bladder (28.6%), prostate (27.9%), and rectum-sigmoid (12.2%) [5]. Hypothesized pathophysiologic pathways leading to malignant priapism include direct tumor cell invasion of the corpora cavernosa, venous occlusion of the penis, and disruption of neural pathways [5].

Patients with penile metastasis do have slightly better survival when they undergo surgical intervention compared to those who undergo conservative measures like radiation and chemotherapy. Despite a greater than 80% mortality rate at one year for those presenting with penile metastasis, partial or total penectomy can be offered for improving short-term quality of life and minimizing local complications [4]. Our patient had new evidence of widely metastatic disease on presentation as depicted via imaging in Figure 2 and likely would not have benefited from further surgical management given his very poor performance status and limited lifespan.

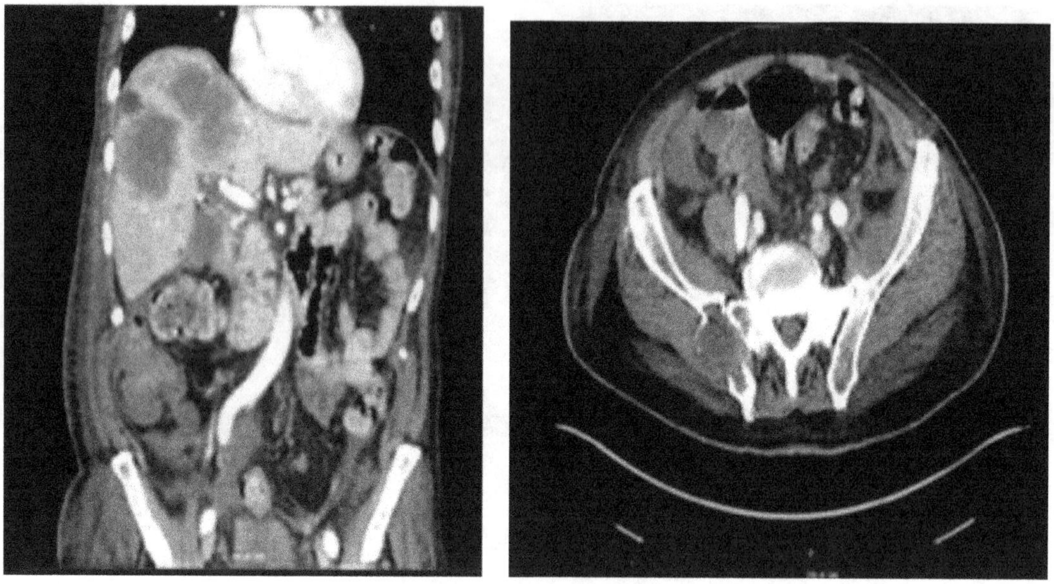

(a) (b)

FIGURE 2: CT of the abdomen and pelvis with IV contrast demonstrating hepatic metastatic disease with an enlargement of the hepatic lobe mass. Right adrenal mass consistent with metastatic disease. Development of portacaval adenopathy consistent with metastatic disease (a). Expansile osteolytic right posterior ilium lesion (b).

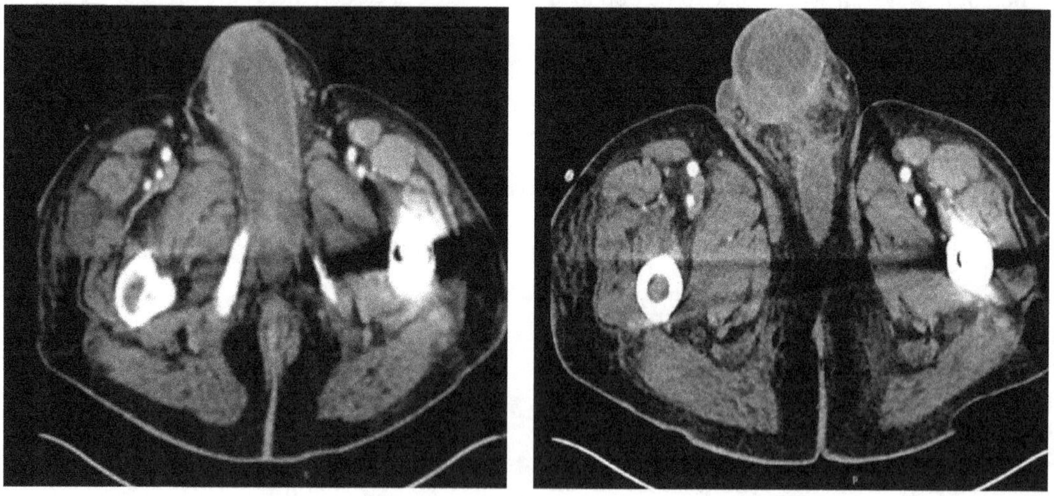

(a) (b)

FIGURE 3: CT of the abdomen and pelvis with IV contrast obtained on postoperative day one demonstrating enlargement of the penis, likely consistent with metastatic, inflammatory, and postsurgical changes (a, b).

Immunohistochemical staining in the setting of a rare disease process can provide valuable information in the determination of disease origin. In our patient's case, intraoperative biopsy of the penis was consistent with poorly differentiated carcinoma with dyscohesive malignant epithelioid cells, which stained positive for pan-keratin, EMA, and PAX-8. The transcription factor, PAX-8, orchestrates embryonic development within Mullerian organs, the kidney, and the thyroid [6]. In one study, PAX-8 was detected in 100% of patients with primary follicular thyroid cancer, and the authors concluded that PAX-8 is both sensitive and specific for cell staining in cases of metastatic tumors of thyroid origin [6]. Another study demonstrated significance in the expression of EMA in patients with follicular thyroid carcinomas [7]. The PAX-8- and EMA-positive staining of the poorly differentiated cells in our patient's penile biopsies suggests that the patient's malignant priapism was a result of his metastatic follicular thyroid cancer. Furthermore, the presence of metastatic thyroid tumor cells within our patient's penile corpora highlights the hematogenous and potentially distant pattern of metastasis that follicular thyroid carcinoma commonly demonstrates [8].

Only one other case of thyroid cancer metastasizing to the penis has been reported in the literature, highlighting

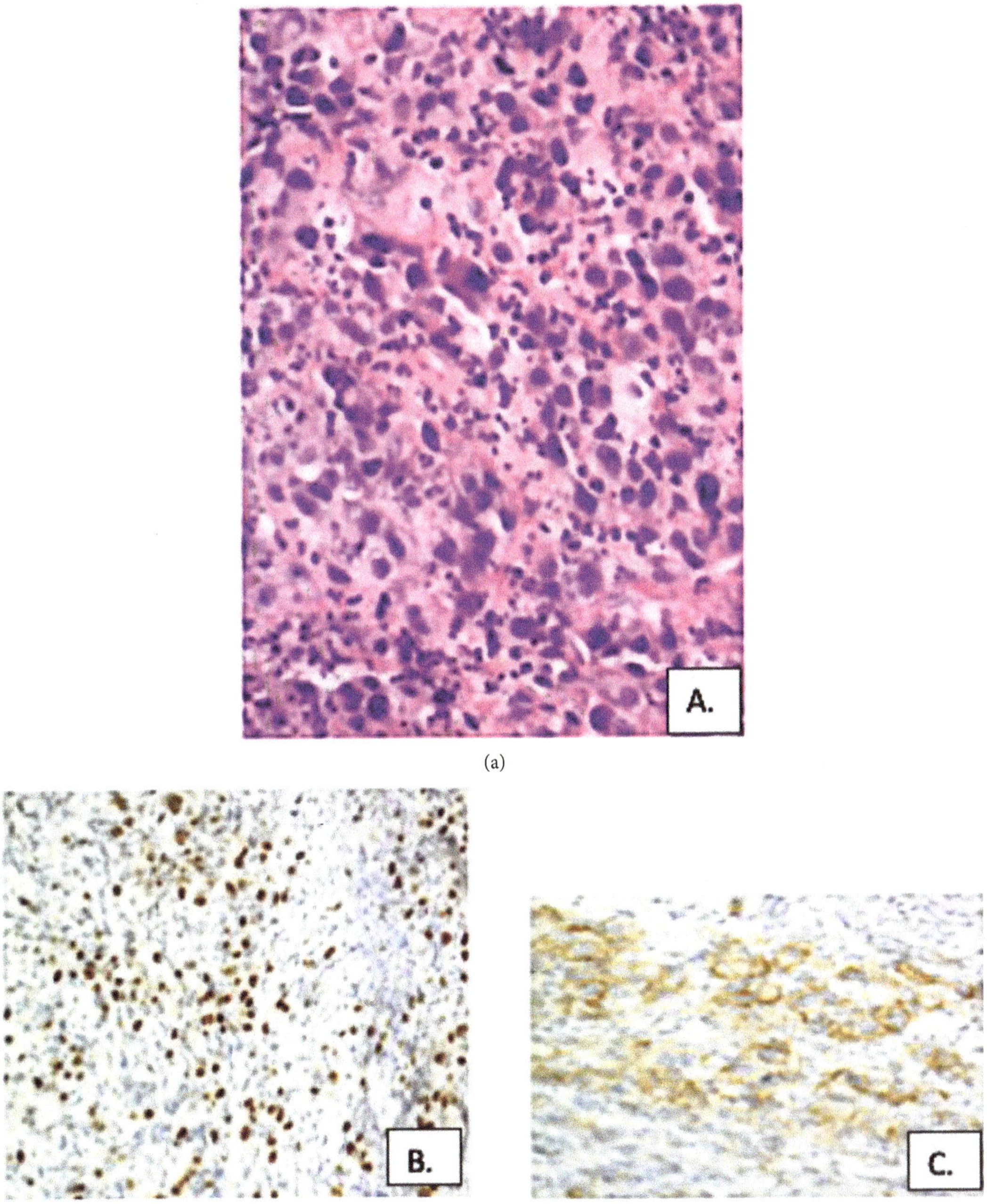

(a)

(b)

(c)

FIGURE 4: Histologic stains demonstrating hematoxylin and eosin stain of penile biopsies showing poorly differentiated carcinoma with dyscohesive malignant epithelioid cells demonstrating pleomorphism in a background of necrosis (a). Positive PAX-8 stain (b). Positive EMA stain (c).

the rarity that is associated with metastasis from a distant organ. That patient had a history of metastatic follicular thyroid cancer that had metastasized to the bone and pelvis. Additionally, the patient developed a nodule on the proximal penile shaft and subsequently underwent total penectomy with the creation of a perineal urethrostomy and ultimately expired secondary to his metastatic disease [4]. With the very limited number of case reports describing metastasis to the penis and only one other case report describing metastasis from follicular thyroid carcinoma, it is difficult to derive an algorithm for clinical and surgical management of these patients. One clinical takeaway is understanding the widespread and terminal nature of a malignancy by the time penile metastasis is identified. In those who present with priapism without a history of malignancy, the clinician should consider metastatic priapism due to an undiagnosed regional or distant organ metastasis.

4. Conclusion

Metastasis to the penis and malignant priapism are very rare phenomena; however, they should be considered especially in a patient with a known history of malignancy. Limited clinical and surgical options exist given the known disseminated nature of disease on presentation.

References

[1] American Cancer Society, "Penile Cancer," https://www.cancer.org/cancer/penile-cancer.html.

[2] C. J. Eberth, "Krebsmetastasen des corpus cavernosum penis," *Archiv für Pathologische Anatomie und Physiologie und für Klinische Medicin*, vol. 51, no. 1, pp. 145-146, 1870.

[3] L. M. Perez, R. A. Shumway, C. C. Carson, S. R. Fisher, and W. R. Hudson, "Penile metastasis secondary to supraglottic squamous cell carcinoma: review of the literature," *The Journal of Urology*, vol. 147, no. 1, pp. 157–160, 1992.

[4] M. O. Grimm, P. Spiegelhalder, H. Heep, C. D. Gerharz, H. D. Röher, and R. Ackermann, "Penile metastasis secondary to follicular thyroid carcinoma," *Scandinavian Journal of Urology and Nephrology*, vol. 38, no. 3, pp. 253–255, 2004.

[5] L. Mearini, R. Colella, A. Zucchi, E. Nunzi, C. Porrozzi, and M. Porena, "A review of penile metastasis," *Oncology Reviews*, vol. 6, no. 1, p. 10, 2012.

[6] A. Ozcan, S. S. Shen, C. Hamilton et al., "PAX 8 expression in non-neoplastic tissues, primary tumors, and metastatic tumors: a comprehensive immunohistochemical study," *Modern Pathology*, vol. 24, no. 6, pp. 751–764, 2011.

[7] N. W. Wilson, H. Pambakian, T. C. Richardson, M. R. Stokoe, C. A. Makin, and E. Heyderman, "Epithelial markers in thyroid carcinoma: an immunoperoxidase study," *Histopathology*, vol. 10, no. 8, pp. 815–829, 1986.

[8] Y. Kushchayeva, Q. Y. Duh, E. Kebebew, A. D'Avanzo, and O. H. Clark, "Comparison of clinical characteristics at diagnosis and during follow-up in 118 patients with Hurthle cell or follicular thyroid cancer," *American Journal of Surgery*, vol. 195, no. 4, pp. 457–462, 2008.

8

Urological Tract Infection with Candida Bezoars in a Woman with Diabetes Type 2

Astrid Van Daele, Johan Schurmans, and Raf Van Reusel

AZ Turnhout, Rubensstraat 166, 2300 Turnhout, Belgium

Correspondence should be addressed to Astrid Van Daele; astridvdaele@gmail.com

Academic Editor: Claudio Simeone

The aim of this report is to describe a case of fungal bezoar obstruction of the kidney and our experience in managing it endoscopically. A 61-year-old woman presented with flank pain. On CT scan, a proximal stone and secondary dilatation was seen. After placing a DJ stent and administering antibiotics, there was persistent pain, sickness, and kidney dilatation on CT scan. URS showed soft tissue bezoars surrounding the stent and the stone. We managed to remove all the fungal balls mechanically and endoscopically. This report showed that endoscopic removal of the bezoars is a good alternative for antifungal installation.

1. Introduction

Urinary tract infections caused by fungi are not rare. The most common species is Candida albicans, which is responsible for over 50% of the cases [1].

The organism exists as a commensal and is most frequently found on the skin. In immunocompromised or debilitated individuals, the fungus may become a pathogen. Hosts with certain risk factors can be susceptible to this opportunistic infection. Urinary tract colonization can be the result of a systemic, disseminated infection or of a local, retrograde infection of the bladder.

Known risk factors include recent or long antibiotic use, diabetes mellitus, indwelling catheter use, urinary tract pathology, malignancy, pregnancy, immunosuppression, renal transplantation, and recent surgery. Also urinary stasis and lithiasis have been reported [2].

Rarely, the fungus can be organized in fungus balls or bezoars, colonizing the drainage system, sometimes leading to obstruction.

2. Case Presentation

A 61-year-old woman, known with diabetes type 2, presented at the emergency department with left flank pain and no fever. White blood cell count (WBC) was 10 000/μL, C-reactive protein (CRP) 32 mg/dL, and glomerular filtration rate (GFR) 58. No imaging was done, and the patient was sent home with Levofloxacin and the diagnosis of an ascending urinary infection.

Two days later, the patient came back to the ER with persisting pain and still no fever. Now the white blood cell count was 11 000/μL and C-reactive protein 8 mg/dL. A CT scan without contrast was done and showed a proximal stone of 6 mm in the left ureter and a secondary dilated pelvicalyceal system. No other aberrant findings were described in the urinary tract. Urinary culture from two days ago showed E. coli, sensitive to the taken antibiotics.

The patient got admitted to the urology department, and a DJ stent was placed. She was discharged on her own initiative the day after with continuation of the antibiotics.

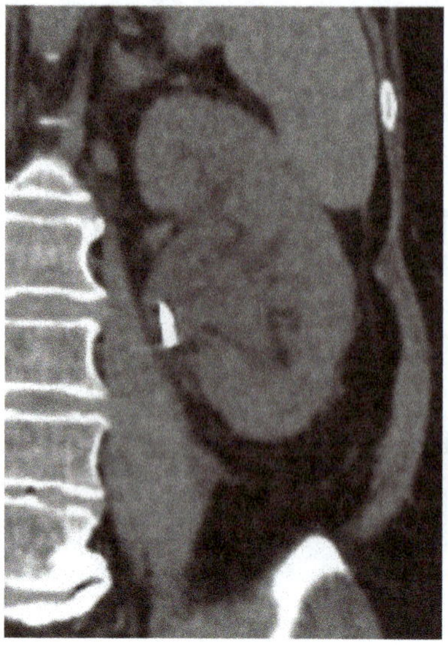

FIGURE 1: CT scan; persistent hydronephrosis despite DJ stent.

Three days after discharge we saw her back at the consultation, earlier than planned. She felt sick, was vomiting, and reported persistent flank pain without fever. Repeat blood sample, urine sample, and blood cultures were taken, and she was admitted. Her WBC was 9000, CRP 200 and GFR 41. A repeat CT scan showed persisting dilation of the left kidney, DJ stent, and stone unchanged in situ (Figure 1).

We decided to perform a diagnostic cystoureteroscopy, thinking the stent was maybe dysfunctional or not well positioned.

On cystoscopy and ureteroscopy, we found soft, spongy masses in the bladder and along the stent (Figure 2). We removed the tissue from the bladder mechanically with small forceps and by rinsing it out through the cystoscope.

In the kidney, we aspirated the mass and pus with syringes through the ureteroscope. We sent this together with the bezoars for culture and microscopy. We removed the stone and the stent and placed no bladder catheter.

Candida albicans was then isolated from the urine, the aspirated fluid and tissue, and her blood. In addition, we isolated E. coli from the urine.

After consulting a microbiologist, we put her on intravenous Diflucan 400 mg/day and Levofloxacin 500 mg twice a day. Two days later, we additionally started her on oral and vaginal antifungal agent because of local Candida infection. Blood cultures were carried out daily. We continued the Diflucan until 14 days after the first negative blood culture.

Fundoscopy and transesophageal ultrasound were carried out to exclude intraocular infection and endocarditis. They were negative.

On outpatient consultation, she did well and blood and urine cultures were negative.

3. Discussion

In our case, the patient was only known with diabetes as the predisposing condition. The trigger for the infection was the proximal ureter stone. On the third admission, her glycaemia was too high. This could be due to the infection she was going through. On the other hand, the uncontrolled glycaemia could have made her susceptible for the Candida infection.

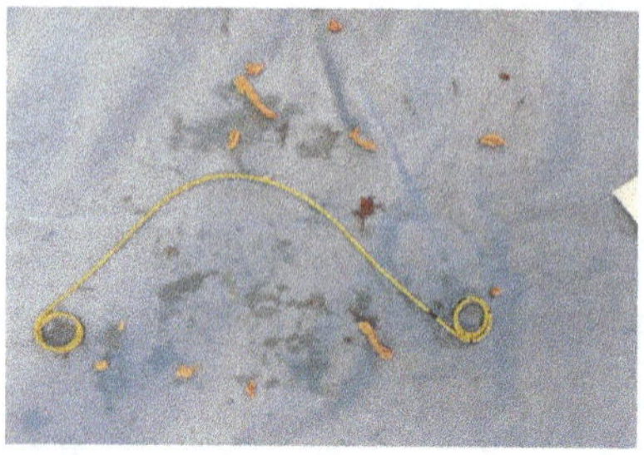

FIGURE 2: DJ stent and surrounding fungal tissue.

In all debilitated or immunosuppressed (septic) patients who have upper urinary tract obstruction with renal filling defect, fungal infection should be considered.

The clinical diagnosis can be confirmed by positive urine or hemoculture. The presence of obstruction and inflammation without lithiasis or after placement of a stent, in the renal collecting system, could be an important clue in the radiological diagnosis. On the ultrasound, an enlarged kidney filled with fungus balls can be seen. On CT, the fungus balls appear as soft tissue masses in the collecting system and, depending on the volume, with mass effect. On contrast-enhanced CT, the tendency of obstruction can be objectivized [3].

Fisher et al. published an algorithm for the treatment of Candida urinary tract infections in general. For bezoars and mycetomas, it is stated that, next to systemic therapy with antifungal agents (fluconazole is preferred), surgical drainage is almost always needed [4].

In the case of presence of fungal balls, several methods have been proposed, such as installation through nephrostomy and percutaneous endoscopic disruption of percutaneous irrigation with streptokinase.

In our case, we managed to physically remove all masses endoscopically, so there was no need for antifungal installation. As Abuelnaga et al. also demonstrated, endoscopic retrieval of the renal tissues by ureteroscopy can be an effective and rapid way to manage fungal balls. The hospital stay and toxicity associated with antifungals can hereby be reduced, in comparison to installation through nephrostomy [5]. Especially in cases where a diagnostic URS is carried out or in cases where a nephrostomy is contraindicated, the URS should be considered as a first line treatment, in combination with systemic antifungal treatment.

4. Conclusion

We described a case of a patient, predisposed with diabetes type 2, who suffered renal obstruction due to a Candida infection with fungal bezoars.

In this case, we managed to physically remove all masses endoscopically, so there was no need for antifungal installation. Especially in cases where a diagnostic URS is carried out or in cases where a nephrostomy is contraindicated, the URS should be considered as a first line treatment, in combination with systemic antifungal treatment.

References

[1] A. G. Dembner and R. C. Pfister, "Fungal infection of the urinary tract: demonstration by antegrade pyelography and drainage by percutaneous nephrostomy," *American Journal of Roentgenology*, vol. 129, no. 3, pp. 415–418, 1977.

[2] J. D. Sobel, C. A. Kauffman, D. McKinsey et al., "Candiduria: a randomized, double-blind study of treatment with fluconazole and placebo," *Clinical Infectious Diseases*, vol. 30, no. 1, pp. 19–24, 2000.

[3] A. Erden, S. Fitoz, T. Karagülle, S. Tükel, and S. Akyar, "Radiological findings in the diagnosis of genitourinary candidiasis," *Pediatric Radiology*, vol. 30, no. 12, pp. 875–877, 2000.

[4] J. F. Fisher, J. D. Sobel, C. A. Kauffman, and C. A. Newman, "Candida urinary tract infections—treatment," *Clinical Infectious Diseases*, vol. 52, suppl_6, pp. S457–S466, 2011.

[5] M. Abuelnaga, S. Khoshzaban, M. Reda Badr, and A. Chaudry, "Successful endoscopic management of a renal fungal ball using flexible ureterorenoscopy," *Case Reports in Urology*, vol. 2019, Article ID 9241928, 4 pages, 2019.

9

Asynchronous Bilateral Ureteric-Arterial Fistula: Diagnosis and Treatment

Pietro Pepe,[1,2] Letterio D'Arrigo,[1,2] Domenico Patane',[1,2] Ludovica Pepe,[1,2] Giuseppe Candiano,[1,2] and Michele Pennisi[1,2]

[1]*Urology Unit-Cannizzaro Hospital, via Messina 829, Catania, Italy*
[2]*Imaging Department-Cannizzaro Hospital, Catania, Italy*

Correspondence should be addressed to Pietro Pepe; piepepe@hotmail.com

Academic Editor: Apul Goel

A 48-year-old woman submitted to anterior exenteration plus ileal-cutaneous conduit for metastatic cervical cancer during the change of the ureteral stent showed massive bleeding in the left ureter. A selective intra-arterial angiography showed a fistula between the ureter and the left common iliac artery that the interventional radiologist quickly repaired by inserting a vascular endoprosthesis. Six months later, gross hematuria secondary to right ureter-iliac fistula occurred again and a second endoprosthesis was inserted. Asynchronous bilateral ureteric stent-related vascular fistula is an uncommon scenario, but it should be suspected in the presence of hematuria following ureteral stent replacement.

1. Introduction

The ureteric-arterial fistula (UAF) is a rare condition characterized by a direct fistulous communication between the ureter and the iliac artery resulting in bleeding into the ureter that was described for the first time by Moschcowitz in 1908 [1]. The UAF frequently can be associated with previous vascular and oncological surgery (bladder, gynecological, or colorectal cancer), aneurysm, or pseudoaneurysm of the common or external iliac artery, radiotherapy, and previous ureteral damage or alteration of the urinary system (stenosis, urinary diversion, or ureteral stent placement). Since these bleedings occur intermittently, the diagnosis is very difficult; in fact, UAF can be life-threatening because of potential massive blood loss, and diagnosis can easily be delayed or even missed because the presence of hematuria could be ascribed to variety of other urologic diseases. The mortality associated with UAF ranges from 7 to 58%, and the clinical outcome is correlated with an early diagnosis [2, 3]. UAF requires a rapid a multidisciplinary approach, including the expertise of the urologist, vascular surgeon, and interventional radiologist, to detect and treat this unusual disease [4, 5].

In this study, we report the clinical management of non-synchronous bilateral ureteric-iliac fistula.

2. Case Presentation

In 2009, a 48-year-old woman underwent radical hysterectomy for cervical cancer followed by adjuvant radiotherapy and chemotherapy. After two years, the patient was submitted to ureter-ileal-cutaneous conduit because of pelvic metastatic disease. During a check-up two years from anterior exenteration, a fibrosis plate in the lower pelvis that compressed both ureters and subsequently caused a hydronephrosis on both sides was diagnosed by abdominal computed tomography (CT). Therefore, at first, the kidneys were drained by percutaneous nephrostomy those later replaced by bilateral ureteral stent.

During a programmed change of the ureteral stent in September 2019, a massive bleeding in the left ureter was showed; through the quick change of the stent, a spontaneous tamponade was made, and after stabilizing the cardiovascular system and correcting the heavy loss of blood, a CT scan followed by a selective intra-arterial angiography in digital technique was carried out. Both examinations showed an

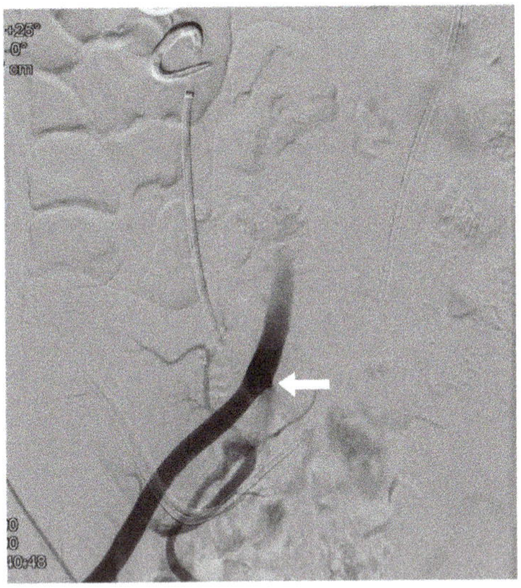

Figure 1: Intra-arterial angiography in digital technique showed a fistula between the common iliac artery and the ureter.

ureteroarterial fistula between the left common iliac artery and the ureter (Figure 1). During the examination, the interventional radiologist successfully repaired the common and the left common iliac artery by inserting a vascular endoprosthesis (stent Bentley BeGraft 10/37 mm). The patient was discharged after five days following CT scan. Six months later, hematuria with anemia occurred again after the programmed bilateral change of the ureteral stent; the patient quickly underwent CT-angiogram that showed the presence of an ureteroiliac fistula of the right side that was repaired by inserting a second endoprosthesis (Figures 2 and 3). The patient was successfully discharged after four day and still today is asymptomatic.

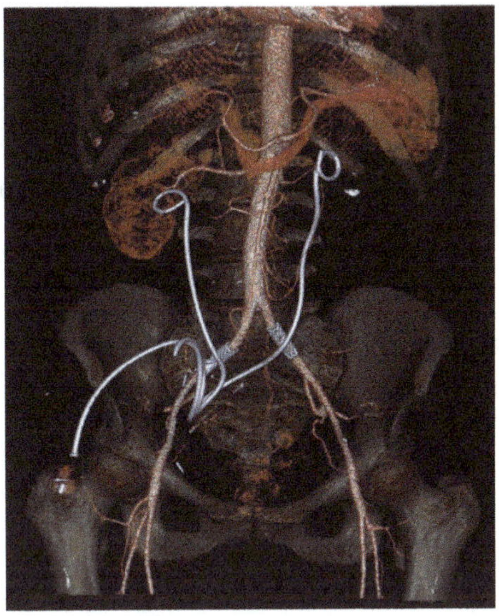

Figure 2: Three-dimensional abdominal CT scan that demonstrated bilateral iliac artery endoprosthesis and ureteral stents (axial evaluation).

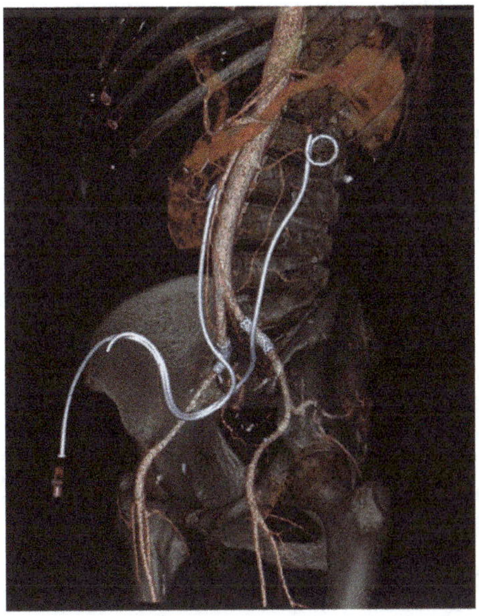

Figure 3: Three-dimensional abdominal CT scan that demonstrated bilateral iliac artery endoprosthesis and ureteral stents (sagittal evaluation).

3. Discussion

Ureteral stent-related UAF are reported in a small number of cases; the causative factor has been attributed to prolonged stent placement varying from 5 months to 15 years before the onset of hematuria [2]. The etiology of UAF is not well understood; a possible mechanism is related to the alteration in the ureteral wall elasticity with eventual pressure necrosis [3]. The other plausible theory is postoperative inflammatory reaction or associated infection leading to inflammatory ureteral fixation to the wall of the arteria leading to erosion. In the majority of ureteric-iliac fistula, the mechanical forces due to the pulsatility of the common iliac artery against the ureter that contribute to the erosion are predisposed by underlying vascular pathology, previous radiation therapy, and previous surgery, including genitourinary, pelvic, vascular operations, or the need of long-term ureteral stents. The hematuria is either intermittent or life-threatening, with some patients presenting spontaneously and others during stent exchange. In fact, most of the patients with a diagnosis of UAF have a history of pelvic malignancy; in addition, the increasing incidence in last decades is related to the increased number of various treatment introduced in clinical practice that predispose the development of a weakness tissue condition. The diagnosis of ureteric-arterial fistula could be elusive and may be delayed depending on the clinical scenario. The sensitivity of the standard angiography examination is 23-41%; but it can be improved to 63% using the "provocative" method, which means mobilizing the ureteral stent during examination. Other diagnostic studies, such as retrograde pyelogram and ureteroscopy, add minimal value in the presence of significant bleeding other than lateralizing the source of the hematuria. Almost 90% of patients with a correct diagnosis are treated successfully; on the other hand, the mortality for patients with an undiagnosed condition is up to 58%.

Multiple treatment options, such as open repair with ligation, embolization of the hypogastric artery or endovascular stenting, are available with various success rates; endovascular stenting has been proven to be effective and provides a faster resolution especially in a setting of massive hemorrhage [4, 5]. To our knowledge, about 140 cases have been described in the literature, but only one paper refers to bilateral ureteric-iliac fistula repair [3]; the mortality rate through UAF has decreased from 69% in 1980 to 7-23% today.

In our case, the patient presented with intermittent hematuria following the ureteral stent replacement; although the initial diagnosis of left ureteric-iliac fistula was delayed because the unusual clinical presentation, conversely, the presence of recurrent hematuria allowed to quickly diagnose the contralateral ureteroiliac fistula that was restored by an interventional radiologist.

4. Conclusion

Ureteric stent-related vascular fistula is an uncommon scenario, but it should be suspected in the presence of early and/or delayed hematuria following ureteral stent replacement; in addition, a multidisciplinary approach (interventional radiologist, vascular surgeon and urologist) is mandatory to achieve the best clinical results.

Ethical Approval

All procedures performed in this study involving human participants were in accordance with the ethical standards of the institutional and/or national research committee and with the 1964 Helsinki Declaration and its later amendments or comparable ethical standards.

Consent

Written informed consent was obtained from the patient for her anonymized information to be published in this article.

References

[1] A. V. Moschcowitz, "Simultaneous ligation of both external iliac arteries for secondary hemorrhage following bilateral ureterolithotomy," *Annals of Surgery*, vol. 48, no. 6, pp. 872–875, 1908.

[2] L. Leone, S. Scarcella, L. Dell'Atti, M. Tiroli, F. Sternardi, and A. B. Galosi, "Uretero-iliac artery fistula: a challenge diagnosis for a life-threatening condition: monocentric experience and review of the literature," *International Urology and Nephrology*, vol. 51, no. 5, pp. 789–793, 2019.

[3] R. C. N. van den Bergh, F. L. Moll, J.-P. P. M. de Vries, and T. M. T. W. Lock, "Arterioureteral fistulas: unusual suspects-systematic review of 139 cases," *Urology*, vol. 74, no. 2, pp. 251–255, 2009.

[4] J. D. Subiela, A. Balla, J. Bollo et al., "Endovascular management of ureteroarterial fistula: single institution experience and systematic literature review," *Vascular and Endovascular Surgery*, vol. 52, no. 4, pp. 275–286, 2018.

[5] A. Massmann, P. Fries, R. Shayesteh-Kheslat, A. Buecker, M. Stöckle, and C. Niklas, "Life-threatening arterioureteral fistula treatment by endovascular complete anatomic iliac artery bifurcation reconstruction," *Journal of Vascular Surgery Cases and Innovative Techniques*, vol. 6, no. 2, pp. 199–204, 2020.

10

Acute Urinary Retention in the Male Child from Urethral Calculi: A Report of Three Cases

L. O. Mbouché ,[1,2] G. Ondobo Andzé,[1,2] A. S. Nwaha Makon,[1] D. Nyanit Bob,[1] E. Njuma Tamufor,[1] A. L. Amenglé,[1,2] F. F. Mouafo Tambo ,[1,2] P. Y. Mure,[3] J. Zé Mikandé,[1,2] and F. F. Angwafo III[1,2]

[1] *Yaounde Gyneco-Obstetric and Pediatric Hospital, Cameroon*
[2] *Faculty of Medicine and Biomedical Sciences of University of Yaoundé I, Cameroon*
[3] *University Teaching Hospital of Lyon, France*

Correspondence should be addressed to L. O. Mbouché; landrymbouche@gmail.com

Academic Editor: Mohamed A. Ghoneim

Urinary stones are uncommon in children. Urethral location of calculi can give rise to various clinical manifestations. We report three cases of urethral lithiasis presenting with acute urinary retention in children.

1. Introduction

Acute urinary retention is commonly encountered in urological practice in adults, mostly from prostatic pathologies. In the male child, lower urinary tract symptoms are usually secondary to congenital uropathy, most often posterior urethral valves, and sometimes neurogenic bladders from spinal dysraphism. Urinary stones can be an obstacle to the normal flow of urine at any level of the lower urinary tract. In Europe, the prevalence of urolithiasis varies from 5 to 9% [1]. It is 20 times rarer in children than in adults [2]. Urolithiasis prevalence varies from 7 to 13% in North America; in Asia its prevalence varies from 1 to 5% [1]. There is a pediatric stone belt that runs from the Philippines, Myanmar, and Thailand in the Far East, extending to Pakistan and Iran in the Middle East and up to Turkey [3].

In sub-Saharan Africa, the prevalence of lithiasis in children is variously appreciated according to the geographical location although literature is sparse and limited to hospital studies. In Cameroon, a series of 123 cases in two hospitals reported a prevalence of 17% in children aged from 7 to 15 years, including 2% of stones located in the urethra [4]. However, no cases of acute retention of urine were reported.

The article presents three cases of acute urine retention from stones located in the male urethra.

2. Presentation

2.1. Case 1. A 2-year-old male was referred to the Pediatric Surgery Department of the Yaoundé Gynaeco-Obstetric and Pediatric Hospital from the Western region of Cameroon, with an enlarged bladder, dribbling urine with overflow incontinence. He presented with progressive dysuria from age 3 months, without fever or hematuria, but with repeated urinary tract infections. *Proteus vulgaris* sensitive to ceftriaxone was isolated in one of the urine samples. He was circumcised at 6 months and there was no family history of urolithiasis.

On clinical examination, the infant was a well-developed, well-nourished male, with a temperature of 37.5°C, a heart rate of 106 beats per minute, a respiratory rate of 25 cycles per minute, and a weight of 12 kg. A tense and sensitive bladder was palpated in the suprapubic region as well as a hard mass, at the base of the penis (Figure 1). There was no costovertebral angle tenderness. An abdominal scout film showed a rounded opacification beneath the pubic symphysis (Figure 2). Voiding radiographs confirmed interruption to flow in the penile urethra with proximal urethral dilatation (Figure 3). The bladder was markedly distended; there was no vesicoureteral reflux. The postvoid residual volume was significant (Figure 4). Ultrasonography of the urinary tract did not reveal abnormalities in the upper unit. Urine culture

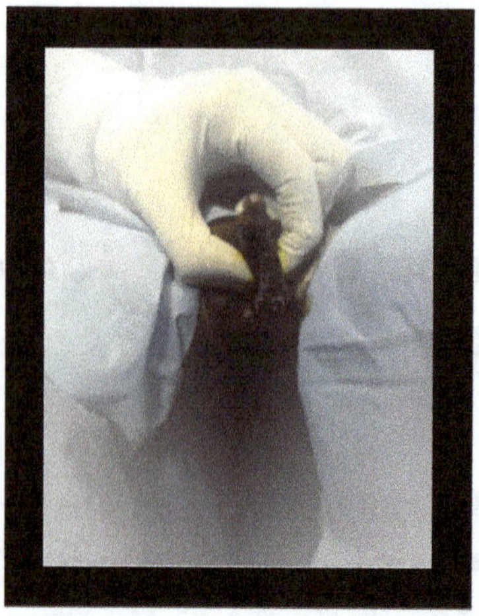

FIGURE 1: Palpation of mass at the base of the penis (case 1).

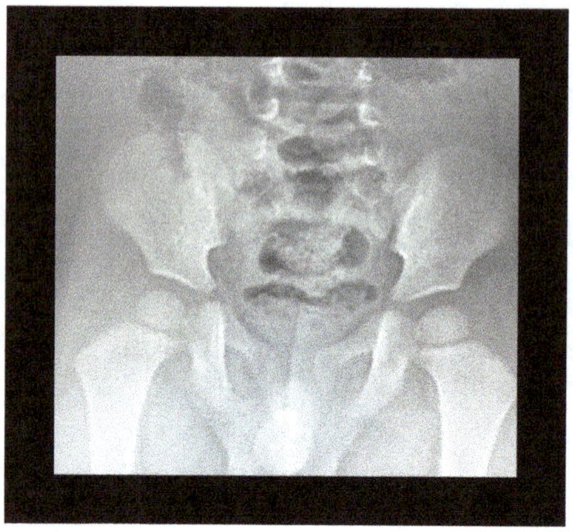

FIGURE 2: Plain abdominal radiograph showing the urethral calculus (case 1).

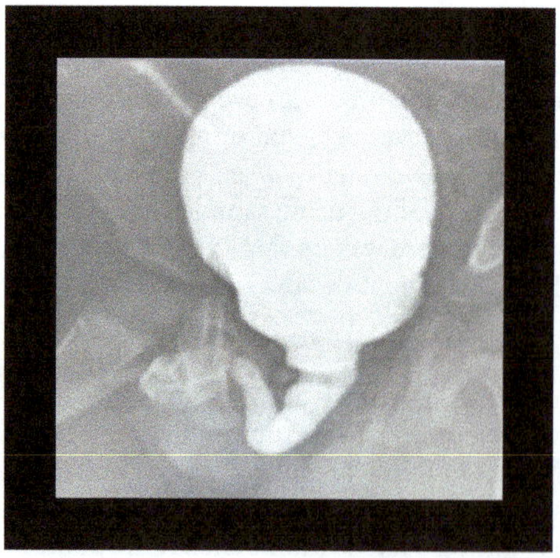

FIGURE 3: VCUG (elongated, dilated urethra) (case 1).

revealed *E. coli* sensitive to ceftriaxone. Blood count, urea, and creatinine were normal.

A suprapubic cystostomy was performed at bedside. At urethroscopy, a stone completely obstructing the lumen and encrusted in the urethral wall, prevented endoscopic extraction (Figure 5). Urethrotomy was therefore performed. An elongated 6 mm x 9 mm lithiasis with a crystalline surface was extracted (Figure 6). A Foley catheter (Ch 10) was left in place for 21 days.

The postoperative period was normal and the infant was discharged from hospital with normal voiding. He has remained asymptomatic at 1-, 3-, and 6-month follow-up visits.

The results of infrared spectrophotometric analysis of the calculus are as follows:

(i) Nucleus: urate ammonium acid (15%), calcium oxalate monohydrate (70%), and calcium oxalate dihydrate (15%)

(ii) Surface: calcium oxalate dihydrate (100%)

A urinary metabolic assessment for hyperoxaluria will complete the work-up as soon as funding is available.

2.2. Case 2. A fourteen-year-old boy presented at the Emergency Department of the Yaoundé Gynaeco-Obstetric and Pediatric Hospital complaining of inability to urinate

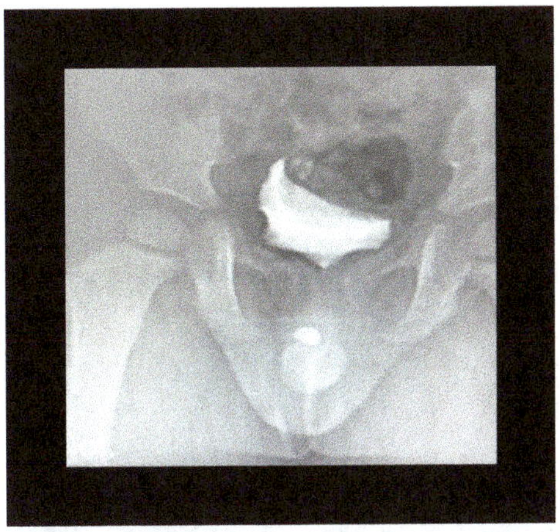

FIGURE 4: Postvoid residue on VCUG (case 1).

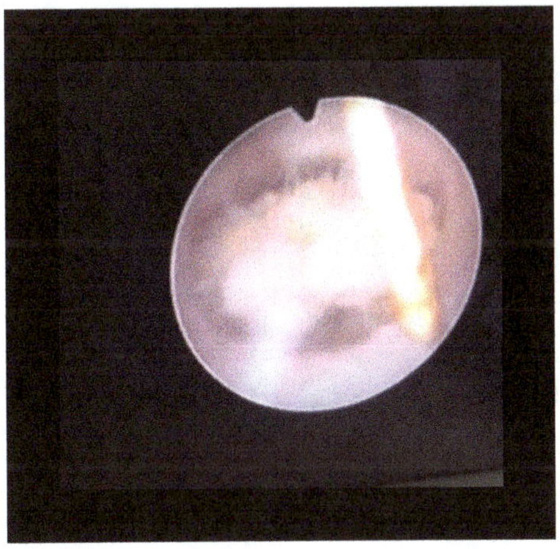

FIGURE 5: Endoscopic view of the calculus (case 1).

for over 20 hours despite the sensation of a full bladder. He was born at term, had normal urine flow at birth, and was treated for a urinary tract infection at 9 months. He was circumcised at 9 years of age without complications. The present symptoms began 1 month previously with pollakiuria and painful micturition with no fever or hematuria. Physical examination revealed an agitated child, writhing with pain in the hypogastric region, and a palpable full bladder (Figure 7). Vital signs were normal. There was no costovertebral angle tenderness. The testes were both descended and the penis presented a stenotic meatus. Palpation of the body of the penis did not reveal any masses. 600 ml of clear urine was drained from an urgent bedside 8 Fr cystostomy (Figure 8). However urinalysis was positive for nitrites and leukocyturia. Blood urea nitrogen and creatinine were normal; there was marked leukocytosis at $11000/mm^3$. An abdominal ultrasound showed grade 2 right ureterohydronephrosis. A scout film confirmed an ovoid calculus in the proximal part of the anterior urethra (Figure 9). A voiding cystourethrogram showed a partially obstructed urethra and absence of passive as well as active vesicoureteral reflux (Figure 10). The patient received amoxicillin-clavulanic acid. Definitive management under general anaesthesia consisted of meatotomy and open perineal urethrostomy. An encrusted urethral stone (13 mm x 6 mm) with a speculated surface was extracted (Figure 10). An indwelling Foley catheter (12 Fr) was left in place for 10 days. The patient was given Oxybutynin for bladder spasms and amoxicillin-clavulanic acid as long as the indwelling catheter was in place.

2.3. Case 3. A patient of 11 years old was referred to the service for acute urinary retention, following repetitive failure to insert urethral catheter two weeks after trauma to the genitalia during a football match. He complained of difficult and painful micturition and eventually urinary retention. A cystostomy was placed in the emergency room. He was circumcised at age 3 and was treated for recurrent UTI in the past. On physical examination, the urethra meatus was normal; there was a hard, round, palpable mass in a tender penile urethra (Figure 11). A scout film of the pelvis showed an image of a urethral stone (Figure 12(a)). Opacification of lower tract during VCUG confirmed the obstruction from the stone but no reflux (Figure 12(b)). There was marked leukocyturia at 17000/mm3. *Citrobacter koseri* was isolated from the urine. We removed the calculus via urethrotomy (Figures 13 and 14). The two urinary catheters were kept on

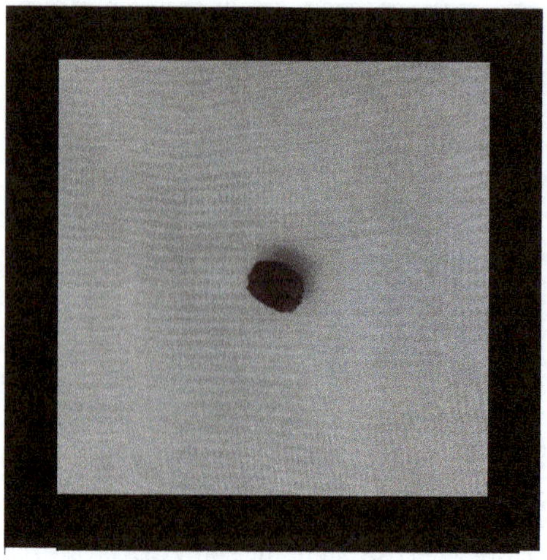

FIGURE 6: Extracted urethral stone (case 1).

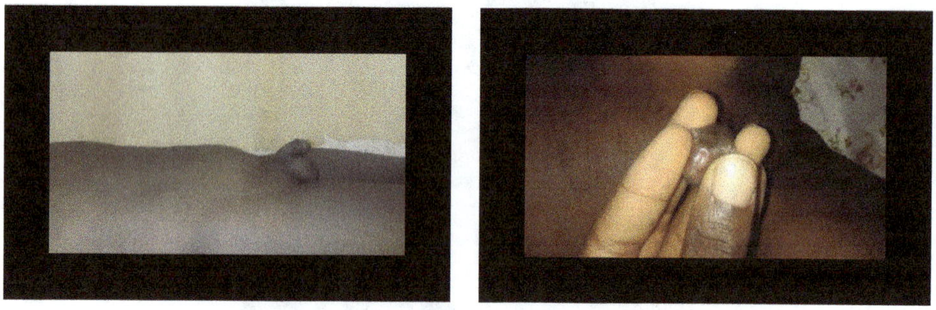

(a) (b)

FIGURE 7: (a) Suprapubic bladder distension (case 2); (b) meatal stenosis (case 2).

the abdomen after dressing (Figure 15). Postoperative follow-up was normal.

3. Discussion

Urolithiasis is rare in children [2]. It accounts for 5 to 15% of urinary stones in developing countries [5, 6]. The series from two geographic zones from Cameroon showed that urate stones are not uncommon as reported in other developing countries. The said series represented a tip of the iceberg as issues of geographical, cultural, and financial access to care limited case recruitment. It generally affects young boys under 5 years of age and bladder calculi are most frequent. Most stones that are impacted in the urethra are indeed of bladder origin. Urethral stones account for 0.3% of all urolithiasis [7]. These stones are constituted mainly of urates and/or triple (Ammonium, Magnesium, and Calcium) phosphates [8, 9].

Pain and a mass in the penis is a common clinical presentation. The signs depend on the location and the size of the stone. Calculi of the posterior urethra are often larger and urine can flow around them. Smaller stones tend to localize at the distal part, most frequently in the fossa navicularis often completely obstructing the passage causing acute retention of urine [10].

Posterior urethral valves are the most common cause of urinary retention in the male child. The cases presented underline the necessity of performing a complete physical examination of the genitalia, including the inspection, percussion, and palpation of the penis in search of a calculus. If urethral lithiasis is suspected, a plain X-ray of the abdomen may be useful to confirm the diagnosis and location of the stone. The sensitivity of pediatric ultrasound for the detection of stones varies from 59 to 78% with a specificity approaching 100% [11–13]. Its use at the level of the urethral is not popular but would certainly be advantageous over standard X-ray which is increasingly proscribed in children.

From a biochemical standpoint, ammonium urate is responsible for nearly half of the calculi observed in developing countries. It constitutes approximately 50% of the nidus of these calculi. In developing countries, a large proportion of urate-nucleated calculi is caused by an infectious process and potentiated by several mechanisms: a gastrointestinal infection that causes diarrheal episodes with loss of electrolytes such as sodium and potassium; an infection of the urinary tract from urease-producing bacteria; or even a mixed infection (both digestive and urinary) [8]. Also, it has been documented that the incidence of urinary stones is higher in countries with warm or hot climates, probably due to low urinary output and scanty fluid intake. These are

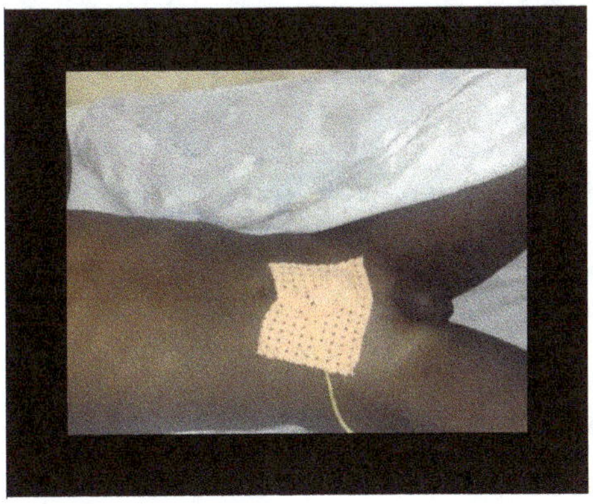

FIGURE 8: Suprapubic cystostomy in place (case 2).

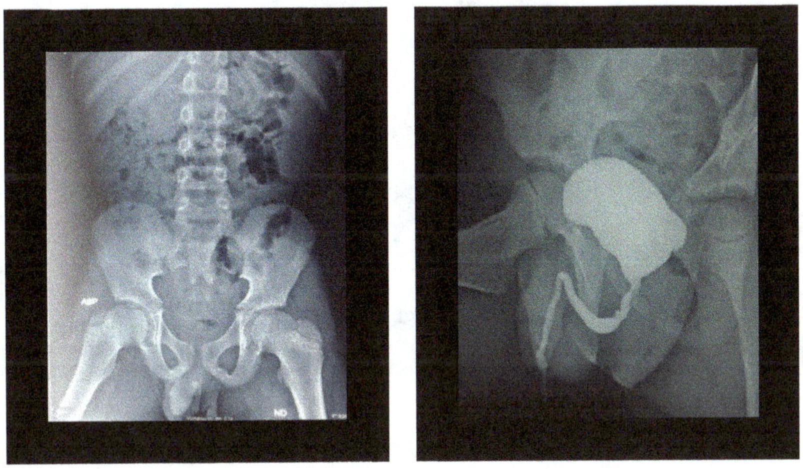

(a) (b)

FIGURE 9: (a) Scout film, stone in the penile midshaft (case 2). (b) VCUG, partial urethral obstruction (case 2).

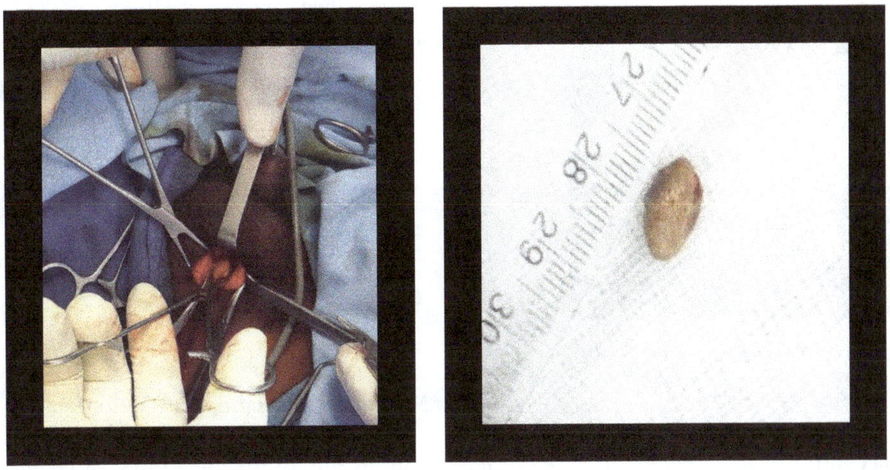

(a) (b)

FIGURE 10: (a) Urethral calculus, in situ (case 2). (b) Extracted calculus (case 2).

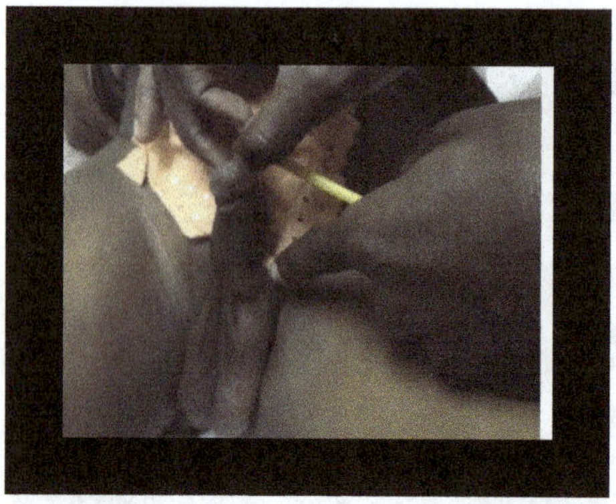

FIGURE 11: Physical exam showing location of stone (case 3).

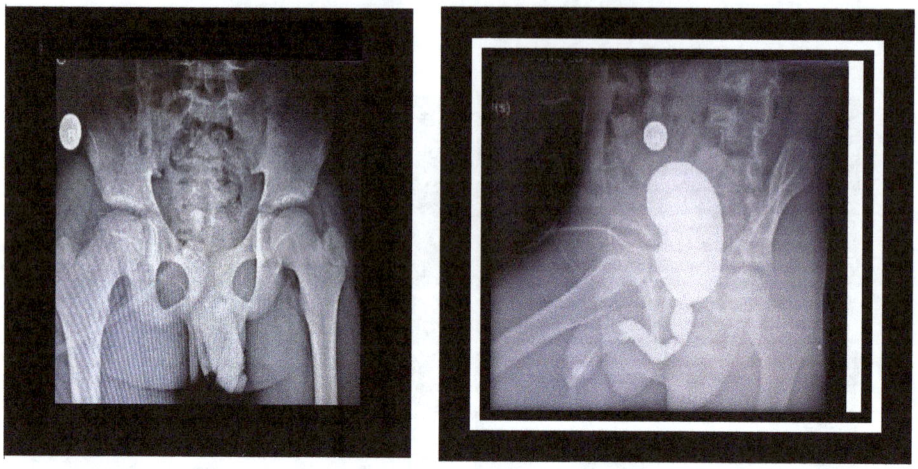

(a) (b)

FIGURE 12: (a) Scout film showing penile stone (case 3). (b) VCUG, interruption of contrast (case 3).

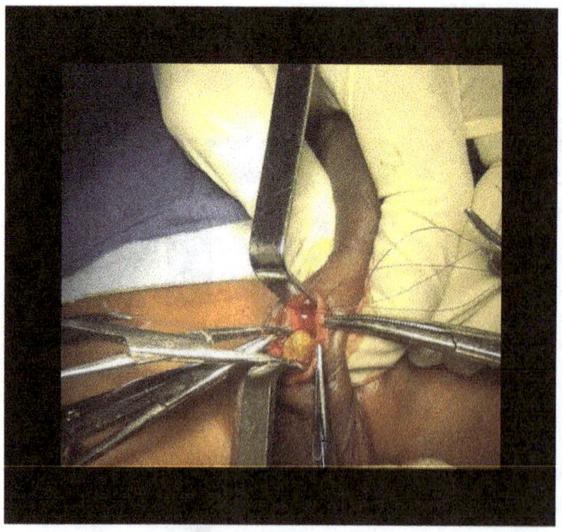

FIGURE 13: Urethral stone extraction (case 3).

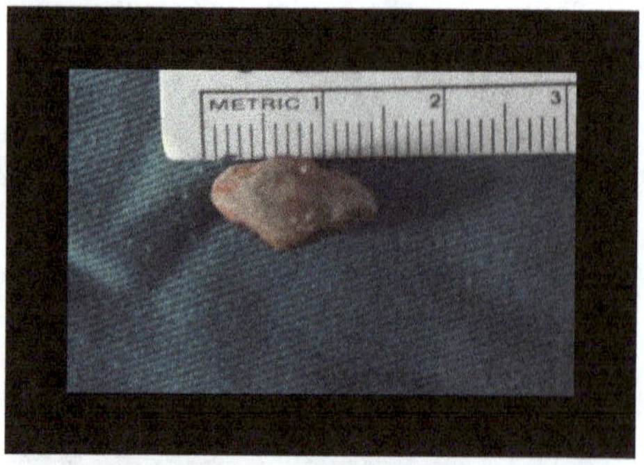

FIGURE 14: Stone removed (case 3).

some of the factors that contribute to the geographical pattern that characterizes the North American and Afro-Asian stone belts [14]. The Afro-Asian stone belt stretches from Sudan, the Arab Republic of Egypt, Saudi Arabia, the United Arab Emirates, the Islamic Republic of Iran, Pakistan, India, Myanmar, Thailand, and Indonesia to Philippines. Within a stone belt, the incidence of urolithiasis varies within the regions due to the local physical geographic conditions and dietary/behavioural practices [15]. The reported prevalence of uncommon stone types could be an underestimation in many developing countries due to the unavailability of qualified manpower and diagnostic tools [15].

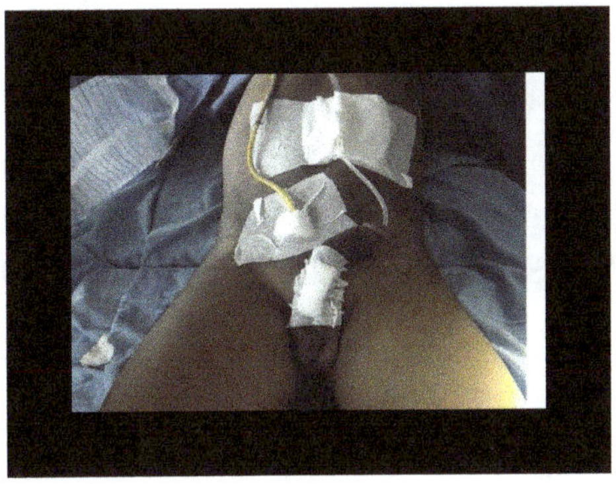

Figure 15: Postoperative dressing with urethral and suprapubic catheter (case 3).

Endoscopic lithotripsy has become the standard treatment in the management of bladder stones and urethral lithiasis. The latter is achieved after pushing back the stone into the bladder with success rates close to 80% [7]. In all three patients, in the absence of lithotripsy and in the presence of large obstructing calculi encrusted in the urethra, open ureterolithotomy was indicated. They all void normally with follow-up that varies from 6 months to 4 years. Lifelong follow-up in respect of recurrent urinary infections and stones but most especially urethral stricture is imperative. North-south collaboration is often necessary for the evaluation of the stone chemical composition in resource limited areas.

4. Conclusion

An underlying congenital or acquired pathology should be sought in the male child presenting with acute urinary retention. The urethra should be examined for an obstructing stone. The association of a plain abdominal X-ray and an ultrasound not only permits the identification of calculi but also appreciates the impact of obstruction on the upper urinary tract. Urgent urinary diversion and removal of the calculus with minimal urethral trauma is recommended treatment.

Acknowledgments

The authors thank the Swiss NGO Children Action for their assistance.

References

[1] I. Sorokin, C. Mamoulakis, K. Miyazawa, A. Rodgers, J. Talati, and Y. Lotan, "Epidemiology of stone disease across the world," *World Journal of Urology*, vol. 35, pp. 1301–1320, 2017.

[2] L. Collard, "Lithiase urinaire de l'enfant et l'adolescent," *Revue Medicale de Liege*, vol. 59, no. 4, pp. 221–226, 2004.

[3] J. Akhtar, S. Ahmed, and N. Zamir, "Management of impacted urethral stones in children," *Journal of College of Physicians and Surgeons Pakistan*, vol. 22, no. 8, pp. 510–513, 2012.

[4] F. F. Angwafo III, M. Daudon, A. Wonkam, P. M. Kuwong, and K. A. Kropp, "Pediatric urolithiasis in sub-Saharan Africa: a comparative study in two regions of Cameroon," *European Urology*, vol. 37, no. 1, pp. 106–111, 2000.

[5] M. Arifi, Y. Halim, M. A. Bouhafs et al., "Traitement par lithotritie extracorporelle des calculs du haut appareil urinaire de l'enfant," *Progrès en Urologie*, vol. 16, pp. 594–597, 2006.

[6] S. Rizvi, S. Naqvi, Z. Hussain et al., "The management of stone disease," *BJU International*, vol. 89, pp. 62–68, 2002.

[7] A. S. Safwat, D. A. Hameed, M. A. Elgammal, Y. M. Abdelsalam, and A. Abolyosr, "Percutaneous suprapubic stone extraction for posterior urethral stones in children: Efficacy and safety," *Urology*, vol. 82, no. 2, pp. 448–450, 2013.

[8] M. Daudon, B. Bounxouei, F. S. Cruz et al., "Composition des calculs observés aujourd'hui dans les pays non industrialisés," *Progrès en Urologie*, vol. 14, pp. 1151–1161, 2004.

[9] S. Aegukkatajit, "Reduction of urinary stone in children from north-eastern Thailand," *Journal of the Medical Association of Thailand*, vol. 82, no. 12, pp. 1230–1232, 1999.

[10] A. B. Salman, "Urethral calculi in children," *Journal of Pediatric Surgery*, vol. 31, no. 10, pp. 1379–1382, 1996.

[11] J. P. Heneghan, K. A. McGuire, R. A. Leder, D. M. DeLong, T. Yoshizumi, and R. C. Nelson, "Helical CT for nephrolithiasis and ureterolithiasis: comparison of conventional and reduced radiation-dose techniques," *Radiology*, vol. 229, no. 2, pp. 575–580, 2003.

[12] W. R. Hendee and M. K. O'Connor, "Radiation risks of medical imaging: separating fact from fantasy," *Radiology*, vol. 264, no. 2, pp. 312–321, 2012.

[13] K. A. Fowler, J. A. Locken, J. H. Duchesne, and M. R. Williamson, "Ultrasound for detecting renal calculi with nonenhanced CT as a reference standard," *Radiology*, vol. 222, no. 1, pp. 109–113, 2002.

[14] M. López and B. Hoppe, "History, epidemiology and regional diversities of urolithiasis," *Pediatric Nephrology*, vol. 25, no. 1, pp. 49–59, 2010.

[15] A. P. Sharma and G. Filler, "Epidemiology of pediatric urolithiasis," *Indian Journal of Urology*, vol. 26, no. 4, pp. 516–522, 2010.

11

Acute Abdomen Revealing an Unusual Case of Intra-Abdominal Testicular Torsion

Maazou Halidou ,[1,2] Amadou Roua,[3] Ibrahim Amadou Magagi ,[2,4] Harissou Adamou ,[2,4] Ousseini Adakal,[5,6] Mohamed Rouga,[5] Soumana Amadou,[7] and Rachid Sani[7]

[1]*Department of Urology, Zinder National Hospital, Zinder, Niger*
[2]*Faculty of Health Sciences, University of Zinder, Zinder, Niger*
[3]*Department of Urology, Regional Hospital Center of Maradi, Maradi, Niger*
[4]*Department of General Surgery, Zinder National Hospital, Zinder, Niger*
[5]*Department of General Surgery, Regional Hospital Center of Maradi, Maradi, Niger*
[6]*Faculty of Health Sciences, Dan Dicko Dankoulodo University, Maradi, Niger*
[7]*Department of Surgery and Surgical Specialties, Faculty of Health Sciences, University of Niamey, Niamey, Niger*

Correspondence should be addressed to Maazou Halidou; halidou3@yahoo.fr

Academic Editor: Tun-Chieh Chen

Introduction. Intra-abdominal testicular torsion is a rare event. We report hereby our experience of the management of a spermatic cord twist on intra-abdominal testis discovered during an acute surgical abdomen. *Case Presentation.* This was a 42-year-old patient admitted to the emergency department for abdominal pain that had been evolving for a week. The physical examination showed tenderness and guarding in the left iliac fossa with an empty ipsilateral hemiscrotum. Complementary examinations led to the discovery of an intra-abdominal left-lateral mass. The laparotomy found a whitish mass with areas of infarction, which was resected. Anatomopathological examination of the operative specimen identified it as a testis with atrophy of germ cells and necrotic areas without evidence of malignancy. *Conclusion.* Intra-abdominal testicular torsion should be considered in case of patients with an acute surgical abdomen with vacuity of one of the bursae.

1. Introduction

The cryptorchidism is defined as an undescended testis into the scrotum [1–5]. It affects 1–5% of term births and between 1.1 and 45% of premature infants [1, 6, 7]. The main complications of this condition are testicular torsion, malignancy, infertility, and exposure to trauma [2, 6, 7]. The intra-abdominal position of the testis is rare and must be evoked ahead of any vacuity of the scrotum with a nonpalpable testis in the inguinal canal [3]. Indeed, in the proportion of impalpable testes (20%), 50–60% are intra-abdominal [1, 3]. Intra-abdominal testicular torsion is a rare surgical emergency involving the functional prognosis of the testis [6, 8]. It is manifested by an atypical clinical picture dominated by an abdominal symptomology which is a source of diagnostic delay [2, 9, 10]. Its management is also controversial when the testis is viable [2]. We report here our experience of the management of spermatic cord torsion on intra-abdominal testis discovered during an acute surgical abdomen.

2. Case Report

A 42-year-old man, married with two children, was admitted to the emergency department for left iliac fossa pain radiating to the flank, which had been evolving for a week without fever. The pain was previously dull, little sensitive to the usual analgesics, with periods of remission. It progressively worsened. After initial care in a peripheral health facility without improvement, the patient was referred to the regional hospital. Clinical examination noted left iliac fossa tenderness with guarding, free hernial orifices, and a vacant left hemiscrotum with a right normal testis; the rectal examination found lateralized pain on the left side of the Douglas pouch. The rest of the somatic examination was unremarkable. The blood count indicated

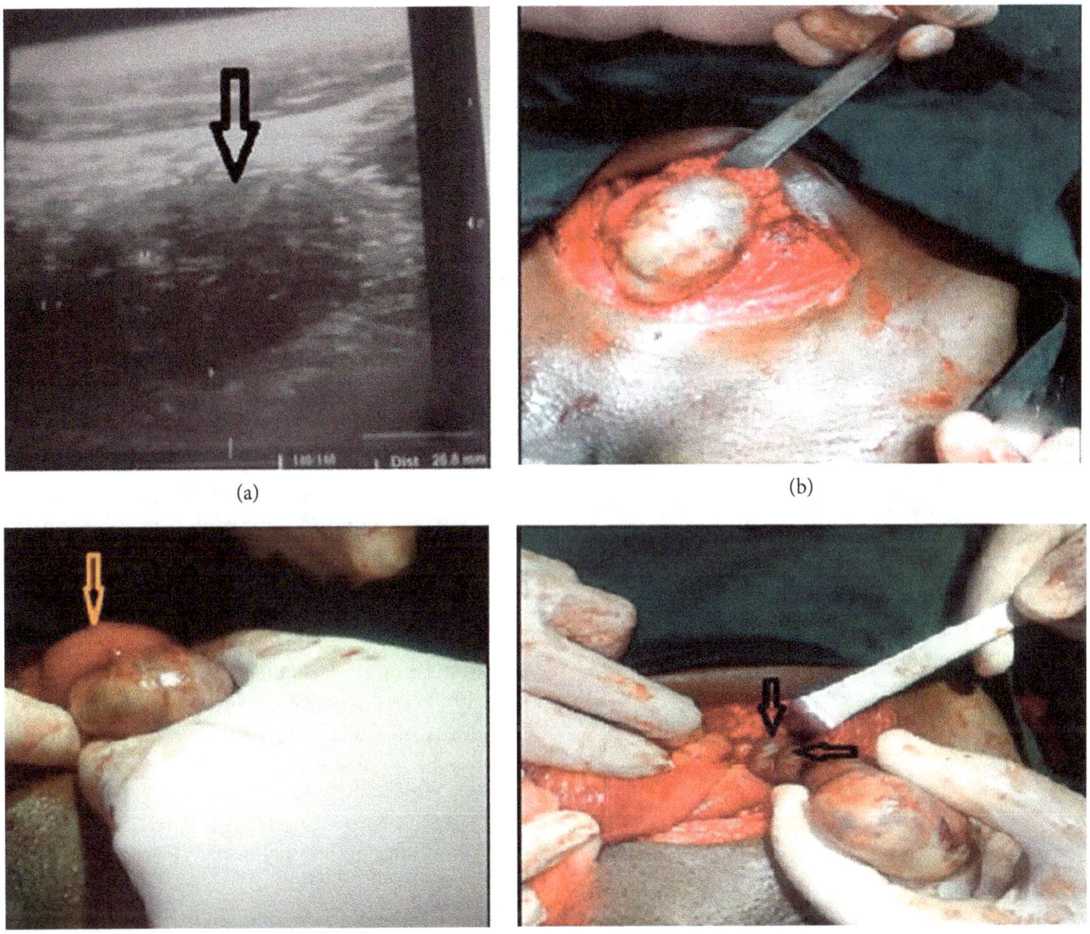

(a) (b) (c) (d)

FIGURE 1: (a) Ultrasound (left lateral vesical mass); (b) mass of externalised testicular appearance; (c) intestinal loop adherent to the mass; (d) pedicle twisting.

leukocytosis at 12,000 elements/mm^3 and a normal hemoglobin level. Ultrasound revealed a heterogeneous left-vesical mass of 43 mm × 32 mm in diameter (Figure 1(a)). After a standard preoperative assessment, surgical exploration by laparotomy was decided. Pfannenstiel incision was made and revealed a pedunculated whitish mass with areas of infarction, testicular-like, adhering to an intestinal loop (Figures 1(b) and 1(c)). The pedicle was twisted twice (Figure 1(d)). Resection of the mass was performed. Considering the elements of the clinical examination, the probable diagnosis of torsion of the spermatic cord on intra-abdominal testis was retained. Histopathological examination of the specimen confirmed the testicular nature of the mass and noted germ cells atrophy with necrotic areas and no malignancy sign. The tumor markers: βHCG (choriogonadotrophic hormone), αFP (alpha fetoprotein), and LDH (Lactodeshydrogenase), measured postoperatively were normal. Postoperative recovery was uneventful. The patient was discharged at postoperative day 5.

3. Discussion

Intra-abdominal testicular torsion is a rare event [5, 9, 10]. Few cases have been described in the literature to date, and the true impact of this entity remains poorly understood [9–11]. Gerster was the first author to report a similar case in 1898 [8, 12, 13]. An intra-abdominal testis has a greater risk of torsion than that which is normally descended, because of lack of anatomical attachment structures, the absence of gubernaculum, the size of the spermatic cord which is not in adequacy with the size of the testicle which is often atrophic [2, 10].

It is well established that both cryptorchidism and testicular ectopia increase the risk of malignant degeneration. The risk of cancer is 35–40 times higher compared to the normal subject due to higher abdominal temperature than scrotal one [8, 9]. Indeed it is reported that 50%–64% of patients with testicular tumors have an undescended testicle [10, 14]. Cancerization also increases the risk of torsion due to increased testicular volume by the neoplastic process [2, 5, 14]. In our observation, the tumor markers were normal and the pathological examination did not find any sign of malignancy.

The torsion of the testis in intra-abdominal position may be asymptomatic or may lead to nonspecific signs including irritability, nausea, and vomiting, constipation, atypical abdominal pain, hematuria, or even shock, which can be misdiagnosed as appendicitis or diverticulitis [7, 9, 11, 12]. Sometimes it can manifest as an abdominal mass [8].

Diagnostic suspicion is stronger when the clinical examination finds vacant bursae associated with acute abdominal pain [5]. The ultrasonography remains insensitive in the detection of the testis in the intra-abdominal position [5, 12], even if in our case the ultrasound was contributive; this is probably due to the large volume of the testis. CT scan or magnetic resonance imaging gives better results in localization of the testis in this situation [5, 13], but those examinations are not available in current practice in our context. The search for impalpable testicles is more relevant to a laparoscopic exploration which is the gold standard in this field or a conventional exploratory surgery [8, 12].

The management of testicular torsion on an intra-abdominal testis remains controversial when the testis is viable; some authors advocate orchiectomy because of the high risk of malignant degeneration [9, 10, 15], while other authors advocate orchidopexy in children under 2 years, or in adults who refuse orchiectomy for psychological or aesthetic reasons [9, 10]. This orchidopexy should be associated with clinical monitoring and regular tumor marker assays [9, 10].

In our Nigerien context with limited resources, the discovery of an intra-abdominal testis is often fortuitous, or in an acute surgical abdomen chart and in adulthood, an orchiectomy should be the treatment of choice, as recommended by experts [1].

4. Conclusion

Intra-abdominal testicular torsion is rare and often presents as a misleading clinical picture. However, this diagnosis should be considered in a subject with acute abdominal pain with one or two vacant bursae. The orchiectomy remains the recommended treatment because of the significant risk of malignant degeneration that increases with age.

Consent

Written informed consent was obtained from the patient's legal guardian(s).

References

[1] C. Radmayr, G. Bogaert, H. S. Dogan et al., *EAU Guidelines on Paediatric Urology*, European Association of Urology, Amhem, pp. 13–18, 2018, https://uroweb.org/guideline/paediatric-urology.

[2] M. Gharbi, N. Amri, W. Chambeh, S. Braiek, and R. E. Kamel, "Les torsions sur testicules cryptorchides," *Canadian Urological Association Journal*, vol. 4, no. 6, pp. 393–396, 2010.

[3] L. H. Braga and A. J. Lorenzo, "Cryptorchidism: a practical review for all community healthcare providers," *Canadian Urological Association Journal*, vol. 11, no. 1-2, pp. 1–2, 2017.

[4] S. Naouar, S. Braiek, and R. El Kamel, "Testicular torsion in undescended testis: a persistent challenge," *Asian Journal of Urology*, vol. 4, no. 2, pp. 111–115, 2017.

[5] A. Q. Khan, P. Hazirah, W. R. Dar, S. Thomas, and I. Ahmad, "Torsedintraabdominal testis mimicking acute appendicitis in a 60 year old male," *International Surgery Journal*, vol. 5, no. 1, p. 336, 2017.

[6] H. Karami, M. Yaghoobi, and A. Hasanzadeh Hadad, "Emergency laparoscopic orchiectomy for intra-abdominal testicular torsion–a case report," *Urology Journal*, vol. 10, no. 3, pp. 1013–1015, 2013.

[7] K. I. Ahmed and M. Aza, "Synchronous bilateral intra-abdominal seminoma presented as acute abdomen," *Clinics in Oncology*, vol. 4, p. 1611, 2019.

[8] A. Papparella, F. Nino, S. Coppola, and P. Parmeggiani, "An unusual case of intra-abdominal testicular torsion: role of laparoscopy," *African Journal of Paediatric Surgery*, vol. 10, no. 1, p. 29, 2013.

[9] S. Hussain, "Torsion of a giant intra-abdominal testicular seminoma presenting as acute abdomen," *Indian Journal of Surgery*, vol. 77, no. S1, pp. 64–65, 2015.

[10] T. Staniuk, Ł. Szymański, and M. Trocha, "Torsed intraabdominal testicular tumor diagnosed during surgery performed due to suspicion of acute appendicitis," *Polski Przegląd Chirurgiczny*, vol. 84, no. 10, pp. 526–530, 2012.

[11] J. S. Aihole, N. M. Babu, D. Haldar, R. Sahadev, and Aihole, J. S., "Acute abdomen caused by torsion of an undescended testis: a rare presentation and its diagnostic dilemma," *Pediatric Urology Case Reports*, vol. 4, no. 5, pp. 369–372, 2017.

[12] M. A. El-Gohary, "Asymptomatic torsion of intra-abdominal testis," *Journal of Pediatric Surgery Case Reports*, vol. 3, no. 1, pp. 30–31, 2015.

[13] R. L. Lewis, M. D. Roller, B. L. Parra, and A. M. Cotlar, "Torsion of an intra-abdominal testis," *Current Surgery*, vol. 57, no. 5, pp. 497–499, 2000.

[14] C. Twiss and M. Grasso, "Abdominal pain associated with an intra-abdominal gonad in an adult," *Reviews in Urology*, vol. 2, no. 3, pp. 178–181, 2000.

[15] O. J. Nickalls, C. L. Tan, and Y. L. Thian, "A torted ruptured intra-abdominal testicular seminoma presenting as an acute abdomen," *Journal of Radiology Case Reports*, vol. 9, no. 12, 2015.

12

Symptomatic IgG4-Related Prostatitis Simultaneously Diagnosed with Aggressive Prostate Cancer

Taisuke Ezaki,[1] Seiya Akatsuka,[2] Tansei Sanjo,[1] and Takeshi Masuda[1]

[1]*Department of Urology, Saitama City Hospital, Saitama, Japan*
[2]*Division of Pathology, Department of Central Laboratory, Saitama City Hospital, Saitama, Japan*

Correspondence should be addressed to Taisuke Ezaki; tezaki@nerima-hosp.or.jp

Academic Editor: Shiou-Sheng Chen

IgG4-related disease is a systemic fibroinflammatory disorder that occasionally affects the prostate. It is usually considered that patients with IgG4-related disease are at high risk of developing malignancies. A 71-year-old man presented to our hospital with a chief complaint of urinary retention. Prostate biopsy revealed concomitant IgG4-related prostatitis and prostate cancer. IgG4-related prostatitis was a possible cause of urinary retention, and the aggressive nature of prostate cancer was the cause of the patient's death 2 years after diagnosis. This is the fourth case report of prostate cancer accompanied by IgG4-related prostatitis; however, there have been no reports of the two diseases coexisting with high clinical significance. Our case report indicates that patients diagnosed with IgG4-related prostatitis should be carefully followed up considering the risk of prostate cancer.

1. Introduction

IgG4-related disease is a rare systemic fibroinflammatory disorder characterized by the enlargement of affected organs, a significant increase in serum IgG4 levels, tissue infiltration with IgG4-positive plasma cells, and fibrosis [1–3]. IgG4-related disease of the genitourinary tract is relatively rare; however, it occasionally affects the prostate [4–8].

Although a complete consensus has not yet been established, patients with IgG4-related disease are typically considered at high risk of developing malignant disease [9–12]. Here, we report a case of prostate cancer accompanied by IgG4-related prostatitis.

2. Case Presentation

A 71-year-old Japanese man presented to our hospital with a chief complaint of urinary retention. He had chronic obstructive pulmonary disease, hypertension, and a history of left femoral head replacement due to osteoarthritis of the hip. Additionally, he had a history of alcohol consumption and cigarette smoking. Prostate volume of 42 cm^3 was defined using transabdominal ultrasonography. Urinary catheterization was performed, and alpha-blocker treatment was initiated. A follow-up examination conducted 1 month later showed serum prostate-specific antigen (PSA) levels of 74 ng/mL, although the last PSA test performed a year ago had revealed normal PSA levels. Blood and urine test results were nearly within normal limits, except that mild anemia and mild hypoalbuminemia were noted. Prostate tissue samples were obtained via transrectal needle biopsy. Digital rectal examination revealed a firm prostate; however, a prostate tissue sample stained with hematoxylin and eosin showed inflammation but no malignant cells. One month after the first biopsy, urinary retention recurred, but 2 weeks of clean intermittent self-catheterization improved the obstructive symptoms. One month later, the patient had elevated PSA levels of 180 ng/mL, and a second prostate biopsy was performed Figure 1. Adenocarcinoma (Gleason score 5 + 4) was detected in 1/12 needle cores Figure 2(c). Computed tomography revealed pelvic lymph node swelling, and multiple bone metastases (lumbar spine, pubic bone,

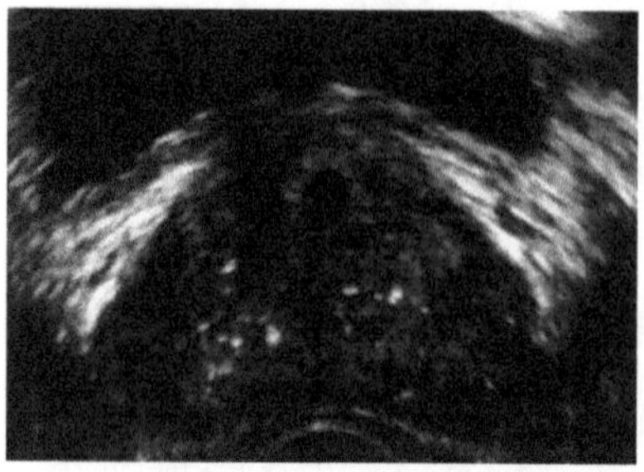

FIGURE 1: Image obtained using transrectal ultrasound at the second biopsy showing an enlarged prostate (axial view). The estimated prostate volume was 49 cm^3. Magnetic resonance imaging was not performed because the patient had undergone femoral head replacement.

and left acetabulum) were detected using bone scintigraphy; therefore, the patient was diagnosed with stage 4 prostate cancer. Moreover, we detected abundant plasma cell infiltration with periglandular storiform fibrosis in prostate tissue samples Figures 2(a) and 2(b). Although plasma cell clonality was not detected, IgG4 immunochemical staining demonstrated IgG4-positive plasma cells Figures 2(d) and 2(e). The ratio of IgG4-positive/IgG-positive plasma cells was >50% Figure 2(f). Given the result of the second biopsy, the initial prostate biopsies were reviewed again, and large numbers of IgG4-positive plasma cells were observed. At this point, the serum IgG4 levels were 1310 mg/dL (normal: <117 mg/dL), and a diagnosis of simultaneous IgG4-related prostatitis and prostate cancer was made. The patient immediately received combined androgen blockade treatment, and his serum PSA levels decreased to 1.7 ng/mL for 4 months. However, he developed castration resistance after 8 months of hormone therapy. Although abiraterone, docetaxel, and cabazitaxel were administered, cancer progressed, and multiple liver metastases appeared. He died 24 months after the diagnosis of prostate cancer. No treatment was given for IgG4-related prostatitis as the patient could urinate without a catheter at the time of diagnosis confirmation. The serum IgG4 levels slightly decreased to 883 mg/dL in the 7th month of hormonal therapy and returned to normal when prednisolone at a dose of 10 mg/day was coadministered with abiraterone in the following month. Notably, he never complained of urinary retention until death.

3. Discussion

IgG4-related prostatitis was first reported by Yoshimura et al. [4], and subsequently, additional studies were conducted on the disease [5–8]. In patients with IgG4-related prostatitis, histological examination of the prostate reveals severe atrophy of the exocrine glands, dense fibrosis, and abundant infiltration of lymphocytes and IgG4-positive plasma cells [4]. IgG4-related prostatitis is occasionally accompanied by IgG4-related disease in other organs [4–8]. Such patients may experience resolution of the urinary symptoms after steroid treatment [5, 6, 8] and exhibit varying levels of serum PSA ranging from 0.1 to 54.0 ng/mL [6–8].

In the present case, acute urinary retention resulted in a hospital visit. Buijs et al. reported that >50% of patients with IgG4-related prostatitis presented with obstructive urinary tract symptoms [8], and we believe that acute inflammation due to IgG4-related prostatitis played an important role in causing urinary retention in our patient. Although prostate cancer can obstruct urine flow in the absence of inflammation, we believe that concomitant inflammation increased the severity of the obstructive symptoms. The observation that the urinary symptoms were ameliorated before cancer treatment suggested that prostate cancer was not the sole cause of urinary retention. As the patient's urinary symptoms were manageable at the time of diagnosis, we did not administer steroid therapy, although steroids have been used to effectively treat the urinary symptoms of IgG4-related prostatitis in previous case reports [5, 6, 8]. Usually, treatment of IgG4-related disease is initiated with 40 mg prednisolone or at a dose of 0.6 mg/kg of body weight/day [2], but spontaneous remission has also been reported [13]. Further, wait-and-see management may be more appropriate in some patients, given the side effects of steroids. In the present case, our strategy appeared reasonable as there was no recurrence of urinary retention.

To the best of our knowledge, only three cases of prostate cancer with IgG4-related prostatitis have been reported to date [6, 14]. The initial serum PSA levels of all three patients ranged from 5.5 to 8.2 ng/mL; two of them underwent radical prostatectomy. Although the case report on one patient did not clearly document prostate cancer treatment, PSA levels were suggestive of nonadvanced cancer. As regards urinary symptoms, symptomatic prostatitis was reported in one patient who presented with dysuria, whereas the other two reports did not provide details on symptoms involving the lower urinary tract. Therefore, this is the fourth case report of prostate cancer with IgG4-related prostatitis. However, inflammation caused by IgG4-related prostatitis was sufficiently severe to cause urinary retention, and prostate cancer was aggressive and life-threatening. No reports have demonstrated the coexistence of two diseases with high clinical significance. Therefore, we consider this case unique and worth reporting.

In our case report, the histopathological characteristics of IgG4-related prostatitis were retrospectively detected in the specimens of the first biopsy. As the patient had no history of IgG4-related disease, the immediate diagnosis of IgG4-related prostatitis was difficult. Nevertheless, an additional careful examination could have led to the diagnosis of IgG4-related prostatitis after the first biopsy. However, if steroid therapy administered for IgG4-related prostatitis had reduced the serum PSA levels, the detection of prostate cancer would have been delayed. Our case report indicates that patients diagnosed with IgG4-related prostatitis based on the symptoms of inflammation should be carefully followed up considering the risk of prostate cancer.

In the present case report, the association between IgG4-related prostatitis and the development of prostate cancer remains unclear. However, a possibility exists that IgG4-related prostatitis and prostate cancer, which manifested

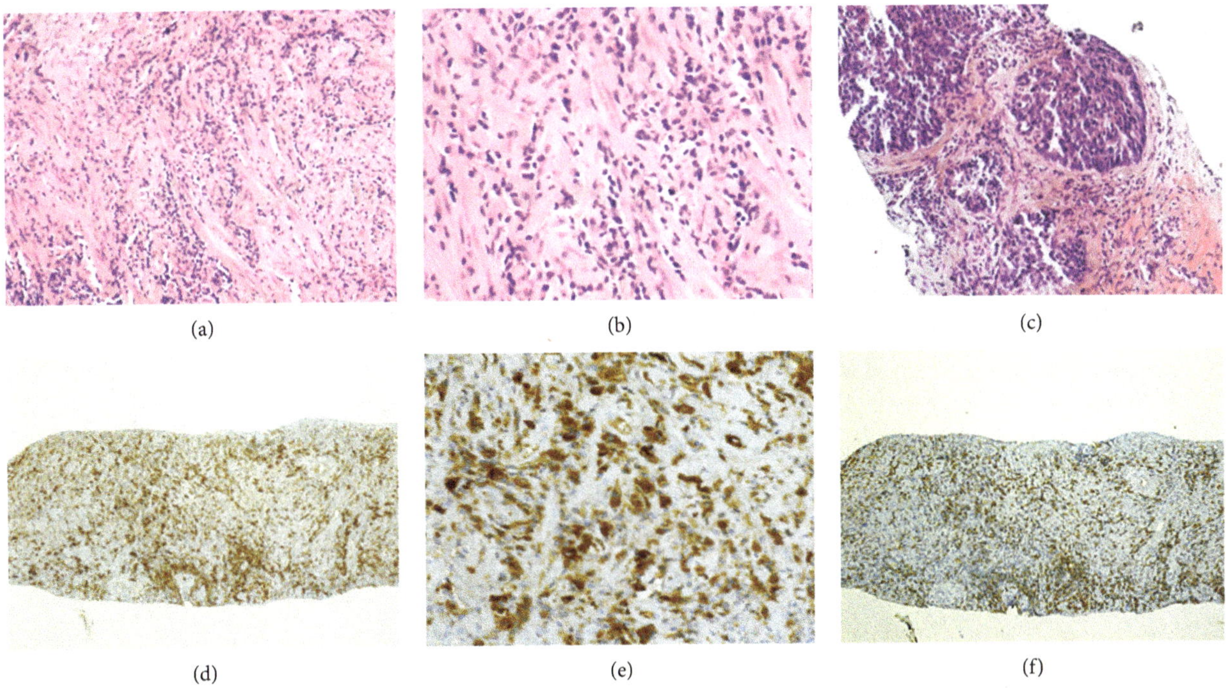

FIGURE 2: Paraffin section of prostate biopsy tissue. (a–c) Hematoxylin and eosin (H&E) staining and immunohistochemical staining for (d, e) IgG4 and (f) IgG. Original magnification: (d, e) ×100; (a, c) ×200; and (b, e) ×400. H&E staining shows storiform fibrosis, exocrine glands with periglandular fibrosis, and lymphoplasmacytic and eosinophilic infiltration (a, b). Adenocarcinoma, Gleason score 5 + 4, was found in 1/12 needle cores, which occupied 10% of the core area, at the second biopsy (c). Indirect immunohistochemical staining for IgG4 revealed multiple IgG4-positive plasma cells (>50/high-power field (HPF)) infiltrating the prostate (d, e). The ratio of IgG4-positive/IgG-positive plasma cells was >50% (the histopathological diagnostic criteria for IgG4-related disease included marked lymphoplasmacytic infiltration, fibrosis, IgG4 positivity in >40% of IgG-positive plasma cells, and >10 IgG4-positive plasma cells/HPF of a biopsy sample).

concomitantly and were diagnosed almost simultaneously, were associated and that their concomitant existence was not a coincidence. However, further investigation is necessary to ascertain the association between these two diseases.

References

[1] H. Umehara, K. Okazaki, Y. Masaki et al., "Comprehensive diagnostic criteria for IgG4-related disease (IgG4-RD), 2011," *Modern Rheumatology*, vol. 22, no. 1, pp. 21–30, 2012.

[2] H. Pieringer, I. Parzer, A. Wöhrer, P. Reis, B. Oppl, and J. Zwerina, "IgG4- related disease: an orphan disease with many faces," *Orphanet Journal of Rare Diseases*, vol. 9, no. 1, p. 110, 2014.

[3] T. Kamisawa, Y. Zen, S. Pillai, and J. H. Stone, "IgG4-related disease," *The Lancet*, vol. 385, no. 9976, pp. 1460–1471, 2015.

[4] Y. Yoshimura, S. I. Takeda, Y. Ieki, E. Takazakura, H. Koizumi, and K. Takagawa, "IgG4-associated prostatitis complicating autoimmune pancreatitis," *Internal Medicine*, vol. 45, no. 15, pp. 897–901, 2006.

[5] I. Nishimori, T. Kohsaki, S. Onishi et al., "IgG4-related autoimmune prostatitis: two cases with or without autoimmune pancreatitis," *Internal Medicine*, vol. 46, no. 24, pp. 1983–1989, 2007.

[6] T. Uehara, H. Hamano, M. Kawakami et al., "Autoimmune pancreatitis-associated prostatitis: distinct clinicopathological entity," *Pathology International*, vol. 58, no. 2, pp. 118–125, 2008.

[7] P. A. Hart, T. C. Smyrk, and S. T. Chari, "IgG4-related prostatitis: a rare cause of steroid-responsive obstructive urinary symptoms," *International Journal of Urology*, vol. 20, no. 1, pp. 132–134, 2013.

[8] J. Buijs, L. Maillette de Buy Wenniger, G. van Leenders et al., "Immunoglobulin G4-related prostatitis: a case-control study focusing on clinical and pathologic characteristics," *Urology*, vol. 83, no. 3, pp. 521–526, 2014.

[9] M. Shiokawa, Y. Kodama, K. Yoshimura et al., "Risk of cancer in patients with autoimmune pancreatitis," *American Journal of Gastroenterology*, vol. 108, no. 4, pp. 610–617, 2013.

[10] J. Asano and T. Watanabe, "Association between immunoglobulin G4-related disease and malignancy within 12 years after diagnosis: an analysis after longterm followup," *The Journal of Rheumatology*, vol. 42, no. 11, pp. 2135–2142, 2015.

[11] A. Schneider, M. Hirth, M. Münch et al., "Risk of cancer in patients with autoimmune pancreatitis: a single-center experience from Germany," *Digestion*, vol. 95, no. 2, pp. 172–180, 2017.

[12] K. Hirano, M. Tada, N. Sasahira et al., "Incidence of malignancies in patients with IgG4-related disease," *Internal Medicine*, vol. 53, no. 3, pp. 171–176, 2014.

[13] P. Brito-Zerón, B. Kostov, X. Bosch, N. Acar-Denizli, M. Ramos-Casals, and J. H. Stone, "Therapeutic approach to IgG4-related disease: a systematic review," *Medicine*, vol. 95, no. 26, article e4002, 2016.

[14] S. A. C. Medlicott, A. Oryschak, and K. Trpkov, "IgG4 prostatitis associated with prostatic adenocarcinoma: a case report and literature review," *Hum Pathol Case Rep*, vol. 14, pp. 8–11, 2018.

13

Idiopathic Scrotal Calcinosis: A Case Report of a Rare Entity

Umesh Jayarajah ,[1] Lalani de Silva,[2] Chandu de Silva,[2] and Sanjeewa Seneviratne [1]

[1]*Department of Surgery, Faculty of Medicine, University of Colombo, Colombo, Sri Lanka*
[2]*Department of Pathology, Faculty of Medicine, University of Colombo, Colombo, Sri Lanka*

Correspondence should be addressed to Umesh Jayarajah; umeshe.jaya@gmail.com and Sanjeewa Seneviratne; sanjeewa@srg.cmb.ac.lk

Academic Editor: Tun-Chieh Chen

Scrotal calcinosis is a benign condition where multiple calcified nodules are found within the dermis of the scrotal skin. It is a rare condition which is usually asymptomatic and has no clear aetiology although several theories have been proposed in the aetiopathogenesis. We report a 55-year-old man with extensive scrotal calcinosis. Surgical excision of the affected scrotal skin was curative.

1. Introduction

Idiopathic scrotal calcinosis is a benign condition involving the scrotal skin defined as presence of multiple calcified nodules confined to the dermis [1]. Although it is believed to be idiopathic, dystrophic calcification of longstanding sebaceous cysts, and degenerative changes of the dartos are postulated to be involved in the pathogenesis [1]. The knowledge regarding this condition is limited only to case reports and series due to the rarity of the disease. Currently, surgery remains the only curative option. We report a 55-year-old man presenting with this rare condition with a review of literature.

2. Case Presentation

A 55-year-old Sri Lankan Sinhalese manual labourer presented with progressively increasing multiple, painless nodules in the scrotum of 4 year duration. He did not have any other medical comorbidities and was otherwise asymptomatic. There was no history of discharge, ulcers, or infection in relation to the scrotal lesions. Physical examination showed multiple, firm, nontender, subcutaneous nodules studded within the scrotal wall (Figure 1). Serum calcium, phosphorous, and parathormone levels were within normal limits. He underwent excision of all the lesions through multiple skin stabs under spinal anaesthesia with a satisfactory cosmetic result.

Pathological examination revealed forty three tan colour nodules, the sizes of which ranged from 23 mm to 5 mm. Microscopy revealed basophilic granular calcified material surrounded by thin fibrotic wall, devoid of an epithelial lining. Foreign body type chronic inflammatory reaction was noted in some areas. There was no evidence of granulomatous reaction (Figure 2). There was no evidence of recurrence at six month follow-up.

3. Discussion

Idiopathic scrotal calcinosis was first described by Lewinski in 1883 [2].The condition usually begins in adolescence or early adulthood. It usually present as yellowish brown, firm, solitary, or multiple nodular lesions on the scrotal skin which are increasing in size and number with time. Usually they are asymptomatic but may produce vague pain, discharge or itching and may also be complicated with infections [2]. Although it involves calcium deposition, there is no association with abnormal calcium metabolism [3]. Indication for surgery is usually cosmetic and in rare occasions, for symptom relief.

Although scrotal calcinosis is believed to be idiopathic in the majority, the pathogenesis is still controversial. Dystrophic calcification secondary to sebaceous cysts, eccrine epithelial cyst, or degenerated dartos muscle are postulated as possible mechanisms by several authors [3–5]. Calcification of sebaceous cysts may occur after an infection that later progresses to a degenerative process and results in the loss of epithelial lining of the cyst wall with calcification of the substance [4]. Ito et al. proposed an eccrine epithelial cyst origin with

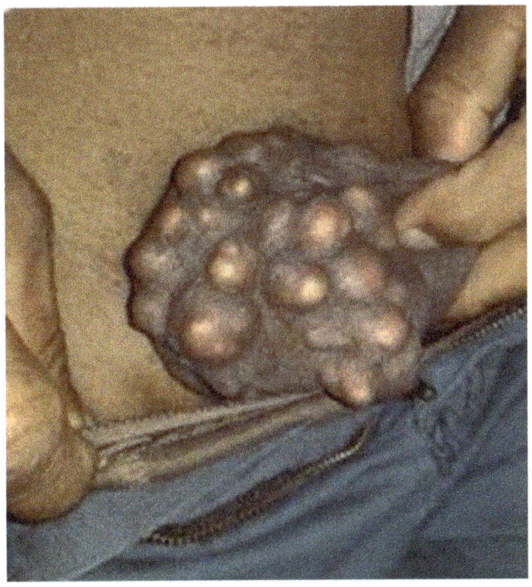

Figure 1: Physical examination showing multiple, firm, nontender, subcutaneous nodules studded within the scrotal wall.

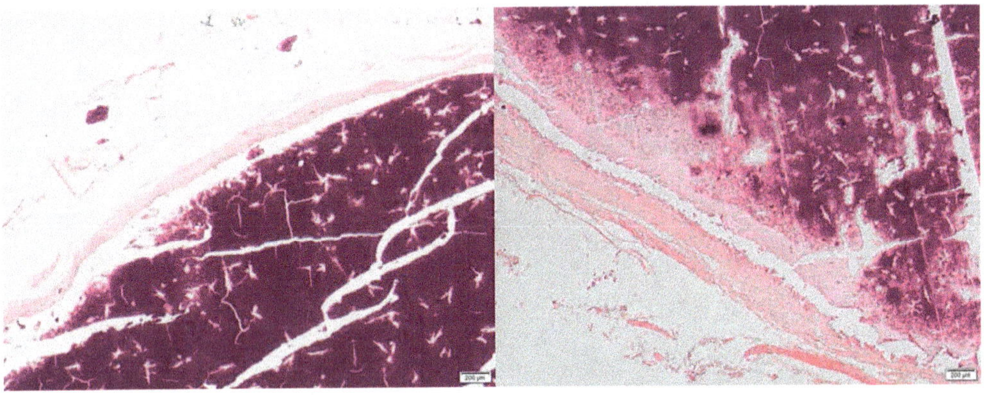

Figure 2: Histology showing calcified granular material surrounded by thin fibrotic wall (H & E ×200).

excessive discharge and collection of debris in the lumen as the possible mechanism following immunohistochemical analyses [5]. If the above features are absent in the histological evaluation similar to the presented case, the origin is considered idiopathic.

Currently, surgery remains the only recommended treatment which provides excellent cosmetic outcomes while enabling the pathological confirmation of diagnosis. As the disease is confined to the scrotal dermis, excision should be limited to the skin. Some authors have used partial scrotectomy and reconstruction in cases with extensive disease [1, 6]. There is lack of data on recurrence however, some authors propose a high incidence of recurrence in the long term [6]. Complete excision including the smallest lesion is believed to be key in minimising recurrence [1, 6].

4. Conclusion

Idiopathic scrotal calcinosis is a rare and benign condition with an unclear pathogenesis. In some cases, the disease is extensive requiring scrotal skin excision. We report a similar case with extensive idiopathic scrotal calcinosis which was excised through multiple stabs. Although the depth of the excision is limited to the dermis, complete excision of even the smallest of lesions is required to minimize recurrences.

Consent

Informed written consent for publication was obtained from the patient prior to collecting data.

References

[1] A. Khallouk, O. El Yazami, S. Mellas, M. F. Tazi, J. El Fassi, and M. H. Farih, "Idiopathic scrotal calcinosis: a non-elucidated pathogenesis and its surgical treatment," *Reviews in Urology*, vol. 13, no. 2, pp. 95–97, 2011.

[2] A. Pompeo, W. Molina, G. Pohlman, D. Sehrt, and F. Kim, "Idiopathic scrotal calcinosis: a rare entity and a review of the literature," *Canadian Urological Association Journal*, vol. 7, no. 5-6, pp. 5–6, 2013.

[3] A. G. Saad and G. S. Zaatari, "Scrotal calcinosis: is it idiopathic?" *Urology*, vol. 57, no. 2, p. 365, 2001.

[4] A. Parlakgumus, E. T. Canpolat, K. Calıskan et al., "Scrotal calcinosis due to resorption of cyst walls: a case report," *Journal of Medical Case Reports*, vol. 2, p. 375, 2008.

[5] A. Ito, F. Sakamoto, and M. Ito, "Dystrophic scrotal calcinosis originating from benign eccrine epithelial cysts," *British Journal of Dermatology*, vol. 144, no. 1, pp. 146–150, 2001.

[6] D. P. Ruiz-Genao, L. Ríos-Buceta, L. Herrero, J. Fraga, M. Aragüés, and A. García-Díez, "Massive scrotal calcinosis," *Dermatologic Surgery*, vol. 28, no. 8, pp. 745–747, 2002.

14

Long-Term Surveillance and Laparoscopic Management of Zinner Syndrome

Niall P. Kelly, Adrian Fuentes-Bonachera, William P. Shields, Ivor M. Cullen, and Padraig J. Daly

Department of Urology, University Hospital Waterford, Waterford, Ireland

Correspondence should be addressed to Niall P. Kelly; niall.p.k@gmail.com

Academic Editor: Apul Goel

Zinner syndrome was first described in 1914 and represents the triad of unilateral renal agenesis and ipsilateral seminal vesicle cyst and ipsilateral ejaculatory duct obstruction. Seminal vesicle cysts are often asymptomatic but can also present with pain, haematospermia, or other lower urinary tract symptoms. Treatment strategies include observation and surgical excision. We present the laparoscopic management of an enlarged seminal vesicle cyst, consistent with Zinner syndrome, 14 years after the initial diagnosis. A 58-year-old male patient was diagnosed with a left-sided seminal vesicle cyst while undergoing assessment for renal transplant due to progressively worsening renal function in his solitary right kidney. The otherwise asymptomatic cyst enlarged from the time of initial diagnosis in 2004 (11.3 cm × 9.7 cm × 13.1 cm) to nearly double the size in 2018 (12.8 cm × 11.9 cm × 14.2 cm). This cyst size ultimately precluded renal transplant, and the patient was referred for excision. Laparoscopic excision of the cyst was performed, histopathology confirmed seminal vesicle cyst tissue, and there has been no recurrence of the cyst to date. The patient remains active on the renal transplant waitlist. Zinner syndrome is a rare syndrome, with the seminal vesicle cysts being managed by observation or surgical excision. We report the longest documented observation of a seminal vesicle cyst, culminating in a safe and successful laparoscopic excision.

1. Introduction

Zinner syndrome was first described in 1914 and represents the triad of unilateral renal agenesis and ipsilateral seminal vesicle cyst and ipsilateral ejaculatory duct obstruction. Often asymptomatic, it can present with haematuria or haematospermia or other lower urinary tract symptoms. The cysts can become markedly enlarged, requiring excision due to symptoms. We present the laparoscopic management of an enlarged seminal vesicle cyst, consistent with Zinner syndrome.

2. Case Report

A 58-year-old male patient with end-stage renal failure (ESRF) due to assumed reflux nephropathy in a solitary right kidney was undergoing assessment for renal transplantation. His past medical history was significant for non-Hodgkin's lymphoma, treated with chemotherapy (completed in 2014) and hypertension. His baseline serum creatinine at the time of initial referral in 2018 was 522 μg/L. Computer tomography (CT) imaging of the abdomen and pelvis (performed in October 2018) revealed a large cystic lesion arising from the area of the left seminal vesicle in 2018 (12.8 cm × 11.9 cm × 14.2 cm, volume approximately 900 cm^3) (Figure 1). The patient was referred to our unit for consideration of excision of the cyst as it was deemed too large to allow renal transplantation by the transplant team.

The seminal vesicle cyst was first diagnosed incidentally following ultrasound examination of the abdomen in 2004 as part of investigations of chronic kidney disease (CKD; serum creatinine in 2004 was 161 μg/L with evidence of proteinuria). This ultrasound identified an absent left kidney and scarring of the right kidney, suggestive of reflux nephropathy, as well as the cyst within the pelvis. The cyst was then assessed with CT, at which time it measured 11.3 cm × 9.7 cm × 13.1 cm (volume approximately 500 cm^3) within the left side of the pelvis, seen to be originating from the seminal

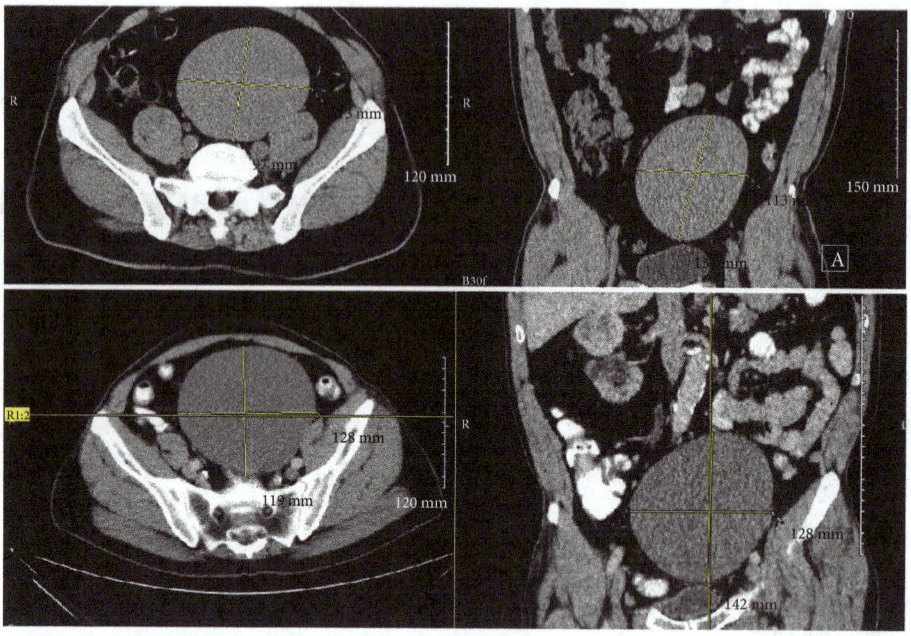

FIGURE 1: CT, axial, and coronal sections of the seminal vesicle cyst from 2004 and 2018. In 2004, the cyst measured 11.3 cm × 9.7 cm × 13.1 cm (volume approximately 500 cm^3), while in 2018, it measured 12.8 cm × 11.9 cm × 14.2 cm (volume approximately 900 cm^3).

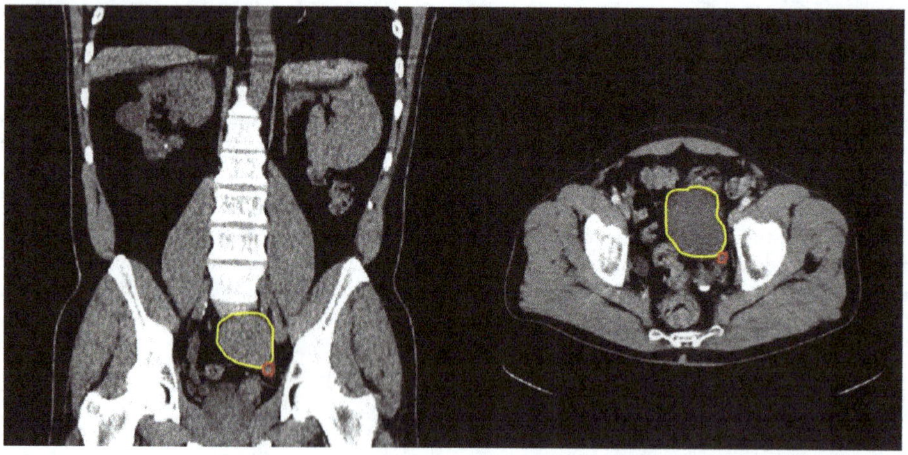

FIGURE 2: CT, axial, and coronal sections from scan in 2004, of a more inferior aspect of the cyst (outlined in yellow), identifying its relationship to the seminal vesicle (outlined in red).

vesicle on that side (Figure 2). This CT also showed some prominence of the right ureter but without a cause for obstruction. Micturating cystourethrogram (MCUG) was not performed during the initial nephrology consultations; thus, reflux could not be absolutely confirmed as the cause of the CKD. As the patient was asymptomatic at the time of initial diagnosis, a decision was taken to defer intervention until only such time that he did become symptomatic. No specific radiological follow-up regimen was followed, although the patient had regular clinical and physical examinations. There was an approximate 80% increase in the volume of the cyst over the 14-year time period, leading to a large lesion occupying the pelvis and precluding safe transplantation of a donor kidney.

The patient underwent laparoscopy with excision of the seminal vesicle cyst in January 2019. A 3-port set-up was used with the patient in a slight Trendelenburg position. The colon was mobilised out of the pelvis, and an impression of the large cyst could be seen in the floor of the peritoneum. The peritoneum was incised and dissected from the cyst. The cyst was incised and drained of approximately 400 mls dark fluid; no organisms grew on the culture of this. Drainage of the cyst allowed for better visualisation of the adherent areas as well as location of the base of the cyst. The specimen was retrieved, and histopathology confirmed that the cyst was of seminal vesicle origin. The patient had an uneventful postoperative stay and was discharged on the first postoperative day. There has been no recurrence of the cyst to date, and he was referred to the nephrological service where he remains active on the renal transplant waitlist.

3. Discussion

Zinner syndrome is a rare syndrome that is often asymptomatic, and thus, the exact incidence is unknown. Some of the symptoms that have been attributed to Zinner syndrome include urinary urgency, bladder outlet obstruction, and haematospermia [1]. Occasionally, there can be flank or groin pain associated with the cysts also [2]. The cysts can grow to be quite large, and the cyst we present in this case is amongst the largest, reported at 14 cm in maximal diameter. Indeed, this is the first reported case whereby renal transplantation has been precluded by the presence of the cyst.

Zinner syndrome arises due to abnormal development of the Wolffian duct, also known as the mesonephric duct. These usually develop into the epididymis, vas deferens, ejaculatory duct, and seminal vesicle, in response to testosterone around the 8th week of foetal life. Abnormalities in the development of the Wolffian duct can lead to seminal vesicle cyst formation, but there are also implications for renal development. The foetal kidney develops from the metanephric mass of intermediate mesoderm following induction by the metanephric diverticulum, or ureteric bud, which is an outgrowth from the Wolffian duct [3].

Management of these seminal vesicle cysts depends on their presentation and symptoms. There have been approximately 200 cases in the literature with marked variation across the reports. Many of the published case reports are of symptomatic seminal vesicle cysts, and most have had some intervention. There are reports of open, laparoscopic, and robotically assisted excision of the cysts [4, 5], and the patients have all experienced a resolution of their symptoms after treatment. Aspiration of symptomatic cysts, however, tends to lead to recurrence of the symptoms, ultimately requiring surgical excision at a later date [6–8]. In patients where infertility was the presenting complaint, transurethral resection of the ejaculatory ducts was attempted [9], with subsequent improvement in semen characteristics.

Observation is advocated for many asymptomatic patients, as was the case in our patient at the time of his initial diagnosis. However, the method and duration of observation are not specified, and indeed, the natural history of these cysts is unclear. The vast majority of cysts are benign in nature, and malignant change has only been documented in a single case [10]. Most papers that report on safe observation have no follow-up documented beyond 1 year, based on clinical follow-up without surveillance imaging. The longest follow-up reported prior to our report was 11 years for a child with a seminal cyst initially diagnosed as a ureterocele at the age of 3 but reclassified as a seminal vesicle cyst at age 14 [11]. There was no change in size of the cyst noted in that report, and annual clinical surveillance is ongoing. Our paper has the longest follow-up of a case of Zinner syndrome in an adult and is also one of the first to document a significant change in the size of the cyst over time, while remaining asymptomatic; our patient's cyst increased in volume by nearly 80%. There may be a role for radiological surveillance of seminal vesicle cysts given the size changes noted in our paper and the potential malignant risk, but prospective studies would be required to elucidate this fact.

In summary, we present the case of a 58-year-old man with the longest documented follow-up of an enlarging yet asymptomatic seminal vesicle cyst as part of a Zinner syndrome diagnosis, which was excised laparoscopically successfully to facilitate renal transplantation.

Consent

The patient provided written informed consent for the preparation of this case report.

Disclosure

2013 Care Checklist has been adhered to in the preparation of this manuscript: https://www.care-statement.org/checklist.

References

[1] M. Kardoust Parizi and N. Shakhssalim, "Management of Zinner's syndrome associated with contralateral seminal vesicle hypoplasia: a case report," *Case Reports in Urology*, vol. 2013, Article ID 494215, 3 pages, 2013.

[2] M. AlArifi, M. Al-Gahwary, and M. Gomha, "The association of renal agenesis and ipsilateral seminal vesicle cyst: Zinner syndrome case report," *Case Reports in Urology*, vol. 2019, Article ID 1242149, 3 pages, 2019.

[3] K. L. Moore and T. V. N. Persaud, *Before We Are Born: Essentials of Embryology and Birth Defects*, Saunders, Philadelphia, 6th edition, 2003.

[4] Z. Tan, B. Li, L. Zhang et al., "Classifying seminal vesicle cysts in the diagnosis and treatment of Zinner syndrome: a report of six cases and review of available literature," *Andrologia*, vol. 52, no. 1, article e13397, 2020.

[5] E. Kord, A. Zisman, A. E. Darawsha, N. Dally, P. H. Noh, and A. Neheman, "Minimally invasive approach for treatment of seminal vesicle cyst associated with ipsilateral renal agenesis," *Urologia Internationalis*, vol. 99, no. 3, pp. 338–342, 2017.

[6] E. P. Kwenda, R. A. Locke, J. S. Archer et al., "Robot-assisted laparoscopic resection of the mesonephric duct remnant in a patient with Zinner syndrome," *Journal of Endourology Case Reports*, vol. 6, no. 3, pp. 198–201, 2020.

[7] T. Maehana, F. Fukuta, K. Kobayashi, M. Hirobe, T. Tanaka, and N. Masumori, "Laparoscopic surgery for seminal vesicle cysts and ureterocele with urination disorder: a case report of Zinner syndrome," *Journal of Endourology Case Reports*, vol. 4, no. 1, pp. 35–38, 2018.

[8] L. Demaeyer, S. Holz, D. Pamart, S. Taylor, and M. Naudin, "Robotic management of painful Zinner syndrome, case report and review of literature," *International Journal of Surgery Case Reports*, vol. 73, pp. 61–64, 2020.

[9] G. Pace, G. P. Galatioto, L. Gualà, G. Ranieri, and C. Vicentini, "Ejaculatory duct obstruction caused by a right giant seminal vesicle with an ipsilateral upper urinary tract agenesia: an embryologic malformation," *Fertility and Sterility*, vol. 89, no. 2, pp. 390–394, 2008.

[10] A. Bhat, I. Banerjee, O. N. Kryvenko, and R. Satyanarayana, "Primary seminal vesicle adenocarcinoma: a lethal yet cryptic malignancy with review of literature," *BML Case Reports*, vol. 12, no. 12, article e232994, 2019.

[11] A. Kanavaki, I. Vidal, L. Merlini, and S. Hanquinet, "Congenital seminal vesicle cyst and ipsilateral renal agenesis (Zinner syndrome): a rare association and its evolution from early childhood to adolescence," *The European Journal of Pediatric Surgery Reports*, vol. 3, no. 2, pp. 98–102, 2015.

15

A Unique Case of Incomplete Bifid Ureter and Associated Arterial Variations

Shivika Ahuja,[1] Hannah Sullivan,[1] Mark Noller,[2] Yun Tan,[1] and Daniel Daly[1]

[1]*Center for Anatomical Science and Education, Department of Surgery, Saint Louis University School of Medicine, Saint Louis, MO 63104, USA*
[2]*Urological Surgeons of Northern California, San Jose, CA 95124, USA*

Correspondence should be addressed to Daniel Daly; daniel.daly@health.slu.edu

Academic Editor: Mohamed A. Ghoneim

Introduction. Urogenital and vascular anomalies, including a left duplex kidney and a left aberrant renal artery that gave rise to the left ovarian artery, were observed in a 77-year-old female cadaver during a routine dissection. *Description.* A left aberrant renal artery, which gave rise to the left ovarian artery, was observed originating from the aorta 4 cm below the left renal artery. Two independent contributions to a bifid ureter were found originating from the hilum of the left kidney. These two contributions descended 12.4 cm and 10.6 cm, respectively, posterior to the left aberrant renal artery and lateral to the left ovarian artery before uniting anterior to the psoas major muscle to descend 12.7 cm to the bladder. *Significance.* While the duplex kidney is a relatively common congenital anomaly that can be asymptomatic, it can also potentially be associated with compression of renal vasculature or the ureter. Ureteral compression can then result in several pathologies including reflux, urinary tract infection (UTI), ureteropelvic junction obstruction, or hydronephrosis. Compression of renal and ovarian vasculature can result in altered blood flow to the kidney and ovary, potentially causing fibrosis, atrophy, or organ failure. Current imaging techniques alone are insufficient for correct diagnostics of such complications, and they must be supplemented with a thorough understanding of the respective anatomical variations.

1. Introduction

Congenital abnormalities of the kidney and urinary tract (CAKUT) that encompass variations in the kidney, ureter, bladder, or urethra range in severity from asymptomatic to significantly contributing to end-stage renal disease [1]. One of the most common CAKUT variations is the duplex kidney, also known as the duplicated ureteral collecting system [2]. A normal ureter travels 25–30 cm from the kidney to the bladder and is divided into three regions—ureteropelvic junction (UPJ), ureterovesicular junction (UVJ), and the point of crossing over the common iliac arteries [3]. A duplex kidney can exist in one of two anatomical variations: complete and incomplete [4]. Complete duplication results in two patent ureters arising from the affected kidney and draining independently into the bladder, while incomplete duplication results in two ureters draining the same kidney but merging prior to reaching the bladder [5]. The incomplete duplication can be further categorized into either a bifid pelvis, which occurs when the two ureteral contributions unite proximal to the UPJ, or a bifid ureter, in which the ureteral contributions merge distally to the UPJ but proximal to the UVJ [5]. Duplex kidneys are more common in women and are usually observed unilaterally, as was observed in the current case [6, 7]. Imaging techniques alone, such as excretory urography, voiding cystourethrography, and CT without contrast, are not always reliable diagnostic tools for this upper urinary tract abnormality due to the positioning of the ureter. Imaging results must be coupled with thorough knowledge of CAKUT anatomical variations to diagnose possible associated complications, such as various types of ureteral reflux and ureteropelvic junction obstruction (UPJO) [8].

The vascular variation of a left aberrant renal artery giving rise to the left ovarian artery could increase the possibility of urogenital complications resulting from ureteral compression. Current literature suggests that because variation in arterial supply to the kidney is more prevalent than previously believed, there is a need to standardize the nomenclature describing additional renal arteries [9, 10]. Various terms, including accessory, aberrant, anomalous, supernumerary, supplementary, multiple, upper/lower polar arteries, and aortic superior and inferior polar arteries, have been used for that purpose [9]. We will use the definition of an aberrant renal artery established by Holden et al. as an artery which enters the kidney outside of the hilum, whereas an accessory renal artery follows the renal artery to enter the kidney at the hilum; both accessory and aberrant renal arteries typically originate from the abdominal aorta, but this can vary [11].

The current case report is of interest due to its clinical importance and novelty, specifically outlining how this unique combination of urogenital and vascular anomalies can exacerbate their individual complications. Accessory renal arteries have been proposed to independently contribute to hypertension, hydronephrosis, or segmental infarcts while also causing or worsening urogenital symptoms associated with a bifid ureter [12]. Similarly, ureteric obstruction of vascular structures can cause ischemia of their target tissues. This case is educationally and clinically valuable as it emphasizes the importance of foundational knowledge of anatomical variations, which, when used in conjunction with imaging studies, could positively impact patient care.

2. Case Presentation

A 77-year-old female body was received through the Saint Louis University Gift of Body Program of the Center for Anatomical Science and Education (CASE) with a signed informed consent form from the donor. The CASE gift body program abides by all the rules set forth by the Uniform Anatomical Gift Act (UAGA).

During routine dissection, the hilum of the left kidney was cleaned and typical anatomical structures were identified, from anterior to posterior, as the renal vein, renal artery, and superior ureteral contribution (Figures 1 and 2). Following the removal of perirenal fat, a second ureteral contribution was found exiting the kidney, slightly inferior to the hilum. The two independent contributions, superior and inferior, descended 12.4 cm and 10.6 cm before they united anterior to the left psoas major muscle to descend over the left common iliac artery to the posterolateral aspect of the bladder (Figure 1).

Further dissection revealed an additional vascular structure, the left aberrant renal artery, entering the inferior pole of the left kidney (Figure 1). Cleaning the structure revealed its origin from the abdominal aorta 4 cm inferior to the left renal artery, which branched from the aorta below the superior mesenteric artery. The aberrant renal artery was then observed travelling in parallel with, but inferior to, the left renal vein and artery toward the left kidney. This artery was also observed passing anterior to the superior and inferior ureteral contributions and bifurcated just prior to reaching the parenchyma of the inferior renal pole of the left kidney. The left ovarian artery was observed branching from the aberrant renal artery nearly halfway to the left kidney. The left ovarian artery then descended medially, but adjacent to the superior ureteral contribution, and more inferiorly, adjacent to the united ureter to supply the left ovary (Figure 1).

3. Discussion

3.1. Left Bifid Ureter. The current case describes a left-sided bifid ureter that united anterior to the psoas major muscle before crossing the left common iliac artery and entering the posterolateral aspect of the bladder. During postmortem examination, duplicated ureters have been observed in 0.8% of cadavers studied [13]. This congenital malformation occurs during the development of the metanephric system which ascends from the sacral to the lumbar region to become the permanent kidney and ureter. The metanephric system is derived from two sources of intermediate mesoderm: the ureteric bud and metanephric blastema. Normally, the metanephric mesenchyme signals the ureteric bud to invade and branch into the mesenchyme, and the ureter reciprocally induces the mesenchyme to differentiate into nephrons [2]. The duplex system arises from a premature splitting of the ureteric bud or the development of two separate buds [14]. This anatomical variation is two times more commonly observed in females as compared to men, but the cause is currently unclear [6]. There have been reports that unilateral duplication is six times more common than bilateral duplication [6, 15]. It has also been reported that there is a one in eight chance for a child with a duplicated ureter to have a parent or sibling with a similar anomaly, thereby suggesting a heritable contribution to the above pathologies [15]. In general, reflux is the most common medical complication associated with a duplex kidney. Ureteroureteric reflux is most closely associated with incomplete duplication with an incidence of 22%, and vesicoureteric reflux is associated with complete duplication [16]. The respective incidences of these types of reflux are 69% and 72% [15, 16]. Other associated urinary tract complications include ureteropelvic junction obstruction and hydronephrosis [8].

3.2. Left Aberrant Renal Artery. Aberrant renal arteries occur in approximately 30% of the population, with left-side predominance, and are more commonly observed supplying the lower renal pole than the upper pole [17, 18]. The developmental mechanism of this variation is unclear, and the embryologic origin of the renal and adrenal arteries is under debate. The most widely held explanation is Felix's ladder theory [19]. This theory states that the blood supply to the developing mesonephros (including the adrenal glands, kidneys, and gonads) differentiates from the nine lateral mesonephric arteries (MAs). These vascular structures originate from the aorta and are divided into three groups: the first and second arteries are cranial, the third through fifth arteries are middle, and the sixth through ninth arteries are caudal. Normally, one middle lateral mesonephric (MLM) artery and one caudal lateral mesonephric artery persist and differentiate into the renal artery and gonadal artery, respectively, while the other vascular structures are obliterated [20]. However, the persistence of an additional MLM artery, for

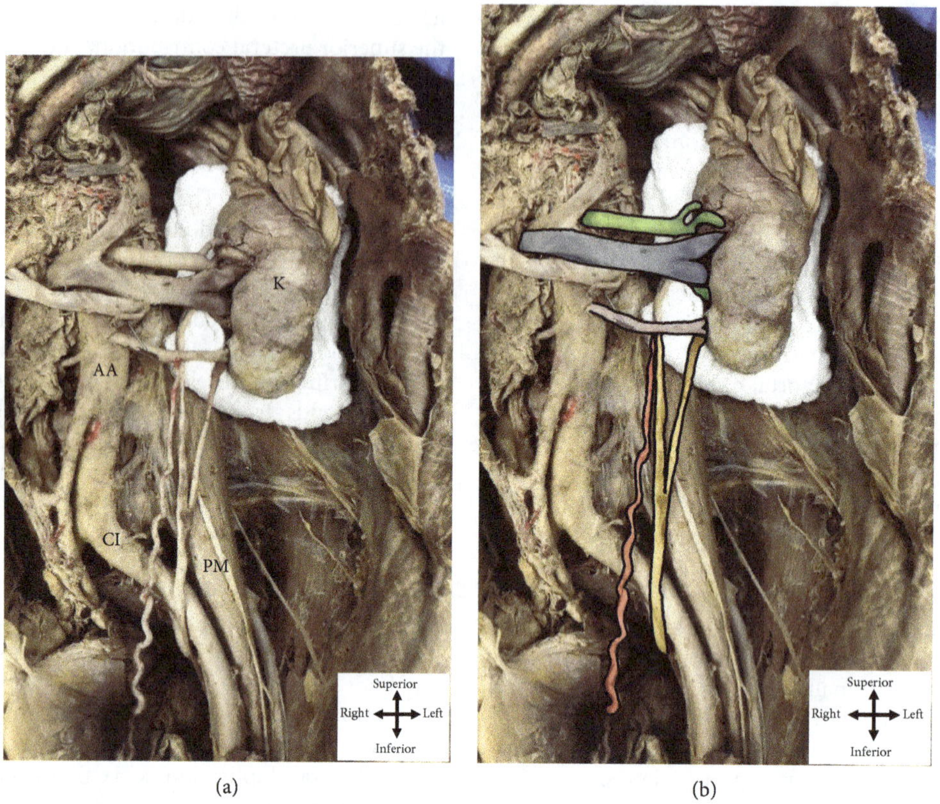

FIGURE 1: The dissected path of the left bifid ureter and aberrant renal artery. (a) depicts the dissected path of the left bifid ureter with labeling of relevant landmarks while (b) depicts relevant structures pseudocolored for ease in visualization. The left renal vein (blue in (b)) is observed as the anterior-most structure in the renal hilum, thereby serving as a reference point for relationships in this region. The left renal artery (green in (b)), located posterior to the renal vein, has upper two segments that can be observed entering the superior pole of the kidney (K in (a)). The left aberrant renal artery (pink in (b)) is observed originating from the abdominal aorta (AA in (a)) and branching before reaching the inferior pole of the kidney. As the aberrant artery courses toward the left kidney, it gives off the highly coiled left ovarian artery (red in (b)) that descends into the pelvis medial to the left ureter. The superior and inferior contributions to the bifid ureter (yellow) emerge from the posterior aspect of the renal hilum and unite to form the left ureter proximal to the bladder and near the anterior surface of the psoas major muscle (PM in (a)). The left ureter crosses over the left common iliac artery (CI in (a)) before entering the pelvis to join the bladder.

unknown reasons, results in the creation of either an accessory or aberrant renal artery, the latter of which is more commonly found entering the kidney at its lower pole [21].

Felix's ladder theory can be applied to developmental malrotation or improper positioning of the kidney to propose an alternative explanation for the left aberrant renal artery. During embryological development, the kidneys medially rotate and ascend to the lumbar region. It is during this ascent that the supplementary lateral mesonephric arteries should regress, but failure to do so could create aberrant renal arteries [22]. However, this is not likely to be the cause of this report's arterial variation because while reported cases did document multiple arterial supplies to the kidney, they also included a truncated ureter, renal arterial supply originating from various sources including the abdominal aorta and common iliac artery, and a pelvic kidney, which were not observed in the current case [23, 24].

In contrast to the ladder theory, Isogai et al. and Nobuyuki et al. recently proposed that the mesonephric arterial ladder is obliterated prior to the metanephric ascent and glomeruli development, meaning that the persistent renal artery is not derived from the mesonephric arterial system but originates from the aorta once the kidney is properly positioned in the posterior abdominal wall [19, 25]. Unlike Felix, these researchers maintain that the embryonic aorta has the potential to further branch after the MAs obliterate, but they also state that the definite renal artery may utilize the MA origins as its own. Nobuyuki et al. also found that the MAs, when observed during weeks 5-6 of embryological development, were segmental but not evenly distributed or symmetrical [25]. Perhaps the existence of more MA buds on the left lateral aspect of the aorta explains why aberrant renal arteries are more commonly found on the left.

The relationship of the ureters to the aberrant renal arteries is significant since the uncommon anatomy of the artery could present an additional risk factor during endoscopic surgery [26]. Damage or occlusion of an aberrant renal artery is known to lead to segmental infarcts and tissue necrosis, which could in turn damage a renal calyx and cause urine extravasation [27]. Vascular anomalies are also a common cause of congenital hydronephrosis, and obstructions at the UPJ can be due to an aberrant renal vessel crossing the ureter anteriorly [28, 29].

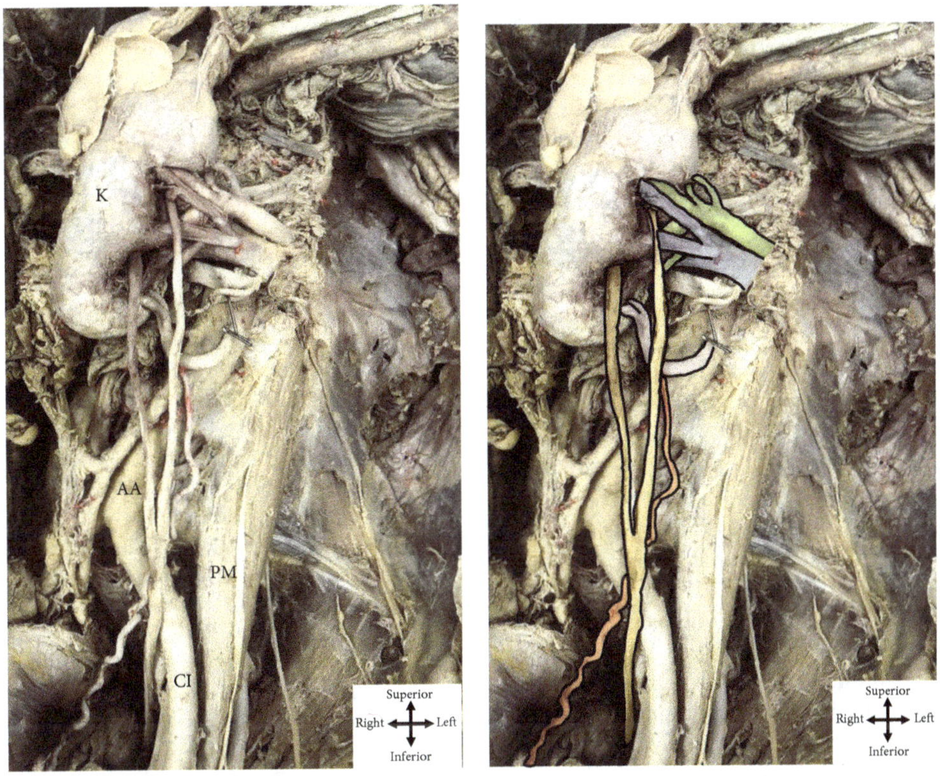

(a) (b)

FIGURE 2: The anatomical presentation of the posterior aspect of the left kidney. (a) depicts the relevant dissected structures associated with labeled landmarks while (b) depicts relevant structures pseudocolored for ease in visualization. The left kidney (K in (a)) has been reflected away from the left posterior abdominal wall to show the posterior aspect of its hilum. The two contributions to the ureter (yellow in (b)) can be observed emerging from the hilum; the superior contribution emerges posterior to the renal vein, and the inferior contribution descends from the renal hilum anterior to the renal vein. The left aberrant renal artery (pink in (b)) is observed branching before entering the substance of the kidney. The left ovarian artery (red in (b)) emerges from the anterior aspect of the aberrant left renal artery. Five segmental arteries and the renal vein are also observed entering the renal hilum (green and blue, respectively, in (b)).

The present case report also addresses the overwhelming volume of vocabulary used to describe variations in the renal arterial supply. Gulas et al. have outlined the variable descriptions regarding additional renal arterial supply beginning with terms that began in the 16th century until today [9]. Per their compilation, the terms "multiple" and "additional" were used most frequently when numerous renal arteries were present [9]. However, these terms lack specificity in that they do not explain the origins of the additional arteries nor how they enter the renal parenchyma. A classification system that accommodates variant renal segmental arteries as well as additional renal arterial supplies must be developed in order to efficiently and clearly share information regarding a patient's condition, thereby decreasing the risk of hemorrhage, segmental ischemia, and renovascular hypertension during renal transplant surgery [30].

3.3. Left Ovarian Artery. The final anomaly observed in this cadaver was the left ovarian artery originating from the left aberrant renal artery. The ovarian artery typically arises anteromedially from the abdominal aorta several centimeters below the renal arteries, while an ovarian artery arising from the renal, lumbar, adrenal, or iliac arteries occurs at a rate of 10-20% [31]. In order to understand why the ovarian artery originates from the aberrant renal artery, it is prudent to first explore the embryological development of the ovary itself.

The gonad develops from the urogenital fold, a structure superior to the developing kidney. As the gonads descend within the elongating body, the ascending kidneys and the aortic mesonephric blood supply pass posterior to the gonads, causing the gonadal vascular supply to also originate from the lateral mesonephric arteries. The lateral mesonephric branches that potentially reach to supply the descending gonads are categorized in one of two ways: the first type is cranial to the renal hilum and the second is caudal to it. Only one of the lateral mesonephric arteries will persist, thereby becoming the gonadal artery. The relationship of the gonadal artery, or in this case the ovarian artery, to the hilum of the kidney paired with the kidney's ascension level (which is higher on the left) will predict the gonadal artery's relationship to neighboring structures, including the renal vein, renal artery, and aorta [32]. While rare, gonadal arteries have been observed to originate from numerous sources due to the anastomoses between the persistent mesonephric arteries as the mesonephric system develops. These sources include the abdominal aorta, renal artery, or accessory renal artery and the variations are often left-sided [32, 33]. The path of this left ovarian artery is consistent with that of an ovarian artery originating from the aorta, so it is unlikely that this left ovarian artery would experience compression. A more likely complication of origination of the ovarian artery from the aberrant renal is an ischemic event due to the reduced caliber of the aberrant artery and the ovarian artery. This ischemia may then lead to infarction or ischemic reperfusion injury to the ovary [34].

4. Conclusion

Postmortem urogenital and vascular anomalies were observed in a 77-year-old female cadaver. No reports were found in the literature documenting the combination of variants observed: left bifid ureter, left aberrant renal artery, and left ovarian artery originating from the aberrant vessel. These findings are clinically important as the aberrant artery reinforces the notion that multiple renal arterial sources are more prevalent than previously believed, meaning that new imaging modalities such as endoluminal ultrasonography, computed tomography angiography (CTA), and magnetic resonance angiogram (MRA) could replace the older methods such as intravenous urography and angiography. Lastly, the acceptance and utilization of a common nomenclature will facilitate the sharing of information between academic, surgical, and radiological fields of study. The aberrant renal vessel can also cause hydronephrosis, which, along with reflux, UPJO, and segmental infarction of the kidney, can manifest itself as a result of a duplex renal system. The knowledge of these potential anatomical variations must be paired with an understanding of their embryological origins and imaging techniques to aid proper clinical diagnosis and treatment.

Acknowledgments

The authors would like to thank Andrey Frolov, PhD, for his assistance in reviewing the manuscript and providing useful insights into the revision process. This study was supported by the Center for Anatomical Science and Education, Saint Louis University School of Medicine.

References

[1] S. Sanna-Cherchi, P. Ravani, V. Corbani et al., "Renal outcome in patients with congenital anomalies of the kidney and urinary tract," *Kidney International*, vol. 76, no. 5, pp. 528–533, 2009.

[2] V. M. Kozlov and A. Schedl, "Duplex kidney formation: developmental mechanisms and genetic predisposition," *F1000Research*, vol. 9, p. 2, 2020.

[3] H. A. Lescay, J. Jiang, and F. Tuma, *Anatomy, abdomen and pelvis, ureter*, in StatPearls, Treasure Island (FL), 2020.

[4] S. Ramanathan, D. Kumar, M. Khanna et al., "Multi-modality imaging review of congenital abnormalities of kidney and upper urinary tract," *World Journal of Radiology*, vol. 8, no. 2, pp. 132–141, 2016.

[5] M. M. Rodriguez, "Congenital anomalies of the kidney and the urinary tract (CAKUT)," *Fetal and Pediatric Pathology*, vol. 33, no. 5-6, pp. 293–320, 2014.

[6] E. Siomou, F. Papadopoulou, K. D. Kollios et al., "Duplex collecting system diagnosed during the first 6 years of life after a first urinary tract infection: a study of 63 children," *The Journal of Urology*, vol. 175, no. 2, pp. 678–682, 2006, discussion 681-2.

[7] J. T. Privett, W. D. Jeans, and J. Roylance, "The incidence and importance of renal duplication," *Clinical Radiology*, vol. 27, no. 4, pp. 521–530, 1976.

[8] S. K. Fernbach, K. A. Feinstein, K. Spencer, and C. A. Lindstrom, "Ureteral duplication and its complications," *Radiographics*, vol. 17, no. 1, pp. 109–127, 1997.

[9] E. Gulas, G. Wysiadecki, J. Szymański et al., "Morphological and clinical aspects of the occurrence of accessory (multiple) renal arteries," *Archives of Medical Science*, vol. 14, no. 2, pp. 442–453, 2018.

[10] K. S. Satyapal, A. A. Haffejee, B. Singh, L. Ramsaroop, J. V. Robbs, and J. M. Kalideen, "Additional renal arteries: incidence and morphometry," *Surgical and Radiologic Anatomy*, vol. 23, no. 1, pp. 33–38, 2001.

[11] A. Holden, A. Smith, P. Dukes, H. Pilmore, and M. Yasutomi, "Assessment of 100 live potential renal donors for laparoscopic nephrectomy with multi-detector row helical CT," *Radiology*, vol. 237, no. 3, pp. 973–980, 2005.

[12] G. Singh, Y. K. Ng, and B. H. Bay, "Bilateral accessory renal arteries associated with some anomalies of the ovarian arteries: a case study," *Clinical Anatomy*, vol. 11, no. 6, pp. 417–420, 1998.

[13] E. Nation, "Duplication of the kidney and ureter: a statistical study of 230 new cases," *Journal of Urology*, vol. 51, no. 5, pp. 456–465, 1944.

[14] A. Bhamani and M. Srivastava, "Obstructed bifid uretereric system causing unilateral hydronephrosis," *Revista de Urología*, vol. 15, no. 3, pp. 131–134, 2013.

[15] J. Whitaker and D. M. Danks, "A study of the inheritance of duplication of the kidneys and ureters," *The Journal of Urology*, vol. 95, no. 2, pp. 176–178, 1966.

[16] G. S. Bisset 3rd and J. L. Strife, "The duplex collecting system in girls with urinary tract infection: prevalence and significance," *American Journal of Roentgenology*, vol. 148, no. 3, pp. 497–500, 1987.

[17] F. T. Graves, "The arterial anatomy of the congenitally abnormal kidney," *The British Journal of Surgery*, vol. 56, no. 7, pp. 533–541, 1969.

[18] B. S. Park, T. K. Jeong, S. K. Ma et al., "Hydronephrosis by an aberrant renal artery: a case report," *The Korean Journal of Internal Medicine*, vol. 18, no. 1, pp. 57–60, 2003.

[19] S. Isogai, M. Horiguchi, and J. Hitomi, "The para-aortic ridge plays a key role in the formation of the renal, adrenal and gonadal vascular systems," *Journal of Anatomy*, vol. 216, no. 6, pp. 656–670, 2010.

[20] W. Felix, Ed.F. M. F. Keibel and M. Hill, "The development of the urinogenital organs," in *Manual of Human Embryology II*, W. Felix, Ed., pp. 752–979, J. B. Lippincott Company The Washington Square Press, Philadelphia, 1912.

[21] F. T. Graves, "The aberrant renal artery," *Journal of Anatomy*, vol. 90, no. 4, pp. 553–558, 1956.

[22] S. Jain and F. Chen, "Developmental pathology of congenital kidney and urinary tract anomalies," *Clinical Kidney Journal*, vol. 12, no. 3, pp. 382–399, 2019.

[23] M. Gülsün, F. Balkanci, S. Çekirge, and A. Deger, "Pelvic kidney with an unusual blood supply: angiographic findings," *Surgical and Radiologic Anatomy*, vol. 22, no. 1, pp. 59–61, 2000.

[24] J. Singh, N. Singh, K. Kapoor, and M. Sharma, "Bilateral malrotation and a congenital pelvic kidney with varied vasculature and altered hilar anatomy," *Case Reports in Medicine*, vol. 2015, Article ID 848949, 3 pages, 2015.

[25] N. Hinata, R. Suzuki, A. Ishizawa et al., "Fetal development of the mesonephric artery in humans with reference to replacement by the adrenal and renal arteries," *Annals of Anatomy*, vol. 202, pp. 8–17, 2015.

[26] C. Giberti, F. Germinale, M. Lillo, P. Bottino, A. Simonato, and G. Carmignani, "Obstetric and gynaecological ureteric injuries: treatment and results," *British Journal of Urology*, vol. 77, no. 1, pp. 21–26, 1996.

[27] J. L. Gutierrez-Calzada, J. Ramos-Titos, J. A. Gonzalez-Bonilla, A. S. Garcia-Vaquero, A. Martin-Morales, and R. Burgos-Rodriguez, "Caliceal fistula formation following renal transplantation: management with partial nephrectomy and ureteral replacement," *The Journal of Urology*, vol. 153, no. 3, pp. 612–614, 1995.

[28] J. Healey, *Surgical Anatomy*, B.C. Decker, Toronto, 2 ed. edition, 1990.

[29] D. Bulmer, *Functional Anatomy of the Urogenital System*, Pitman Medical, 6 ed edition, 1974.

[30] F. J. Sampaio and M. A. Passos, "Renal arteries: anatomic study for surgical and radiological practice," *Surgical and Radiologic Anatomy*, vol. 14, no. 2, pp. 113–117, 1992.

[31] U. Borell and I. Fernstrom, "The ovarian artery: an arteriographic study in human subjects," *Acta Radiologica*, vol. - Original Series, Volume 42, no. 4, pp. 253–265, 1954.

[32] H. Notkovich, "Variations of the testicular and ovarian arteries in relation to the renal pedicle," *Surgery, Gynecology & Obstetrics*, vol. 103, no. 4, pp. 487–495, 1956.

[33] S. R. Kotian, A. K. Pandey, S. Padmashali, J. Jaison, S. G. Kalthur, and Manipal University, India, "A cadaveric study of the testicular artery and its clinical significance," *Jornal Vascular Brasileiro*, vol. 15, no. 4, pp. 280–286, 2016.

[34] A. Eser, D. Hizli, H. Haltas et al., "Effects of curcumin on ovarian ischemia-reperfusion injury in a rat model," *Biomedical Reports*, vol. 3, no. 6, pp. 807–813, 2015.

16

Complete Penoscrotal Transposition with Other Extragenital Anomalies in a Neonate Delivered at Term

Ali Mahamudu Ayamba,[1,2] Raymond Saa-Eru Maalman,[1] Yaw Otchere Donkor,[1] and John Noah Anyorigiya[3]

[1]*Department of Basic Medical Sciences, School of Medicine, University of Health and Allied Sciences, Ho, Volta Region, Ghana*
[2]*Consultant Urologist, Department of Surgery, School of Medicine, University of Health and Allied Sciences, Ho, Volta Region, Ghana*
[3]*Medical Officer, Margaret Maquart Catholic Hospital, Kpando, Volta Region, Ghana*

Correspondence should be addressed to Raymond Saa-Eru Maalman; rmaalman@uhas.edu.gh

Academic Editor: Claudio Simeone

A complete penoscrotal transposition (CPST) is a very uncommon congenital maldevelopment that is always associated with other abnormal body variations (malformations). We report a rare case of a term neonate delivered with CPST, which had a flaccid penis and an intact scrotum with unilateral limb and digital deformity, imperforate anus, cardiac malformation a facial deformity. Neonate died two hours after delivery. The foetal abnormality was not detected through routine antenatal services received by the mother.

1. Introduction

There is a rare occurrence of congenital scrotal anomalies categorized as penoscrotal transposition (PST), bifid scrotum, ectopic scrotum, and accessory scrotum [1]. This report describes the case of PST which is an uncommon external genitalia malformation present at birth where the penis is located inferior and posterior to the scrotum [1–3]. PST is generally associated with hypospadias and can either be described as complete or incomplete based on the location of the penis and scrotum [2]. Commonly reported form is the incomplete PST in which the penis is located in the middle of the scrotum, while in the complete PST, the penis that arises from the perineum covers completely by the scrotum [2].

The aetiology for the abnormal embryological sequence responsible for PST is still unclear [3, 4]. The genital tubercle and the labioscrotal swellings are the embryological origins of the penis and scrotum, respectively [5]. During normal embryonic development, in the 9th–11th week, the scrotal swellings migrate infero-medially and fuse in the midline caudal to the genital tubercle that forms the penis by the 12th week of gestation [4]. This is usually achieved under the influence of androgens and therefore PST arises from abnormal or arrested migration due to poor response to androgens [5]. Somoza et al. [4] and Park et al. [6] suggested that an abnormal positioning of the genital tubercle at the 6th gestation week concerning the scrotal swellings or a defective gubernaculum leads to PST.

Complete penoscrotal transposition (CPST) is frequently characterized by major and often life-threatening associated anomalies involving the urogenital, cardiovascular, gastrointestinal, and skeletal systems [4]. Common genital anomalies include hypospadias and chordee, and 100% of cases have a renal defect [5]. Several urogenital, cardiovascular, gastrointestinal, and skeletal system anomalies are, however, widely acknowledged associates, which very often present a major life-threatening situation in utero or in vivo. This suggests that penoscrotal transposition is often part of a wider group of embryonic malformations that should be investigated prenatally for an informed decision on the progress of pregnancy and route of delivery [7]. Such a case of CPST is described below.

2. Case Report

We attended to a 21-year-old gravida one para zero woman who was referred to Margaret Marquart Catholic Hospital, Kpando, Ghana, on account of the prolonged first stage of labour with poor progress. A 2.4 kg newborn male was delivered at a gestation age of 41 weeks 3 days by a first-trimester scan and last menstrual period (LMP) via caesarean section on the account of nonassuring foetal heart rate. On physical examination, he was noticed to have a complete transposition of the external genitalia with cryptorchidism, hypoplastic penis from the perineum just above the blind anal position, and caudal to the scrotum (Figure 1(a)). Further examination revealed imperforate anus (Figure 1(b)), unilateral limb and digital deformity (Figure 2), and cardiac malformation and facial deformity.

The APGAR scores were 2 at the first and fifth minutes. Neonate died two hours after delivery. Other externally associated abnormalities included a laterally rotated left lower limb, which had four digits with a cleft between the third and fourth digits and low set ears. The mother had a booking visit to a hospital at the 11th-week gestation and a regular attendant for antenatal reviews at a primary care facility. Routine laboratory investigations during antenatal care (ANC) such as blood count indices, blood grouping, urinalysis, stool examination and microscopy, fasting blood sugar, retroviral status, and blood film for malaria parasites results were done and essentially normal. Record of the only ultrasound scan taken at 11th-week gestation did not indicate any anomaly. Throughout the pregnancy, she was on routine antenatal medications prescribed at the primary attending clinic, and she had no chronic illness. There was no evidence of the mother being exposed to teratogens during pregnancy.

The woman's 35-year-old husband has a 4-year-old daughter from a previous relationship who was delivered with an imperforate anus. History indicated that both parents of the 4-year-old daughter drink alcohol. Thus, the mother, a housewife, and the father, a driver of a local alcoholic beverage company, drink local alcoholic bitters with the intent to boost their appetite before and during the pregnancy period. However, the mother of the case being reported is a trader that do not drink alcohol. The 4-year-old daughter had a successful surgical reconstruction and currently living a normal life.

3. Discussion

Penoscrotal transposition (PST) is a congenital urogenital anomaly described first in 1923 by Appleby [7]. Its manifestations vary greatly from a slightly caudally displaced penis implanted within a bifid scrotum (incomplete) to an entirely transposed posterior penis originating from the perineum [5–7]. In this case report, there is a complete swap of position with cephalic scrotum and caudally located penis (Figures 1(a) and 1(b)). Also, there presents a hypoplastic penis located beneath the scrotum and directly cephalic to the blind anal position which makes it a complete penoscrotal transposition or a major type of external genital malposition as opposed to the commonly reported partial transposition and bifid scrotum.

CPST is a rare heterogeneous condition that could result from abnormal genital tubercle development around the 6th week of gestation. It could also be associated with a delay in the midline fusion of the urethral folds [8]. Human sex development is broadly divided into the genetic determination stage for which the presence of the Y-chromosome specify male, the stage of gonadal development (testes and ovaries), and the phenotypic stage which is largely influenced by specific hormonal secretion. The male external genitalia which differentiates during the phenotypic stage develops from a bipotential Anlagen, the genital tubercles, labioscrotal folds (urogenital folds and urogenital swellings). Up to the 9th week, the external genitalia are indifferent in both sexes. Under the influence of androgens, the penis and scrotum develop and attain their final position with full differentiation of the organ at the end of the 12th week. The embryological sequence responsible for malformations involving the genitourinary largely remains unclear.

Complex genitourinary positional anomalies are often associated with other systems abnormalities that may present as life-threatening during pregnancy, delivery, or postnatal.

Previous investigations have reported that anomalies associated with PST such as chordee and hypospadias could be found in 90% of patients, whereas imperforate anus, cardiologic, and gastrointestinal anomalies may be found in 30–60% of victims [5, 9].

The lessons we learnt from both the major and minor reported cases of varied combinations of these organ defects are a mostly functional and aesthetic outcome from surgery [4]; however, the perinatal outcomes are mixed [8]. The commonly associated anomalies noted in most reports include vertebral-, anal-, cardiac-, tracheoesophageal-, renal-, and limb (VACTERL) anomalies [5]. These congenital anomalies are conventionally viewed as compatible with intervention or incompatible with life. Surgical intervention may be challenging and worsening in resolving PST due to delay in performing the surgery to within age 12 months and 18 months. In order not to cause further harm to the penile, spongy is very delicate and great caution is needed to achieve a fully developed penis at puberty.

Clinical examination, prenatal obstetric imaging by skilled sonographers/radiologist using standard ultrasound scan machines as a start, and magnetic resonance machines or other modalities of investigations for the purpose enable the identification, classification of degree of anomaly, and monitoring of the progress of these pregnancies. This aims at offering intervention when necessary as well as planning for an appropriate and safe delivery route. Unfortunately, most antenatal clinics currently either lack these skilled labours, the equipment, or both in most developing countries including Ghana to detect organ and skeletal malformations.

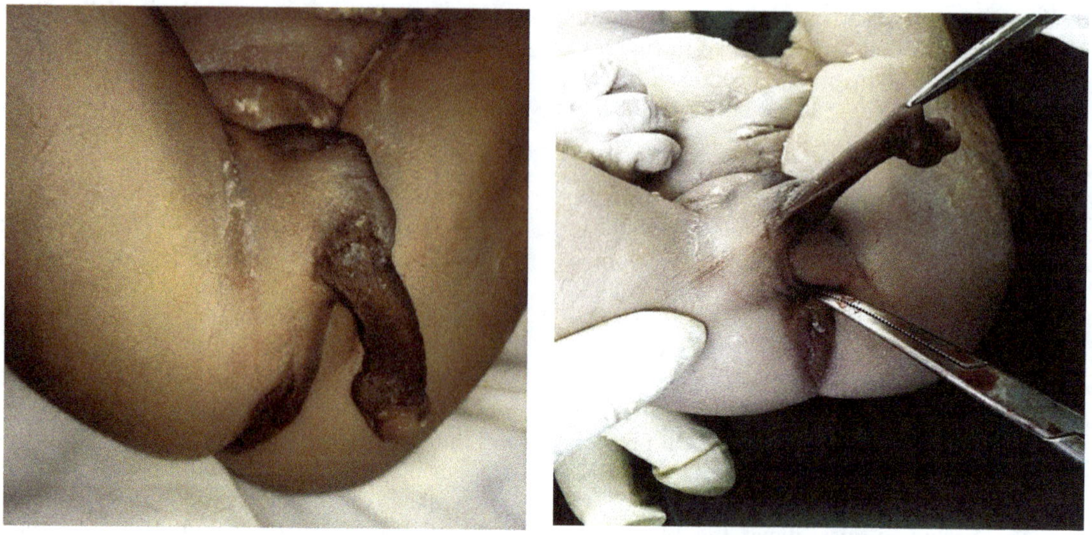

(a) (b)

Figure 1: (a) Showing transposition of the hypoplastic penis and scrotum cephalically (b) showing the perineum and the root of the penis.

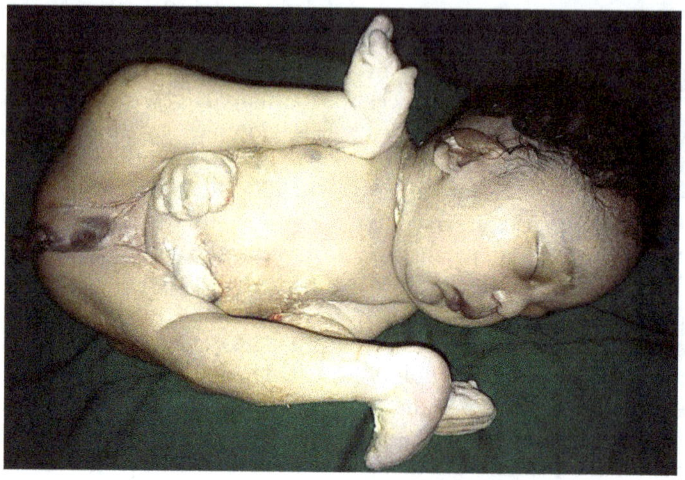

Figure 2: Lateral rotation of the left leg and 4 digits on the right foot.

4. Conclusion

A case of complete penoscrotal transposition was presented with major or life-threatening anomalies, which were not detected prenatally. This case illustrates the underutilisation of detection in utero as well as organ characterization, which is possible at the first trimester of pregnancy. It also informs us that there is much emphasis on maternal factors in the causes of congenital malformation, with a little investigation on the paternal contributory factors. In this case, the anomalies were incompatible with life and hence required psychological counselling to the parents.

It is, therefore, recommended that there is a need for pregnant women to have a complete skeletal scan before the end of the first trimester. There should also be in-depth psychological counselling on postdelivery trauma to parents of babies with such anomalies and perinatal death.

References

[1] H. K. Moorthy, B. S. Pillai, R. S. Rathore, and N. Mehta, "Ectopic scrotum: a unique case report," *Canadian Urological Association Journal*, vol. 9, no. 9-10, p. 665, 2015.

[2] F. Beyazıt, E. Pek, and H. Aylanç, "A rare case of complete penoscrotal transposition with hypospadias in a newborn," *Turk Jinekoloji ve Obstetrik Dernegi Dergisi*, vol. 14, no. 1, pp. 74-75, 2017.

[3] J. S. Rajkumar, A. Rajkumar, S. Akbar et al., "Acquired penoscrotal transposition—a rare complication of fournier's gangrene—Case Report," *Indian Journal of Surgery*, vol. 81, no. 3, pp. 284–286, 2019.

[4] I. Somoza, M. G. Palacios, R. Mendez, and D. Vela, "Complete penoscrotal transposition: a three-stage procedure," *Indian Journal of Urology*, vol. 28, no. 4, pp. 450–452, 2012.

[5] L. A. Pinke, S. R. Rathbun, D. A. Husmann, and S. A. Kramer, "Penoscrotal transposition: review of 53 patients," *Journal of Urology*, vol. 166, no. 5, pp. 1865–1868, 2001.

[6] N. C. Park, S. W. Kim, and D. G. Moon, *Penile augmentation*, Springer Berlin Heidelberg, 2016.

[7] D. M. Rodin, C. J. Koh, and A. B. Retik, "Sacral ectopic phallus in a case of extreme penoscrotal transposition and bladder agenesis," *Journal of Pediatric Urology*, vol. 2, no. 1, pp. 55–58, 2006.

[8] S. D. Naren, C. Soren, and P. V. Subbarao, "Penoscrotal transposition: a case report," *The Indian Journal of Surgery*, vol. 75, no. 1, pp. 64-65, 2013.

[9] D. Buyukkayhan, S. Kurtoglu, E. Koklu, N. Hatipoglu, and M. Akcakus, "Complete penoscrotal transposition associated with aortic stenosis in a newborn," *Journal of Pediatric Endocrinology and Metabolism*, vol. 20, p. 881, 2007.

17

Gubernaculum Sparing Laparoscopic Orchiopexy in Cryptorchidism with Ipsilateral Congenital Absence of the Vas Deferens: Unique Outcome

Ebtehal Althobaiti,[1] Hattan Badr,[2] Maryam Aloqalaa,[1] Raghdah Alsharif,[1] and Naif Alqarni[3]

[1]*Faculty of Medicine, Umm Al-Qura University, Makkah, Saudi Arabia*
[2]*Department of Urology, King Abdullah Medical City, Makkah, Saudi Arabia*
[3]*Pediatric Urology Division, Pediatric Surgery Department, Maternity and Children Hospital, Makkah, Saudi Arabia*

Correspondence should be addressed to Naif Alqarni; alqarni11@hotmail.com

Academic Editor: Shiou-Sheng Chen

Congenital absence of the vas deferens (CAVD) is an uncommon anomaly that occurs in up to 1% of the male population. It can be associated with various other anomalies, including cryptorchidism and renal anomalies, such as renal agenesis. We here present a case of cryptorchidism with ipsilateral congenital absence of the vas deferens and renal agenesis and used the Stephen-Fowler technique for Orchiopexy depending on gubernacular vessels. A 7-month-old boy was referred to our center with left grade 2 hydronephrosis, right renal agenesis, and right impalpable, undescended testis. Examination under anesthesia and laparoscopic exploration with staged Stephen-Fowler orchiopexy were performed. The patient was followed up at 3, 6, and 12 months and had an excellent outcome. Cryptorchidism with congenital ipsilateral absence of the vas deferens and renal agenesis is a rare diagnostic entity. Our case supports the suggested theory that the gubernacular vessels can increase the blood supply to the testis, although further studies are needed to confirm this hypothesis.

1. Introduction

Congenital absence of the vas deferens (CAVD) is an uncommon anomaly that occurs in only about 1% of the male population [1]. Since the development of the genital and renal systems are closely integrated, renal agenesis and other renal anomalies often coexist with CAVD, in about 30.2% of cases [2]. Although the exact spectrum of causes is unknown, it involves a defect in the developmental process before the complete separation of the Wolffian duct (mesonephric duct) and ureteric bud during the 5th week of gestation [3]. Such anomalies are usually found incidentally in the evaluation of various conditions, including undescended testis, which is considered one of the most common congenital anomalies in boys [4].

In 1976, a laparoscopic procedure was initiated for the diagnosis of impalpable, undescended testis; this has now become the gold standard as a diagnostic and therapeutic procedure [4]. One of the most commonly used laparoscopic procedures for high intra-abdominal testes is the staged Stephen-Fowler orchiopexy which has had a success rate reaching up to 100%, as reported by Agrawal et al. [5]

We here present a case of cryptorchidism with ipsilateral CAVD and renal agenesis and used the Stephen-Fowler technique for Orchiopexy depending on the gubernacular vessels, with an excellent outcome.

2. Case Presentation

A 7-month-old boy was referred to the Maternity and Children Hospital in Makkah for further management of left grade 2 hydronephrosis, right renal agenesis, and right impalpable, undescended testis. The patient presented to the

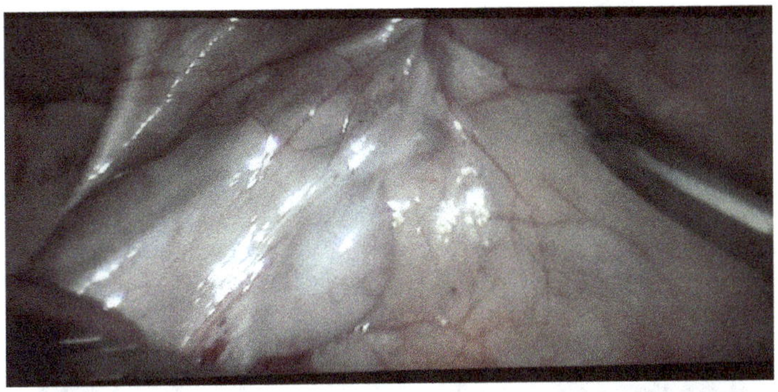

FIGURE 1: Absence of the right vas deferens in laparoscopic surgery.

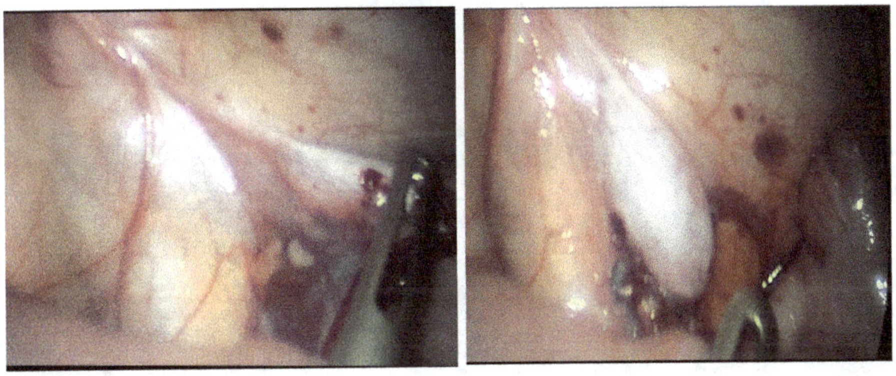

FIGURE 2: Thicker gubernacular vessels in the 2nd stage Stephen-Fowler compared to the 1st stage.

outpatient department (OPD) for assessment. Genital examination revealed a normal-size, circumcised penis, sizable left testis in the scrotum, and an impalpable, undescended right testis. The patient was booked for examination under anesthesia and laparoscopic exploration.

Laparoscopic exploration was performed on February 13, 2017, and revealed a sizable right testis proximal to the internal inguinal ring by 4 cm with short spermatic vessels, and an absent right vas deferens and epididymis (Figure 1). This left the choice of performing either Orchiectomy or Orchiopexy. For the sake of hormone generation, we decided to perform Orchiopexy depending on the gubernacular vessels. We therefore performed first-stage Stephen-Fowler Orchiopexy by clipping the spermatic vessels.

After 6 months, the patient was admitted for second-stage Stephen-Fowler orchiopexy on September 11, 2017. Intraoperative findings showed that the testis was the same size. We performed peritoneal dissection lateral to the testis; the medial peritoneal aspect and the gubernaculum remained untouched (Figure 2). The testis was brought through the inguinal canal into the right hemiscrotum, where a dartos pouch was created (Figure 3) and the testis was fixed in this position. The dimension of the testis was 12 × 5 mm.

At three-month follow-up, the right testis was assessed in the OPD; both testes were present in the scrotum with normal sensation, and the right testis was comparable in size to the left. Six months after the 2nd stage procedure, ultrasound of the scrotum was performed to assess the size, echogenicity, and vascularity of the testis; this revealed a normal anatomical location of both testicles, with a homogenous echo pattern and normal vascularity. The right testis measured 13 × 6 mm and the left testis measured 16 × 8 mm (Figure 4).

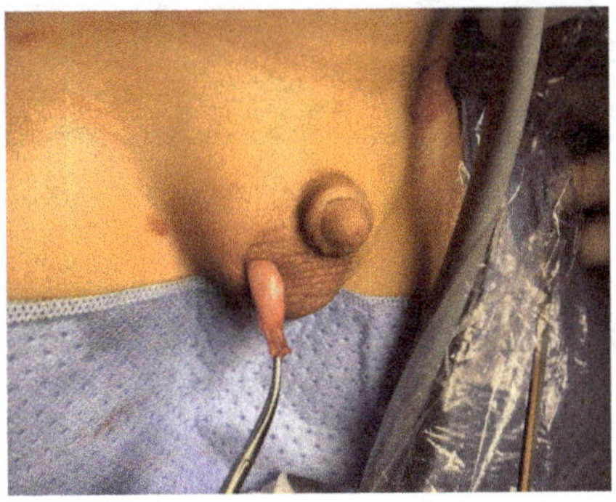

FIGURE 3: Fixation of the right testis into the scrotum.

At the 12-month follow-up, both testicles appeared to have a normal anatomical location and parenchymal echogenicity. The right testicle measured 10 × 7 × 8 mm, and the left testicle measured 15 × 8 × 10 mm (Figure 5). Vascularity was good according to doppler ultrasound.

3. Discussion

The renal and genital systems codevelop. During the 5th week of gestation, the mesonephric duct gives rise to the ureteric bud, which forms the metanephric duct that later forms the

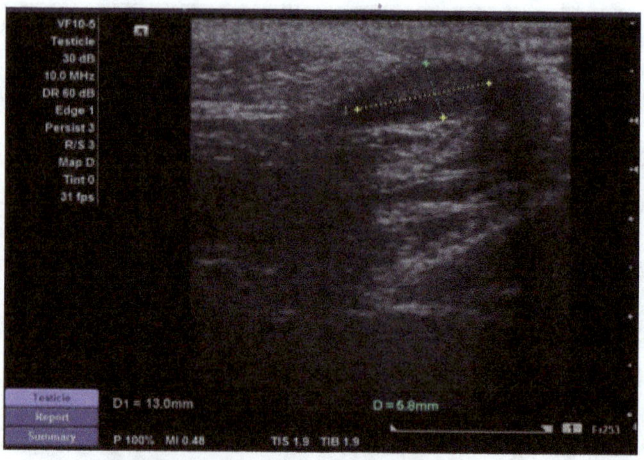

FIGURE 4: US of the right testis at six-months follow-up.

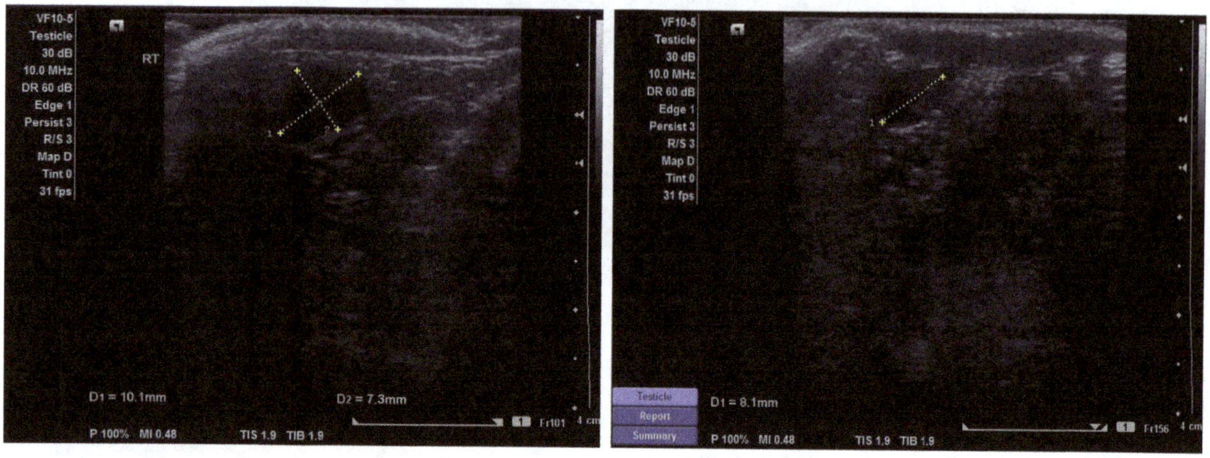

FIGURE 5: US of the right testis at twelve-months follow-up.

ureter and the metanephric blastema, which produces the standard lobulated feature of the kidney [6]. The mesonephric duct regresses in females but persists in males to outline the genital duct system, which consists of the seminal vesicle, the ductus deferens, and the distal two-thirds of the epididymis [7]. Any interference before the complete division of the mesonephric duct and the ureteric bud during the 7th week or earlier can result in a congenital unilateral absence of the vas deferens (CUAVD) and renal agenesis, as in our case [2, 3].

In 1737, John Hunter first described CUAVD, and Reverdin described the association between agenesis of the vas deferens and the ipsilateral kidney in 1870 [3]. This association is found in 73.3% of cases of CUAVD [2]. Undescended testis has an incidence of up to 3% [4]. The combination of CUAVD and renal agenesis in cryptorchidism in a single case, such as ours, is considered a very rare entity [8].

The Stephen-Fowler procedure reflects a forward extension of the diagnostic laparoscopy and is considered the gold standard, as it is safe, achievable, effective and has a good outcome overall [4]. The procedure is divided into single-stage or two-stage procedures, depending on the location of the undescended testis. Our patient underwent a two-stage Stephen-Fowler orchiopexy, which is used when the testis is close to the iliac vessels or 2 cm away from the internal inguinal ring [9]. In the first stage, the testicular vessels are isolated and clipped at the furthest point from the testis; then the second stage takes place after at least 4 months, in which the peritoneum is dissected around the vessels up to the testis, keeping the testis attached only to the vas deferens which eases the mobilization of the testis as far as the length of the vas will allow [9]. Since our patient had cryptorchidism with ipsilateral absence of the vas deferens, we could not depend on the collaterals from the vasal artery, as would normally be the case. A similar case report was published by Dong et al. who performed laparoscopic orchiectomy due to the short length of the spermatic cord structure, unlike our case, who underwent laparoscopic orchiopexy with dependence on the collaterals from the gubernacular vessel [6]. Lane et al. reported the case of an 18-month-old boy with left renal agenesis, left cryptorchidism, and left absence of the vas deferens; a 6-month follow-up after Orchiopexy showed that the testis reascended into the groin and left Orchiectomy was then performed [7]. Kulkarni et al. reported a 12-year-old boy with right renal agenesis, right cryptorchidism, and right absence of the vas deferens, for whom open Orchiopexy was performed; no follow-up results were described [8].

A study published in 2007 reported an outcome of laparoscopic two-stage Stephen-Fowler Orchiopexy preserving the gubernacular vessels in the presence of vas deferens and stated that the gubernaculum is thick and well vascularized and thus could theoretically increase the blood supply to the testis. They recorded a testicular survival rate close to 90% [10]. We applied this theory to our case and achieved an excellent outcome over the follow-up period.

A recent study first compared gubernaculum sparing laparoscopic orchiopexy (GSLO) and the conventional laparoscopic orchiopexy (CLO). This study prospectively reviewed 212 intra-abdominal testes managed in either way. They reported an overall rate of testicular atrophy of 6.6%, 0.6% in the GSLO group, and 28.3% in the CLO group [11].

4. Conclusion

CAVD is a rare anomaly that is associated with other genitourinary malformations. In our case, we depended on the gubernaculum vessels to at least offer the chance for Orchiopexy rather than proceed directly to Orchiectomy. The outcome of our patient supports the theory of Robertson et al. that the gubernacular vessels are able to increase the blood supply to the testis. Further cases should be studied to confirm this hypothesis.

References

[1] G. Shepherd and A. Rajimwale, "Embryology of the absent vas supported by 2 cases of congenital unilateral absence of vas with varied associations," *Urology Case Reports*, vol. 2, no. 2, pp. 49-50, 2014.

[2] E. C. Akinsal, N. Baydilli, M. E. Dogan, and O. Ekmekcioglu, "Comorbidity of the congenital absence of the vas deferens," *Andrologia*, vol. 50, no. 4, Article ID e12994, 2018.

[3] B. Mo, V. Garla, and L. M. Wyner, "A case of congenital unilateral absence of the vas deferens," *International Medical Case Reports Journal*, vol. 6, no. 1, pp. 21–23, 2013.

[4] R. Kumar, K. C. Mandal, P. Halder, M. Hadiuzzaman, M. Mukhopadhyay, and B. Mukhopadhyay, "Laparoscopy in the evaluation of impalpable testes and its short-term outcomes: a 7 years' experience," *Journal of Indian Association of Pediatric Surgeons*, vol. 22, no. 4, pp. 232–236, 2017.

[5] A. Agrawal, M. Joshi, P. Mishra, R. Gupta, B. Sanghvi, and S. Parelkar, "Laparoscopic stephen-fowler stage procedure: appropriate management for high intra-abdominal testes," *Journal of Laparoendoscopic & Advanced Surgical Techniques*, vol. 20, no. 2, pp. 183–185, 2010.

[6] Y. D. Yu and Y. K. Hong, "A case of cryptorchidism with ipsilateral congenital unilateral absence of the vas deferens and contralateral renal agenesis," *Case Reports in Urology*, vol. 2016, Article ID 2379793, 3 pages, 2016.

[7] V. A. Lane, S. Scammell, N. West, and G. V. Murthi, "Congenital absence of the vas deferens and unilateral renal agenesis: implications for patient and family," *Pediatric Surgery International*, vol. 30, no. 7, pp. 733–736, 2014.

[8] V. D. Kulkarni, N. A. Deshpande, P. N. Deshpande, and M. Phanse, "Undescended testis with congenital unilateral absence of the vas deferens," *Sri Lanka Journal of Surgery*, vol. 32, no. 3, p. 40, 2015.

[9] V. Mehendale, S. Shenoy, R. Shah, N. Chaudhari, and A. Mehendale, "Laparoscopic management of impalpable undescended testes: 20 years' experience," *Journal of Minimal Access Surgery*, vol. 9, no. 4, pp. 149–153, 2013.

[10] S. A. Robertson, F. D. Munro, and G. A. MacKinlay, "Two-stage Fowler-Stephens orchidopexy preserving the gubernacular vessels and a purely laparoscopic second stage," *Journal of Laparoendoscopic & Advanced Surgical Techniques*, vol. 17, no. 1, pp. 101–107, 2007.

[11] L. H. Braga, F. Farrokhyar, M. McGrath, and A. J. Lorenzo, "Gubernaculum testis and cremasteric vessel preservation during laparoscopic orchiopexy for intra-abdominal testes: effect on testicular atrophy rates," *The Journal of Urology*, vol. 201, no. 2, pp. 378–385, 2019.

18

Management of Groin Pain using an Iliohypogastric Nerve Block in a Patient with Inguinal Hernia due to Persistent Müllerian Duct Syndrome

Takanori Sekito,[1] Takuya Sadahira,[1] Masahiro Sugihara,[2] Kohei Edamura,[1] Motoo Araki,[1] and Yasutomo Nasu[1]

[1]*Department of Urology, Dentistry and Pharmaceutical Sciences, Okayama University Graduate School of Medicine, 2-5-1 Shikata-cho, Kita-ku, Okayama 700-8558, Japan*
[2]*Division of Surgery, Nishi Fukuyama Hospital, 340-1 Matsunagacho, Fukuyama City, Hiroshima 729-0104, Japan*

Correspondence should be addressed to Takuya Sadahira; t.sadahira@gmail.com

Academic Editor: Tun-Chieh Chen

Persistent Müllerian duct syndrome can cause an inguinal hernia, although this is a rare occurrence; recurrent inguinal hernias can, in turn, cause ongoing groin pain. Management of groin pain plays an important role in patients' quality of life. We present our experience with a 43-year-old man who had a 2-week history of left-sided groin pain. The patient underwent laparoscopic surgery for a left inguinal hernia via the transabdominal preperitoneal approach. Right-sided cryptorchidism was noted during surgery, with a solid structure—thought to be a uterus—extending into the left inguinal canal. The diagnosis was persistent Müllerian duct syndrome, and the groin pain was relieved after a laparoscopic right orchiectomy with a bilateral preperitoneal hernia repair using a mesh. Four years later, magnetic resonance imaging performed for new-onset left groin pain showed a left inguinal hernia caused by the uterine structure. We diagnosed the recurrent hernia as the cause of his pain. Prior to performing any invasive surgical procedures, an iliohypogastric nerve block was performed using 1% lidocaine. Short-term analgesia was provided by the block, improving his quality of life. He has been followed since then and has declined surgical neurectomy. An iliohypogastric nerve block can be an effective method of controlling groin pain caused by an inguinal hernia resulting from persistent Müllerian duct syndrome; the effectiveness of the nerve block will help determine whether surgical neurectomy is indicated for permanent pain control.

1. Introduction

Persistent Müllerian duct syndrome (PMDS) is characterized by the presence of Müllerian remnants in patients with a 46,XY karyotype and normal male external genitalia [1]. The diagnosis of PMDS is usually made when the Müllerian structures are detected incidentally during investigation or treatment for inguinal hernia, with or without cryptorchidism [2]. Surgical management and follow-up for patients with PMDS remain controversial and challenging because of 2 major complications: infertility and malignant degeneration of the testis.

There are rare reports of groin pain induced by an inguinal hernia resulting from PMDS [3]. Pain management is an important aspect of care for patients with PMDS. We report our experience with a patient who had a recurrent inguinal hernia caused by PMDS, resulting in persistent groin pain. We successfully managed this patient's pain with an iliohypogastric nerve block. This effective management technique will help clinicians to decide whether surgical neurectomy will be indicated as the next step for pain control.

2. Case Presentation

A 43-year-old man presented to our institution with a 2-week history of left-sided groin pain. He was married but had no children and had initiated treatment for infertility at another institution three years prior. The semen analysis revealed oligozoospermia. His brother had a history of cryptorchidism and eventually developed testicular cancer and underwent orchiectomy. On physical examination, the right testis was not palpable in the scrotum, and there was a nonreducible swelling at the left groin. Computed tomography demonstrated herniation in the left groin and right cryptorchidism. The patient desired removal of the right-sided cryptorchidism because of his family history of testicular cancer.

We performed herniorrhaphy using the transabdominal preperitoneal approach for the left inguinal hernia. We confirmed right cryptorchidism (Figure 1(a)) at the time of surgery. We also noted a solid structure resembling a uterus that extended into the left inguinal canal (Figure 1(b)). We performed a laparoscopic right orchiectomy with bilateral preperitoneal hernia repair using a mesh. The structure that resembled a uterus was not removed to preserve the remaining internal male genitalia. Histopathology of the right testis showed no evidence of malignant degeneration. The patient was discharged without groin pain or any other complications after surgery and was advised of his diagnosis of PMDS.

Four years later, he returned with new-onset left groin pain that had persisted for 3 weeks, accompanied by left lower quadrant abdominal pain. The pain was causing difficulty with his occupation as a truck driver. Magnetic resonance imaging (MRI) showed a left inguinal hernia, with uterine and vaginal structures extending from the left inguinal canal into the scrotum. The Müllerian duct derivatives were continuously connected to the prostate on the dorsal side (Figure 2). At the time of his arrival, the patient eventually did not conceive a child even after in vitro fertilization for several times as fertility treatment; therefore, the patient already decided to discontinue the fertility treatments.

We diagnosed the recurrent hernia as the cause of his pain. Prior to performing any invasive surgical procedures, we performed an iliohypogastric nerve block using 1% lidocaine. This nerve block relieved his pain. He has had an uneventful course since the block and has been able to return to work. Two weeks after the nerve block, the patient returned to our hospital for follow-up care and had no complaint of groin pain. We discussed how to manage recurrent groin pain in the future. Our plan for any future recurrence was to perform surgical neurectomy of the iliohypogastric nerve for long-term pain control and better quality of life. However, the patient did not agree to undergo the procedure at this most recent appointment.

3. Discussion

The rare condition of PMDS occurs when there is either a deficiency of antimüllerian hormone (AMH) activity or an abnormality in AMH receptors. Sertoli cells in the fetal testicle produce AMH, causing the involution of embryonic Müllerian structures in normal male fetuses [4]. The 3 main clinical presentations of PMDS are bilateral cryptorchidism, hernia uteri inguinalis, and transverse testicular ectopia. One review notes that 59% of patients present with bilateral cryptorchidism, 19% with hernia uteri inguinalis, and 22% with transverse testicular ectopia [5].

Hernia uteri inguinalis occurs when a single testis remains in the abdomen while the other is in the inguinal canal, along with the uterus and ipsilateral fallopian tube, resulting in unilateral cryptorchidism with a contralateral inguinal hernia [4]. This type occurs in 14% of patients with idiopathic PMDS and approximately 20% of patients with mutations involving the AMH pathway [5]. Although our patient had this presentation, we did not perform karyotype analysis to detect mutations in the AMH pathway.

Malignant degeneration and infertility are major potential complications of PMDS. We performed a laparoscopic orchiectomy of the undescended testicle, considering our patient's family history of testicular cancer. However, because he was also trying to father a child at the time of the surgery, it was important to leave the remaining, correctly positioned, testis in place [6].

How to manage fertility in a patient with PMDS is important. In one review, intracytoplasmic sperm injection may be helpful in some cases with PMDS as fertility treatment [5], like what was performed to our patient. Infertility in PMDS can be related to the structural abnormalities caused by the Müllerian organs or long-term cryptorchidism [1]. However, an attempt to remove the Müllerian structures can damage the male excretory ducts enclosed in the Müllerian derivatives [5]. Minimizing risk to damage vital structures for fertility should be considered before a complete excision of the Müllerian organs. To the best of our knowledge, although there are no reports describing about freezing sperm in patients with PMDS before surgery, a patient can also be advised to freeze sperm before the Müllerian organs will be removed.

In PMDS, the histology of the testes is usually normal. The incidence of malignant degeneration in these testes is 18%, whose rate is the same as the rate of malignancy in abdominal testes in men without PMDS [4]. Concerning resection outcomes of Müllerian organs, Müllerian malignancies are much less frequent than testicular malignancies [1]. Literature on this topic is rare, with a few reports describing uneventful recovery after surgery in a small number of patients [2–4].

Groin pain induced by an inguinal hernia, itself caused by PMDS, has been rarely reported [7]. The inguinal region receives sensory innervation from the iliohypogastric, ilioinguinal, and genitofemoral nerves [8], as shown in Figure 3. The iliohypogastric nerve predominantly originates from L1 [9] and supplies the skin of the pubic area and the upper part of the thigh and buttock. Our patient experienced groin pain when his internal uterine and vaginal structures extended into the left inguinal canal. When the structures were released from the inguinal canal for some reason, e.g., body movement, he experienced spontaneous relief. However, when the structures extending into the left inguinal canal became incarcerated, they caused persistent groin pain accompanied by left lower quadrant abdominal pain; this pain resulted from compression of the iliohypogastric nerve.

It is also possible that entrapment neuropathy caused our patient's pain. The pain caused by entrapment neuropathy starts within weeks, and neurological symptoms may occur. Repeated nerve blocks are usually needed until the pain

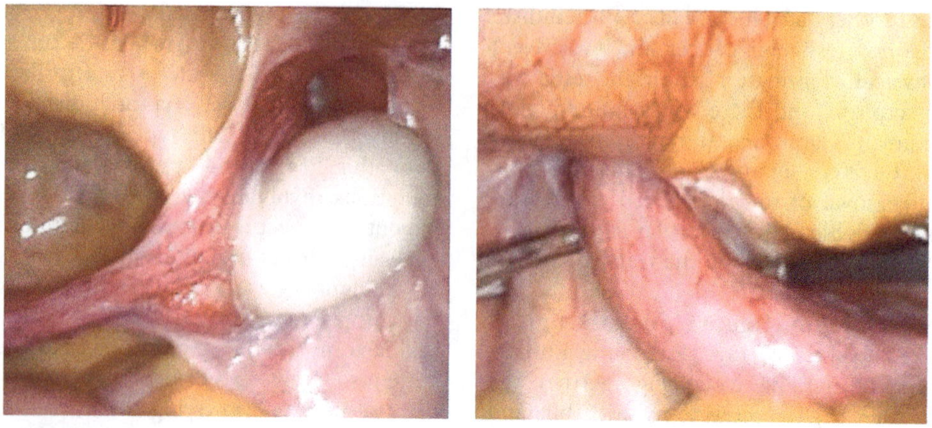

(a) (b)

Figure 1: (a) Right-sided cryptorchidism is seen during laparoscopic surgery for a left inguinal hernia. (b) Laparoscopic inspection reveals a solid structure, resembling a uterus, extending into the left inguinal canal.

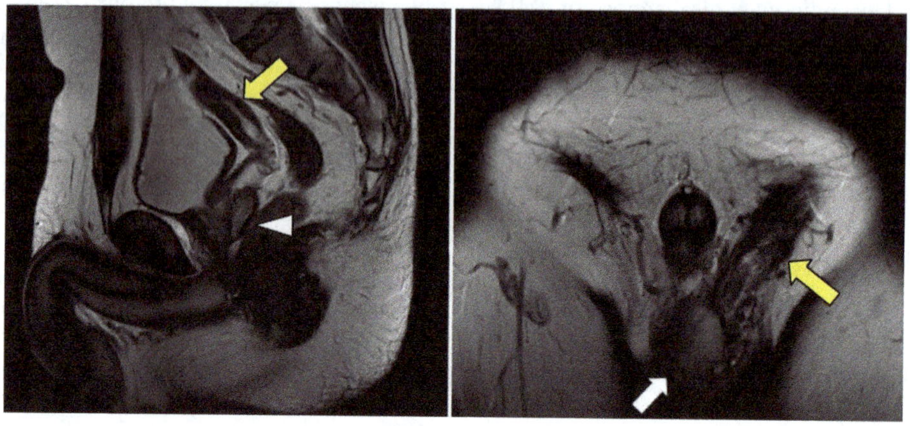

Figure 2: Magnetic resonance imaging shows a left inguinal hernia containing uterine and vaginal structures extending from the left inguinal canal into the scrotum (yellow arrows). There is a normal testis in the left hemiscrotum (white arrow). Müllerian duct derivatives are connected to the prostate on the dorsal side (white arrowhead).

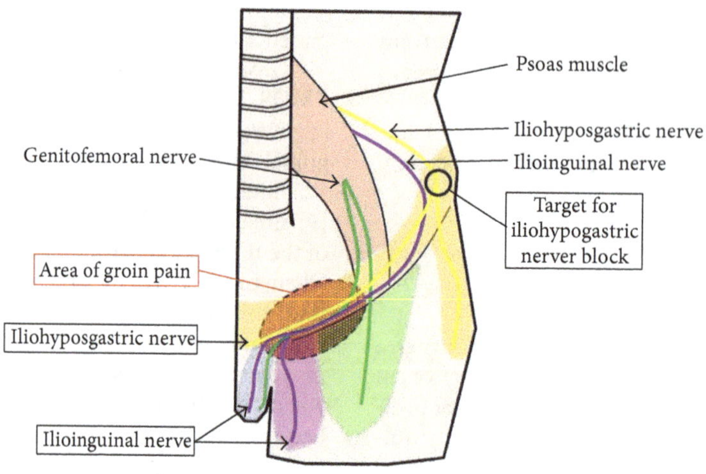

Figure 3: Sensory nervous distribution in the groin area. The dashed ellipse represents the area of our patient's groin pain. The circle represents the area of iliohypogastric nerve block placement.

resolves [10]. Our patient's pain started 4 years after his orchiectomy and hernia repair, and he had no neurological symptoms. Additionally, given the MRI findings, we suspected that his pain was caused by a hernia resulting from PMDS.

Previous studies show that the branches of the iliohypogastric, ilioinguinal, and genitofemoral nerves communicate freely and that there is great variation in the sensory innervation of the inguinal region [8]. One report demonstrates that the iliohypogastric nerve communicates with accessory branches of the ilioinguinal nerve (55%) [9]. The ilioinguinal nerve runs parallel to the spermatic cord; therefore, an iliohypogastric nerve block may have some effect in improving groin pain in the sensory innervation region of the ilioinguinal nerve. Performing a simultaneous ilioinguinal and iliohypogastric nerve block could be an even better option to control groin pain.

The use of an iliohypogastric nerve block provided good pain control for our patient, but this relief will most likely be temporary. Definitive surgical treatment would involve resection of the Müllerian organs, i.e., hysterectomy and salpingectomy. Resection of Müllerian organs is an invasive procedure and carries the risk of damaging the vas deferens and disrupting the blood supply to the testes [11, 12]. Our plan was to offer surgical neurectomy of the iliohypogastric nerve as a less invasive alternative to control recurrent groin pain, since we confirmed that the iliohypogastric nerve block was effective. However, our patient did not agree to this plan. To appropriately manage pain resulting from PMDS, it is extremely important to take a patient's full clinical picture into consideration. Nerve blocks can be helpful in providing immediate pain control, and they provide information when considering subsequent optimal treatment.

4. Conclusion

Management of groin pain is an important element of quality of life for patients with inguinal hernias due to PMDS. Use of an iliohypogastric nerve block can be a helpful option to control this pain, and the effectiveness of the nerve block will help clinicians to decide whether surgical neurectomy will be indicated as subsequent treatment for pain control.

References

[1] J. Farikullah, S. Ehtisham, S. Nappo, L. Patel, and S. Hennayake, "Persistent Müllerian duct syndrome: lessons learned from managing a series of eight patients over a 10-year period and review of literature regarding malignant risk from the Müllerian remnants," *BJU International*, vol. 110, no. 11c, pp. E1084–E1089, 2012.

[2] M. Shamim, "Persistent Mullerian duct syndrome with transverse testicular ectopia presenting in an irreducible recurrent inguinal hernia," *The Journal of the Pakistan Medical Association*, vol. 57, no. 8, pp. 421–423, 2007.

[3] K. Tanabe, S. Mori, Y. Kita et al., "A rare case report of bilateral recurrent inguinal hernia due to persistent Müllerian duct syndrome treated by transabdominal preperitoneal repair," *Medicine (Baltimore)*, vol. 99, no. 7, article e19079, 2020.

[4] M. M. Sichani, M. Heidarpour, A. Dadkhah, and M. Rezvani, "Persistent Mullerian duct syndrome with an irreducible inguinal hernia," *Urology Journal*, vol. 6, no. 4, pp. 298–300, 2009.

[5] J. Y. Picard, R. L. Cate, C. Racine, and N. Josso, "The persistent Müllerian duct syndrome: an update based upon a personal experience of 157 cases," *Sexual Development*, vol. 11, no. 3, pp. 109–125, 2017.

[6] F. Bugrul, Z. Y. Abali, T. Kirkgoz et al., "Persistent Müllerian duct syndrome: a rare but important etiology of inguinal hernia and cryptorchidism," *Sexual Development*, vol. 13, no. 5-6, pp. 264–270, 2020.

[7] J. Y. Picard and N. Josso, "Persistent Müllerian duct syndrome: an update," *Reproduction, Fertility, and Development*, vol. 31, no. 7, pp. 1240–1245, 2019.

[8] N. Sasaoka, M. Kawaguchi, K. Yoshitani, H. Kato, H. Furuya, and A. Suzuki, "Evaluation of genitofemoral nerve block, in addition to ilioinguinal and iliohypogastric nerve block, during inguinal hernia repair in children," *British Journal of Anaesthesia*, vol. 94, no. 2, pp. 243–246, 2005.

[9] Z. Klaassen, E. Marshall, R. S. Tubbs, R. G. Louis Jr., C. T. Wartmann, and M. Loukas, "Anatomy of the ilioinguinal and iliohypogastric nerves with observations of their spinal nerve contributions," *Clinical Anatomy*, vol. 24, no. 4, pp. 454–461, 2011.

[10] A. S. Seid and E. Amos, "Entrapment neuropathy in laparoscopic herniorrhaphy," *Surgical Endoscopy*, vol. 8, no. 9, pp. 1050–1053, 1994.

[11] V. J. Nayak, S. K. Bylappa, A. S. Kamath, and M. H. Krishnappa, "Persistent Mullerian duct syndrome: a case report and review of the literature," *International Journal of Applied & Basic Medical Research*, vol. 4, no. 2, pp. 125–127, 2014.

[12] M. Wuerstle, T. Lesser, R. Hurwitz, H. Applebaum, and S. L. Lee, "Persistent Mullerian duct syndrome and transverse testicular ectopia: embryology, presentation, and management," *Journal of Pediatric Surgery*, vol. 42, no. 12, pp. 2116–2119, 2007.

19

Penile Hair Tourniquet Syndrome (PHTS): A Case Report of a Two-Year-Old Boy

Alhareth Baarimah[1] **Latif Dar,**[2] **Rayan Dashnan,**[3] **Saeed Alshahrani,**[2] **Mohammed Beaiti,**[3] **and Khaled ALDhabaan**[3]

[1]*Department of Urology, International Medical Center (IMC), Jeddah, Saudi Arabia*
[2]*Department of Pediatric Urology, Abha Maternity and Child Hospital (AMCH), Abha, Saudi Arabia*
[3]*Department of Pediatric Urology, Khamis Mushayt Maternity and Children Hospital, Khamis Mushayt, Saudi Arabia*

Correspondence should be addressed to Alhareth Baarimah; alhareth.adnan@gmail.com

Academic Editor: Tun-Chieh Chen

Penile hair tourniquet syndrome (PHTS) is an unusual phenomenon. A physician should have a high index of suspicion when a circumcised child presents with glans swelling and inflammation. It must be considered a surgical emergency, as early diagnosis and treatment can prevent complications (e.g., urethra-cutaneous fistula, complete urethral transection, penile gangrene, and penile amputation). We report a case of two-year-old boy to highlight the importance of early diagnosis and prompt treatment.

1. Introduction

Hair tourniquet syndrome (HTS) is a condition seen mostly in circumcised children. It is characterized by a constriction caused by hair around an appendage, clitoris, or penis, and its clinical picture is akin to a compartment syndrome. When it involves the glans penis, it is referred to as penile hair tourniquet syndrome (PHTS) or hair coil penile strangulation [1]. The hair gets wrapped around the coronal sulcus of a circumcised child, leading to a spectrum of clinical situations ranging from mild swelling and redness of the glans to more serious complications such as urethro-cutaneous fistulas, gangrene, and penile amputation [2]. We are reporting this case because a delay in diagnosis—due to a lack of awareness among general practitioners, or uncareful examination—can lead to devastating complications [3].

2. Case Presentation

A two-year-old boy was admitted to the ER with a painful swelling of the penis, which his mother had first recognized three days prior. A pediatrician had prescribed a local antibiotic cream and analgesic, but the condition had not improved. The boy had begun to have difficulty passing urine.

Upon arrival at the ER, the patient's general physical examination was normal. Upon local examination, the penis was found swollen, edematous, and tender to the touch. The glans penis was somewhat dusky. A constriction band was noticed at the base of the penis (Figure 1). The boy was reexamined using a loupe, and a hair coil was found embedded within the constriction mark. A local anesthetic spray was applied. The hair was held with a blunt-tipped probe and cut using microscissors. After removing the constricting hair coil, the area was carefully examined. The skin and subcutaneous tissue appeared eroded—and more so on the ventral aspect of the penis. An 8F Foley catheter was passed, and the urethra was found intact. The catheter was kept in place, and the patient was administered oral antibiotics and anti-inflammatory medication.

The patient was discharged home on postoperative day three with the catheter still in place (Figure 2). After removal of the catheter five days later, the patient passed urine freely

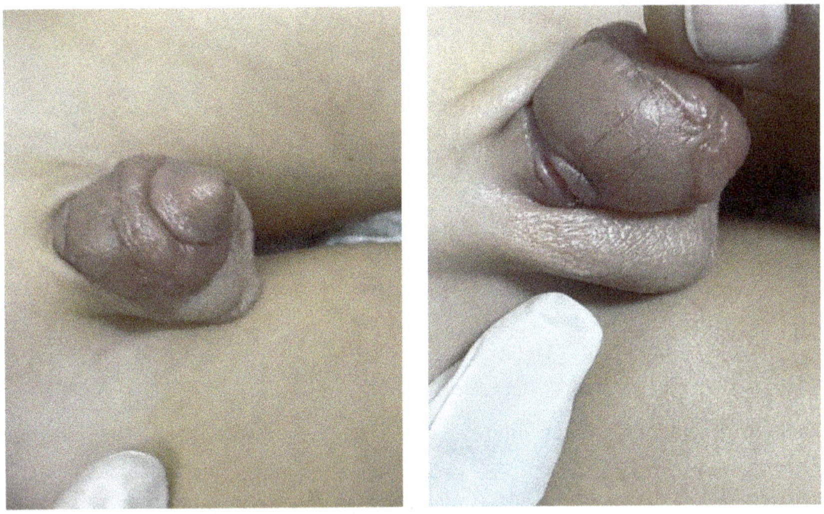

(a) (b)

FIGURE 1: (a) Appearance of penile hair tourniquet syndrome at time of diagnosis. (b) Causative factor: hair strand of mother.

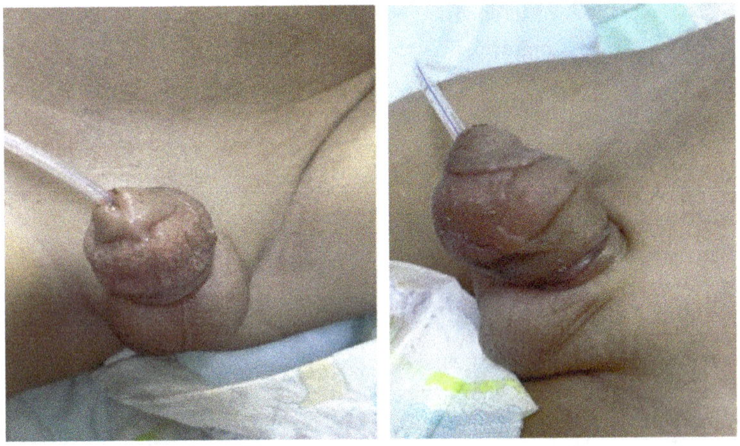

FIGURE 2: Postoperative day three with the catheter in place.

without any difficulty. At one month, the wound had completely healed without any complications (Figure 3).

3. Discussion

PHTS is a well-established phenomenon that affects children. It is characterized by strangulation of the glans penis by a constricting hair coil. Although frequently described in relation to the penis in circumcised boys, the penis is not the only affected organ: HTS can involve any appendage with an end artery, including fingers, toes, and the clitoris. Cases affecting the vulva, labia minora, and ear lobules have also been reported [4, 5].

If it goes unrecognized, the condition can lead to devastating complications [2]. It is easily preventable, and when recognized early, it can be treated simply by removal of the coil under local anesthesia [3]. The problem is lack of awareness: PHTS usually goes unnoticed because most primary care providers, such as pediatricians, emergency pediatric physicians, and pediatric surgeons, are not fully aware of the condition [1, 4].

The first case was reported as early as 1832, but, surprisingly, the condition still has not received the recognition it deserves. It is barely mentioned in textbooks, although numerous case reports have been published in the literature [3–5].

PHTS is almost exclusively seen in children—and most frequently among those between one and eight years of age. Infants are especially vulnerable [4]. Cases have been reported in toddlers, school-age children, and even later in life [1]. Circumcision is an important predisposing factor [1–3]. The usual culprit is the mother's hair, which can get into a baby's diaper and become wrapped around the penis [3]. This is usually accidental, but some cultural beliefs may also play a part, as hair may be intentionally placed around the penis in the belief that it will improve sexual performance in adult life, treat enuresis, or get rid of evil spirits [2–5].

Once the coiled hair dries, it constricts and strangulates the distal penis. Initially, lymphatic and venous backflow is affected, leading to edema and swelling of the distal penis. This progresses and eventually affects arterial flow, resulting

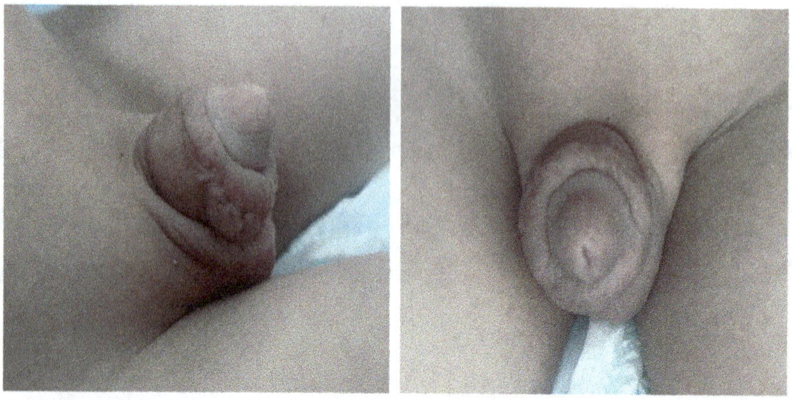

Figure 3: At one month, the wound had completely healed without any complications.

Table 1: Classification of the degree of penile injury.

Grade	Description of the injury
Grade 0	Constriction of skin, without urethral injury
Grade I	Partial division of the corpus spongiosum and occurrence of a urethrocutaneous fistula
Grade II	Complete division of the corpus spongiosum and constriction of the corpus cavernosum
Grade III	Gangrene, necrosis, and complete amputation of the glans penis

in ischemia, necrosis, gangrene, and amputation of the affected part of the penis [1, 3]. In 1980, Bashir and El-Barbery described the morphological characteristics of PHTS and classified its degrees of injury into four grades (Table 1) [4]. In our case, the injury falls into grade 0.

The diagnosis of PTHS is not straightforward, especially in the presence of swelling and edema. The hair becomes buried in the skin and is difficult to detect with the naked eye. A high degree of suspicion and awareness is therefore essential [3, 4]. Magnifying glasses or loupes are useful aids for detecting the constricting hair coil [3].

Once the diagnosis is made, treatment involves removing the constricting band of hair by cutting or unwinding it [4]. While using a magnifying glass or a loupe, the hair is held with a blunt-tipped probe and cut using microscissors [3]. The procedure can be performed in the ER or the outpatient clinic using a local anesthetic spray [3]. Depilatory hair-removal creams have also been used. If removal fails, a surgical exploration under anesthesia becomes necessary [3].

4. Conclusion

PHTS is an unusual phenomenon. Early recognition and prompt treatment are necessary to prevent devastating, serious complications. This condition frequently goes unrecognized due to a lack of awareness among primary caregivers. A high degree of suspicion and raised awareness will go a long way to ensuring early diagnosis, prompt treatment, and prevention of PHTS complications.

Consent

Written consent was obtained from the father for publication of this case report and the accompanying images.

References

[1] H. Badawy, A. Soliman, A. Ouf, A. Hammad, S. Orabi, and A. Hanno, "Progressive hair coil penile tourniquet syndrome: multicenter experience with 25 cases," *Journal of Pediatric Surgery*, vol. 45, no. 7, pp. 1514–1518, 2010.

[2] K. Zengin, M. Y. Ozdamar, S. Albayrak et al., "Hair coil penile tourniquet syndrome in an unusual age," *Case Reports in Urology*, vol. 2015, Article ID 642547, 2 pages, 2015.

[3] W. F. Rawls, J. T. White, A. Mohamed, D. Peppas, and E. Rosenberg, "Case report: penile strangulation secondary to hair tourniquet," *Frontiers in Pediatrics*, vol. 8, no. 8, p. 477, 2020.

[4] B. Özçift and K. Ağras, "Hair tourniquet syndrome of penis: a rare situation in boys with serious complications if not recognized," *Turkish Journal of Urology*, vol. 45, no. 4, pp. 322–324, 2019.

[5] M. S. Sheikh Andalibi, A. Azarfar, M. Esmaeeli, N. Sheykh Andalibi, A. Alizadeh, and Y. Ravanshad, "Penile hair tourniquet syndrome due to a coil of hair: first report in Iran," *Nephro-Urol Mon.*, vol. 9, no. 4, article e59788, 2017.

20

Recurrent Testicular Torsion of a Fixed Testis

Ibrahim Alnadhari, Ausama Abdulmuhsin, Omar Ali, Ahmad Shamsodini, Morshed Salah, and Osama Abdeljaleel

Division of Urology, Department of Surgery, Al Wakra Hospital, Hamad Medical Corporation, Doha, Qatar

Correspondence should be addressed to Ibrahim Alnadhari; ibrahimah1978@yahoo.com

Academic Editor: Giorgio Carmignani

Recurrent testicular torsion after previous orchiopexy is rare and needs high index of suspension to avoid misdiagnosis and delayed management. This case showed that this diagnosis can occur even when the testis is still fixed to the scrotal wall. A 31-year-old male who had previous testicular fixation for testicular torsion with a single stitch to the lower pole before 6 years presented with recurrent testicular torsion and missed diagnosis. This case confirm that recurrent testicular torsion after previous fixation should be included in the differential diagnosis of acute scrotum and emphasis on the testicular fixation with nonabsorbable suture in at least two points to prevent recurrent torsion.

1. Introduction

Testicular torsion is considered one of the important causes of acute scrotum condition. It is most common just after birth and during puberty. It occurs in about 1 in 4,000 to 1 per 25,000 males per year before 18 years of age [1]. Although its overall incidence is not high, it remains the most common cause of testicular loss in these age groups. Yet, torsion may occasionally occur in men of 40-50 years old.

Testicular torsion is mainly diagnosed by history and physical examination then immediate surgical exploration is indicated but scrotal ultrasonography can be useful diagnostic tool if it is available and there is doubt in diagnosis [2]. Late presentation to hospital and delay due to hospital transfer were the major risk factors for delayed management and orchiectomy in such patients [3]. Recurrent testicular torsion after previous orchiopexy is rare and needs high index of suspension to avoid misdiagnosis and delayed management. Hereby we present a case of missed recurrent testicular torsion after previous orchiopexy.

2. Case Report

A 31-year-old male patient presented to the emergency complaining of left testicular pain for 5-day duration since the onset of pain, continuous pain associated with swelling, gradually increased. He had previously undergone bilateral orchidopexy before 6 years for left testicular torsion. Patient visited general practitioner on the same day of onset of pain and was diagnosed as epididymitis and given antibiotics with analgesics and discharged. On examination the entire left hemiscrotum was swollen and tender and appeared as a confluent mass without identifiable landmarks. Scrotal ultrasonography showed hypoechoic left testis without intrinsic vascularity (Figure 1) and moderate to gross left hydrocoele is noted with internal echoes and septation.

Urgent surgical exploration of left side revealed intact tunica vaginalis with moderate hydrocele, left testis delivered which was black, torsed, and attached with old stitch from lower pole to the side wall of scrotum (Figure 2). Old stitch was removed and the testis was detorsed but it was gangrenous so orchiectomy done.

The right testis was explored and it was attached with single stitch to the lower pole; old stitch was removed and fixation with three stitches 3/0 vicryl to the scrotal wall was done (Figure 3). Patient was discharged on the first postoperative day and he had uneventful postoperative course. He was given clear instructions to avoid trauma to his single testis and to report to the emergency in case of testicular pain.

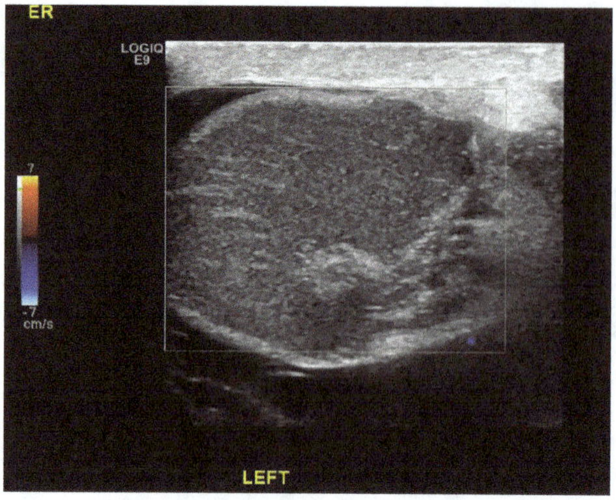

FIGURE 1: Scrotal ultrasonography showed absent testis blood flow.

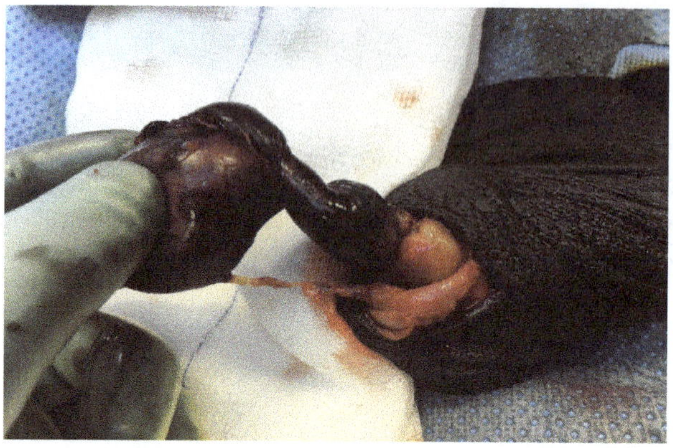

FIGURE 2: Black, torsed left testis attached with old stitch from lower pole to the side wall of scrotum.

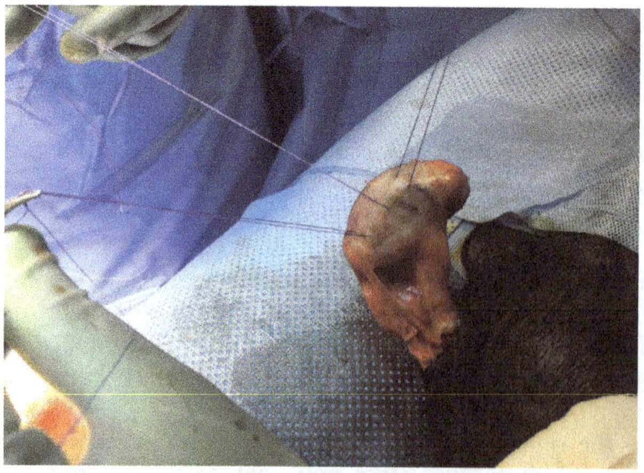

FIGURE 3: Fixation of the right testis with three stitches.

3. Discussion

Early diagnosis and management of testicular torsion is important to save the testis. Correction within 4-6 hours gives good testicular preservation but if it is done after 12 hours there is high risk of testicular atrophy [2].

The diagnosis of testicular torsion after previously fixed testicles is rare but it should be included in the differential diagnosis of acute scrotum.

There have been reported cases of recurrent testicular torsion after the previous [4–14]. Some of them were diagnosed early and second time orchiopexy was done [4–7, 9, 12–14] and others were delayed in the diagnosis and underwent orchiectomy [8, 10, 11]. In most of the cases, they used absorbable suture and during exploration the testicle was found freely hanging and lost its attachment to the scrotal wall or tunica vaginalis.

As in our case, only two reported cases with torsion occurred while the testis is attached to the scrotum through the stitch in the lower pole [13, 14]. Single lower pole stitch makes the testis hanged "like a hammock" which increase its risk of rotation and torsion.

Fixation of the detorsed testis and the contralateral testis using nonabsorbable suture is recommended to prevent metachronous or recurrent torsion [15]. Fixation of the testis in at least two points theoretically prevents torsion.

Testicular torsion leading to orchidectomy is a major catastrophe for the patient and previous history of orchiopexy does not exclude the diagnosis.

4. Conclusion

Recurrent testicular torsion after previous orchiopexy is rare but should be included in the differential diagnosis of acute scrotum. Testicular fixation with nonabsorbable suture and in at least two points can help to prevent recurrent torsion.

References

[1] V. J. Sharp, K. Kieran, and A. M. Arlen, "Testicular torsion: diagnosis, evaluation, and management," *American Family Physician*, vol. 88, no. 12, pp. 835–840, 2013.

[2] AUA, *Acute Scrotum*, vol. 36, American Urological Association, 2017.

[3] A. P. Bayne, R. J. Madden-Fuentes, E. A. Jones et al., "Factors associated with delayed treatment of acute testicular torsion—do demographics or interhospital transfer matter?" *The Journal of Urology*, vol. 184, supplement 4, pp. 1743–1747, 2010.

[4] R. E. May and W. E. Thomas, "Recurrent torsion of the testis following previous surgical fixation," *British Journal of Surgery*, vol. 67, no. 2, pp. 129-130, 1980.

[5] A. S. Kossow, "Torsion following orchiopexy," *New York State Journal of Medicine*, vol. 80, Article ID 1136e7, p. 80, 1980.

[6] P. M. Naughton and D. G. Kelly, "Torsion after previous orchiopexy," *British Journal of Urology*, vol. 55, no. 5, p. 578, 1983.

[7] S. J. Hulecki, J. P. Crawford, and B. Broecker, "Testicular torsion after orchiopexy with nonabsorbable sutures," *Urology*, vol. 28, no. 2, pp. 131-132, 1986.

[8] E. A. Tawil and J. G. Gregory, "Torsion of the contralateral testis 5 years after orchiopexy," *The Journal of Urology*, vol. 132, no. 4, pp. 766-767, 1984.

[9] D. R. McNellis and H. H. Rabinovitch, "Repeat torsion of "fixed" testis," *Urology*, vol. 16, no. 5, pp. 476-477, 1980.

[10] J. F. Redman and J. W. Walt Stallings, "Torsion of testicle following orchiopexy," *Urology*, vol. 16, no. 5, pp. 502-503, 1980.

[11] P. W. Johenning, "Torsion of the previously operated testicle," *The Journal of Urology*, vol. 110, no. 2, pp. 221-222, 1973.

[12] B. Vorstman and D. Rothwell, "Spermatic cord torsion following previous surgical fixation," *The Journal of Urology*, vol. 128, no. 4, pp. 823-824, 1982.

[13] J. A. Morgan and L. B. Mellick, "Testicular torsion following orchiopexy," *Pediatric Emergency Care*, vol. 2, no. 4, pp. 244–246, 1986.

[14] A. Thurston and R. Whitaker, "Torsion of testis after previous testicular surgery," *British Journal of Surgery*, vol. 70, no. 4, p. 217, 1983.

[15] L. Palmer and J. Plamer, "Management of Abnormalities of the External genitalia of boys," in *Campbell-Walsh Urology*, A. J. Wein, L. R. Kavoussi et al., Eds., pp. 4497-4498, Philadelphia, Pennsylvania, 11th edition, 2016.

Zinner's Syndrome: A Rare Diagnosis of Dysuria Based on Imaging

Ahmed Ibrahimi,[1,2] **Abdelmoughit Hosni,**[2,3] **Idriss Ziani,**[1,2] **Fatima Zahra Laamrani,**[2,3] **Hachem El Sayegh,**[1,2] **Laila Jroundi,**[2,3] **Lounis Benslimane,**[1,2] **and Yassine Nouini**[1,2]

[1]*Department of Urology A, Ibn Sina University Hospital, Rabat, Morocco*
[2]*Faculty of Medicine and Pharmacy, Mohammed V University in Rabat, Morocco*
[3]*Emergency Radiology Department, Ibn Sina University Hospital, Rabat, Morocco*

Correspondence should be addressed to Ahmed Ibrahimi; ahmed.ibrahimi@um5s.net.ma

Academic Editor: Apul Goel

Zinner's syndrome is a rare congenital malformation of the seminal vesicle and ipsilateral upper urinary tract, due to developmental arrest in early embryogenesis of the Müllerian duct. Clinical presentation is nonspecific and includes voiding symptoms such as dysuria, ejaculatory disorders, and hypogastric or perineal pain. The diagnosis is made with imaging techniques, notably Magnetic Resonance Imaging (MRI) which remains the gold standard exam for diagnosis confirmation and therapeutic management. Treatment options depend on the severity of symptoms, the size of the cyst, and the complications. Herein, we report a rare case of a 33-year-old young patient who presented recurrent dysuria and ejaculatory disorders for the last 5 years. Imaging studies revealed an empty left renal fossa, with cystic pelvic mass related to the seminal vesicle and which was compatible with the diagnosis of Zinner's syndrome. The patient underwent successful laparoscopic removal of the cyst and seminal vesicle, with total disappearance of urinary and sexual complaints with a 3-year follow-up.

1. Introduction

Zinner's syndrome is a rare congenital malformation of the seminal vesicle and ipsilateral upper urinary tract [1, 2]; it is characterized by the simultaneous association of unilateral renal agenesis, ipsilateral seminal vesicle cyst, and ipsilateral ejaculatory duct obstruction. It is often diagnosed in the second and third decades of life and can lead to serious complications, particularly infertility [3, 4]. Clinical presentation is nonspecific, thus often making the diagnosis delayed or missed, and the majority of patients remain asymptomatic until beginning sexual activity [1]. Magnetic Resonance Imaging (MRI) occupies a prominent place in the diagnostic arsenal and remains the examination of choice to make the diagnosis [5].

We herein, through this rare case of a 33-year-old man diagnosed with Zinner's syndrome, aimed to discuss the hierarchy and the results of different imaging techniques that are employed in order to reach the correct diagnosis, as well as the different clinical, etiological, and therapeutic aspects of this uncommon condition.

2. Case Presentation

A 33-year-old patient, father of three children, without past medical or surgical history presented to the urology department for apyretic recurrent dysuria, with episodes of hematospermia and painful ejaculation evolving for 5 years.

Physical examination revealed no palpable pelvic mass, with normally developed external genitalia. Digital rectal examination (DRE) was painless and found a renitent mass facing the anterior wall of the rectum, with normal prostate volume and consistency. Routine blood and urine laboratory tests, including urine culture, were normal.

Abdominal ultrasonography revealed an empty left renal fossa, associated with a left retrovesical liquid mass. A transrectal ultrasonography was performed, showing a large left retrovesical hypoechoic mass with a posterior enhancement

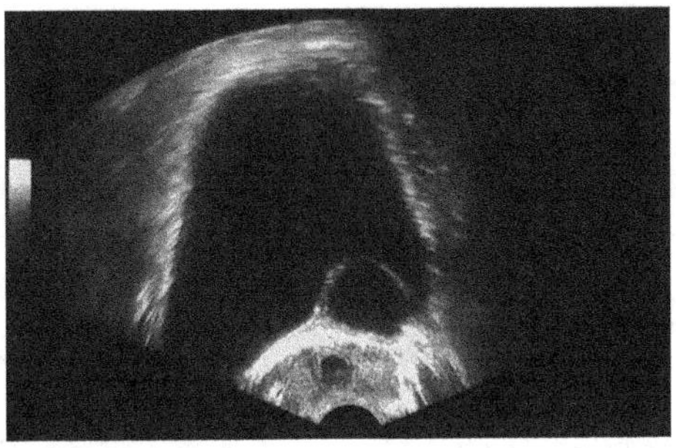

Figure 1: Transrectal ultrasonography showing a large left retrovesical cyst compressing the urinary bladder and protruding into the bladder lumen.

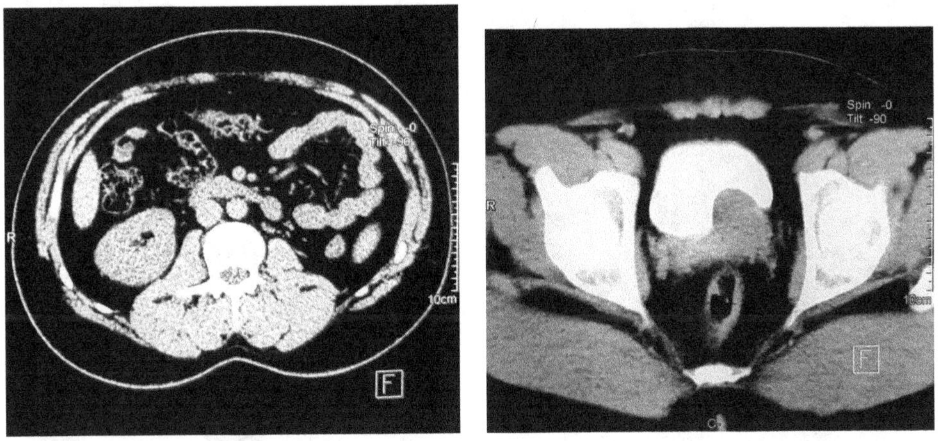

(a) (b)

Figure 2: (a) Axial view of CT scan showing a single right kidney with empty left renal fossa; (b) CT scan of the pelvis revealing a homogeneous liquid mass retrovesical compressing the urinary bladder and protruding into the bladder lumen.

and impure content, compressing the urinary bladder and protruding into the bladder lumen (Figure 1).

Abdominal and pelvic computed tomography (CT) showed left renal agenesis (Figure 2(a)), associated with the presence of a large left retrovesical mass without contrast enhancement, suggesting a cystic mass and compressing the posterior bladder wall (Figure 2(b)).

A pelvic MRI was performed to identify precisely the origin of the cystic mass using a T1-weighted, T1-weighted with gadolinium injection, and T2-weighted sequences in the axial and coronal plans (Figures 3 and 4). We found then a unique cystic-to-tubular structure in the seminal vesicle appearing hyperintense on T2W images and hyperintense on T1W images (due to hemorrhage and a high proteinaceous concentration on the seminal fluid), measured to 20 × 35 × 40 mm. From its posterolateral side emerges a tubular structure crossing the iliac vessels anteriorly, which was considered an ectopic ureter (Figures 4 and 5). The right seminal vesicle did not show any abnormality. CT findings were reviewed, and the presence of the ectopic ureter was noticeable within the multiplanar reconstructions.

Urethrocystoscopy showed no lesions in the urethra or bladder, revealing a large intraluminal protruding mass at the left lateral trigonal area and partially obstructing the bladder neck (Figure 6).

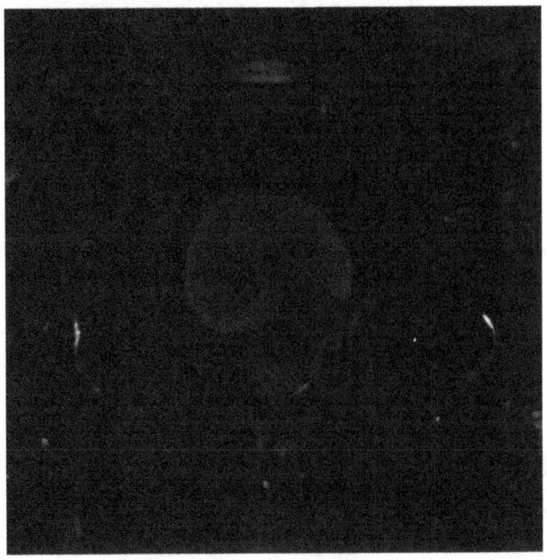

Figure 3: MRI coronal image in the T2-weighted sequence showing a seminal vesicle lesion which is separated from the prostate by its capsule.

Imaging findings and cystoscopic examination lead to the diagnosis of Zinner's syndrome, and surgical management was planned.

The patient underwent laparoscopic removal of the cyst and seminal vesicle. The postoperative course was

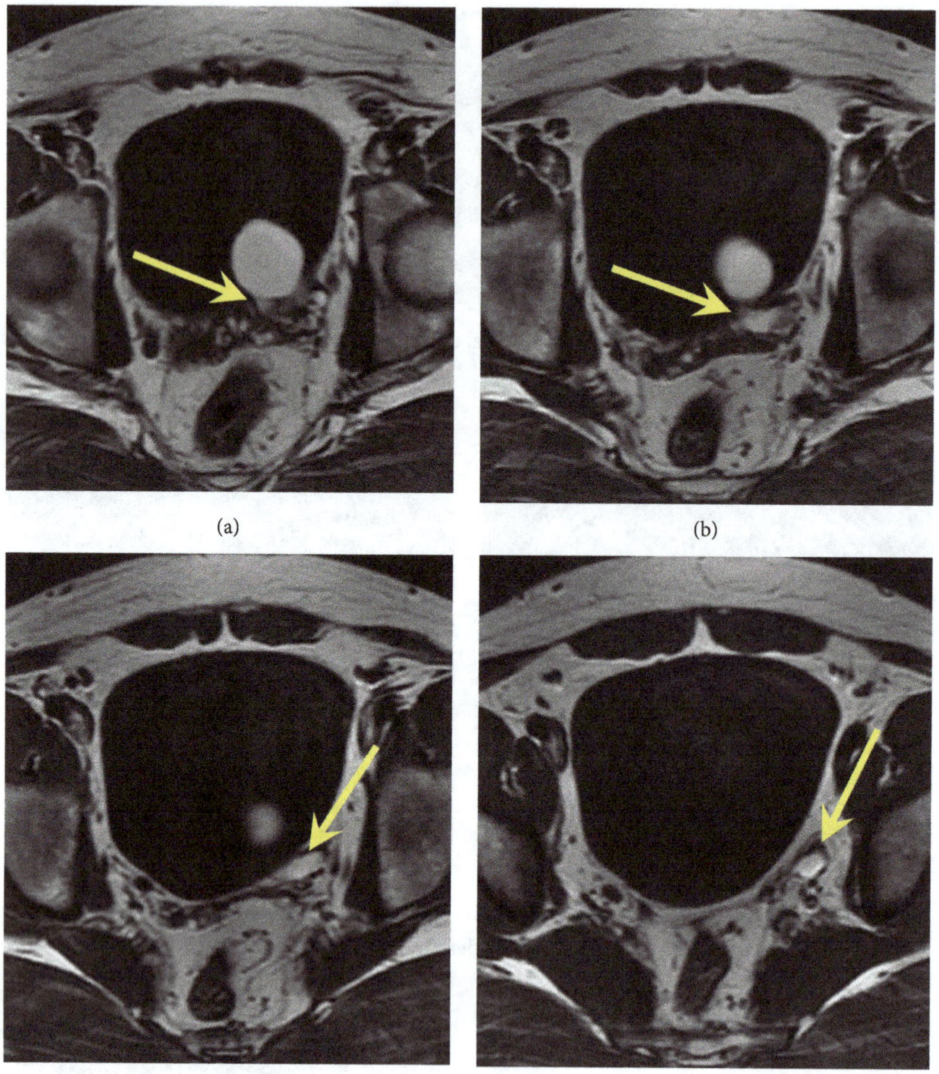

(a) (b) (c) (d)

FIGURE 4: MRI axial superposed images on the seminal vesicle cyst in the T1-weighted sequence. Yellow arrow showing the tubular structure linked to the seminal vesicle cyst considered an ectopic ureter.

uneventful, and the patient was discharged from the hospital on the 4th day without any complication. The follow-up was marked by total disappearance of urinary and sexual complaints.

3. Discussion

Zinner's syndrome was first described in 1914 by Zinner. It is defined as the association of a seminal vesicle cyst, an ipsilateral renal agenesis, and an ejaculatory duct obstruction [1, 4]. The ipsilateral ureter can be absent or incomplete or may have an abnormal course towards the seminal vesicle. This last situation, which was found in our case, concerns 36% of the cases [5, 6]. Zinner's syndrome remains a rare congenital malformation with only 200 cases reported in the available literature [1, 4, 5]. The association of abnormalities is frequently found on the right side, with a right-sided ratio of 2 : 1. Bilaterality is found in only 2% of cases [7]. Otherwise, a contralateral renal agenesis was reported in 4 cases of seminal vesicle cysts [8].

Symptoms depend mainly on the cyst's size; commonly, cysts less than 5 cm are asymptomatic. Symptoms are usually present at the second or third decade, with a mean age at presentation of 30 years; this age corresponds to a significant increase in the size of the cyst, as well as the beginning of sexually active life. Symptoms reported in the literature are usually related either to micturition which includes dysuria, obstructive urination, frequency, urgency, and hematuria; to perineal, scrotal, hypogastric, or defecation pain; or in some cases to ejaculatory disorders such as pain following ejaculation, infertility, and hematospermia. Complications such as epididymitis or prostatitis represent a considerable form of revelation [6, 7, 9]. Rarely, giant cysts can lead to bladder or colon obstruction [5].

Infertility is frequently associated; its pathogenesis is unclear, but it is more likely due to the associated ejaculatory duct obstruction. Examination of seminal fluid should be

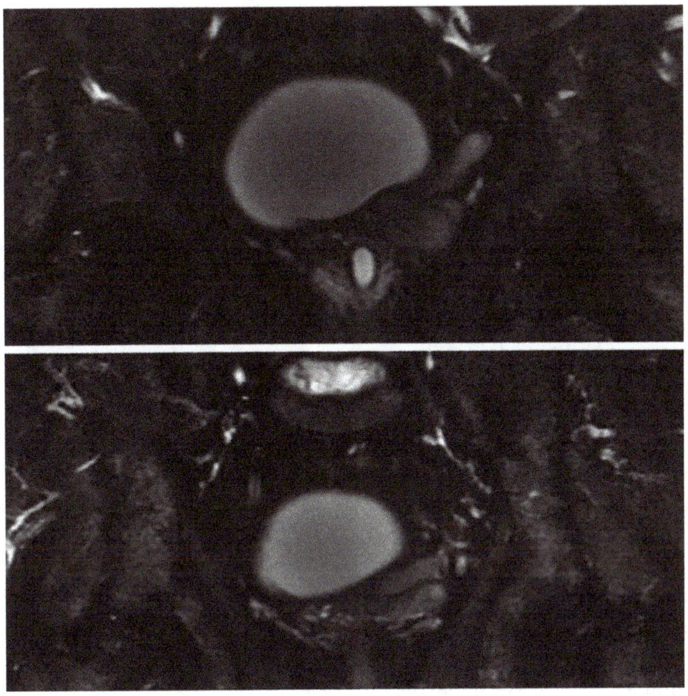

FIGURE 5: MRI coronal slices showing the communication between the seminal vesicle cyst and ectopic ureter.

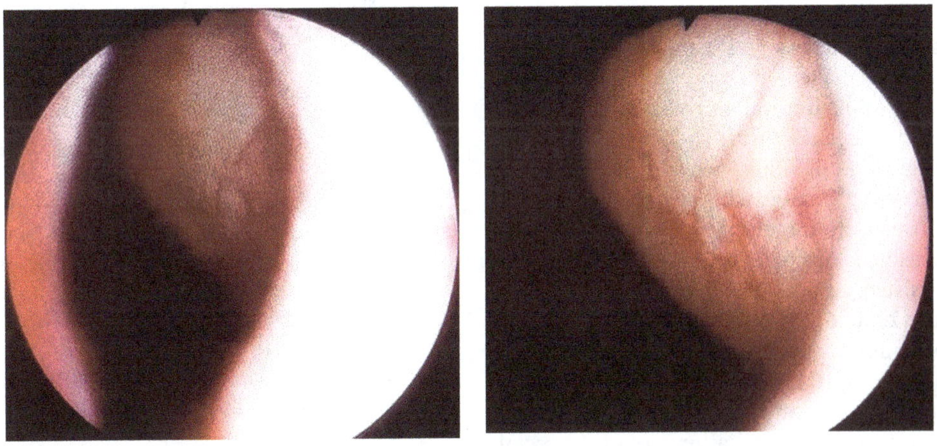

(a) (b)

FIGURE 6: (a, b) Urethrocystoscopy showing a large intraluminal protruding mass at the left lateral trigonal area and partially obstructing the bladder neck.

systematic in the presence of Zinner's syndrome; results can show a low ejaculatory volume, azoospermia, alkaline pH, low concentration of carnitine and fructose in the seminal plasma, and high citrate level [7, 9]. In our patient, the symptoms were troublesome despite the small size of the cyst, which did not exceed 4 cm, probably because the cyst is protruding in the bladder lumen and thus causing voiding complaints; fertility was conserved in our patient, and none of the cited complications did happen.

Imaging remains the key to diagnosis. Transrectal ultrasonography (US) shows the seminal vesicle cyst as an anechoic pelvic mass with a thick wall; infection or hemorrhage from the cyst may appear as cystic mass containing internal echos [5].

CT is superior to ultrasonography, and reported findings are of a retrovesicular cystic pelvic mass arising from an enlarged seminal vesicle associated with ipsilateral renal agenesis, but it may be insufficient to confirm the diagnosis [1, 3].

MRI is considered superior to CT scan in the analysis of these conditions [5]. With its invasiveness, multiple pulse sequences, multiplanar capability, and high soft-tissue resolution, it is considered a "gold standard" for diagnosis and surgical planning. Images from MRI provide a better characterization of the cyst content, a precise detection of associated genitourinary abnormalities, and an evaluation of the anatomic relationship with the pelvic structures. Unilocular cystic masses are more commonly found than tubular and multilocular features. Typically, the cyst content is described as a homogeneous hyposignal on T1-weighted sequences and homogeneous hypersignal on T2-weighted sequences. However, some cysts may have a hypersignal on both T1- and T2-weighted sequences related to an old hemorrhage and a high proteinaceous concentration on the seminal fluid [1, 10]. Intracystic vegetations can be a sign of malignancy, although malignant degeneration remains exceptional with only 3 reported cases in the literature [11, 12].

The differential diagnosis of pelvic cysts in male patients includes prostatic utricle cystic dilatation, prostatic utricle cysts (previously known as Müllerian duct cysts), ejaculatory duct cysts, prostatic cysts, diverticulosis of the ampulla of the deferens canal, ectopic ureterocele, and abscess [13]. Diagnosis criteria of seminal vesicle cysts are the cyst position (median, paramedian or lateral, and intra- or extraprostatic), associated abnormalities (renal agenesis, anomalies of the external genitalia), and imaging aspects on MRI [14].

Once diagnosed, management of seminal vesicle cysts depends on their size and symptomatology, as well as the presence of complications [2, 4]. A wide variety of treatment modalities and techniques have been reported including conservative management represented by percutaneous drainage and transurethral or transrectal aspiration, but both are associated with a greater risk of recurrence [3]. Surgical procedures are the mainstay in the management of symptomatic, complicated, or recurrent patients based on open surgery or minimally invasive surgery, with laparoscopic transperitoneal approaches or, recently, robotic-assisted approaches which guarantee a successful outcome [2, 4, 6]. Nevertheless, the challenge of different treatment approaches is preserving the fertility of the patient and relieving the symptoms.

In our case, laparoscopic removal of the cyst and seminal vesicle was performed after failure of transrectal ultrasonography-guided aspiration of the cyst, which was complicated by hemorrhage, with inability to evacuate the cyst content completely. Conservative treatment was attempted in our patient 6 months ago, and since then, the cyst has increased in size and the symptoms became worse, affecting the patient's quality of life, thus requiring recourse to surgical treatment.

4. Conclusion

Zinner's syndrome is an uncommon cause of dysuria in men; its diagnosis is based on imaging techniques. Ultrasonography is a noninvasive exam and could provide valuable information, CT scan could be sufficient to make the diagnosis if it defined the origin of the pelvic mass, and MRI is the exam of choice for a precise lesional statement and successful therapeutic management.

Authors' Contributions

All authors have read and approved the final version of the manuscript.

References

[1] S. Florim, V. Oliveira, and D. Rocha, "Zinner syndrome presenting with intermittent scrotal pain in a young man," *Radiology Case Reports*, vol. 13, no. 6, pp. 1224–1227, 2018.

[2] M. Kardoust Parizi and N. Shakhssalim, "Management of Zinner's syndrome associated with contralateral seminal vesicle hypoplasia: a case report," *Case Reports in Urology*, vol. 2013, 3 pages, 2013.

[3] M. AlArifi, M. Al-Gahwary, and M. Gomha, "The association of renal agenesis and ipsilateral seminal vesicle cyst: Zinner syndrome case report," *Case Reports in Urology*, vol. 2019, Article ID 1242149, 3 pages, 2019.

[4] B. J. Pereira, L. Sousa, P. Azinhais et al., "Zinner's syndrome: an up-to-date review of the literature based on a clinical case," *Andrologia*, vol. 41, no. 5, pp. 322–330, 2009.

[5] R. Sundar and G. Sundar, "Zinner syndrome: an uncommon cause of painful ejaculation," *Case Reports*, vol. 2015, bcr2014207618 pages, 2015.

[6] D. van den Ouden, J. H. M. Blom, C. Bangma, and A. H. V. C. de Spiegeleer, "Diagnosis and management of seminal vesicle cysts associated with ipsilateral renal agenesis: a pooled analysis of 52 cases," *European Urology*, vol. 33, no. 5, pp. 433–440, 1998.

[7] S. Khanduri, G. Katyal, H. Sharma, A. Goyal, N. Singh, and H. Yadav, "Unique association of multiple seminal vesicle cysts with contralateral renal agenesis: a rare variant of Zinner syndrome," *Cureus*, vol. 9, no. 7, article e1415, 2017.

[8] Y. Aswani, R. Varma, P. Choudhary, and R. B. Gupta, "Wolffian origin of vagina unfolds the embryopathogenesis of OHVIRA (obstructed hemivagina and ipsilateral renal anomaly) syndrome and places OHVIRA as a female counterpart of Zinner syndrome in males," *Polish Journal of Radiology*, vol. 81, pp. 549–556, 2016.

[9] S. E. Hannema and I. A. Hughes, "Regulation of Wolffian duct development," *Hormone Research*, vol. 67, no. 3, pp. 142–151, 2007.

[10] M. Matsuki, M. Matsuo, Y. Kaji, and N. Okada, "Ectopic ureter draining into seminal vesicle cyst: usefulness of MRI," *Radiation Medicine*, vol. 16, no. 4, pp. 309–311, 1998 Jul-Aug.

[11] J. P. Trigaux, B. Van Beers, and F. Delchambre, "Male genital tract malformations associated with ipsilateral renal agenesis: sonographic findings," *Journal of Clinical Ultrasound*, vol. 19, no. 1, pp. 3–10, 1991.

[12] H. M. Shebel, H. M. Farg, O. Kolokythas, and T. El-Diasty, "Cysts of the lower male genitourinary tract: embryologic and anatomic considerations and differential diagnosis," *Radiographics*, vol. 33, no. 4, pp. 1125–1143, 2013.

[13] B. H. Lee, J. W. Seo, Y. H. Han, Y. H. Kim, and S. J. Cha, "Primary mucinous adenocarcinoma of a seminal vesicle cyst associated with ectopic ureter and ipsilateral renal agenesis: a case report," *Korean Journal of Radiology*, vol. 8, no. 3, pp. 258–261, 2007.

[14] Y. Kim, H. W. Baek, E. Choi, and K. C. Moon, "Squamous cell carcinoma of the seminal vesicle from Zinner syndrome: a case report and review of literature," *Journal of Pathology and Translational Medicine*, vol. 49, no. 1, pp. 85–88, 2015.

22

Zinner Syndrome with Ectopic Ureter Emptying into Seminal Vesicle

M. Hevia Palacios,[1] M. Álvarez-Maestro,[2] J. Gómez Rivas,[3] A. Aguilera Bazan,[4] and L. Martínez-Piñeiro[5]

[1]Member of Urology Department, Ramon y Cajal Hospital, Spain
[2]Member of Urology Department, La Paz Universitary Hospital, Spain
[3]Member of Urology Department, Clinico San Carlos Hospital, Spain
[4]Section Chief, La Paz Universitary Hospital, Spain
[5]Chief Urology Department, La Paz Universitary Hospital, Spain

Correspondence should be addressed to M. Hevia Palacios; manuel.hevia.palacios@gmail.com

Academic Editor: Fumitaka Koga

A 66-year-old male patient in follow-up in the urology department for a non-muscle-invasive bladder cancer was detected by ultrasound to have absence of the left kidney and a cystic, multilobed image at the location of the seminal vesicle. Magnetic resonance imaging reveals left renal agenesis and the existence of multiple cysts in the ipsilateral seminal vesicle that reaches a size of 6.9 × 3.7 cm, as well as a ureteral remnant that opens into the seminal vesicle. The patient does not present urinary symptoms, neither pain with ejaculation nor hematuria. A triad of seminal vesicle cyst, ipsilateral renal agenesis, and ipsilateral ejaculatory duct obstruction is known as Zinner syndrome. Congenital anomalies of the seminal vesicles are rare; some of them are associated with malformations of the upper urinary system. Seminal vesicle cysts are associated with ipsilateral renal agenesis and ectopic or dysplastic ureter. Patients may remain asymptomatic and be diagnosed incidentally or may present with symptoms such as increased urinary frequency, dysuria, recurrent infections, pain with ejaculation, and perineal discomfort.

1. Introduction

Zinner syndrome, known as the triad of renal agenesis, cysts in the ipsilateral seminal vesicle, and ejaculatory duct obstruction, was described by A. Zinner in 1914 [1] and around 200 cases have been reported in the literature [2]. Congenital anomalies of the seminal vesicles are infrequent, most of them have cystic malformations and some are associated with malformations of the upper urinary system. The common embryological origin of the urinary and genital tracts (mesonephros or Wolf ducts and the ureteric bud) can produce, in the presence of an anomaly, an alteration in the development of both systems [3].

2. Case Report

A 66-year-old male patient with no comorbidities, ex-smoker, on follow-up for a non-muscle-invasive bladder cancer operated resulting in T1G2 in the pathological examination, is subsequently receiving treatment with BCG and without recurrences during follow-up. The patient remains asymptomatic and does not report pain with ejaculation or perineal discomfort.

Physical examination and blood tests, including kidney function and PSA, did not show any abnormalities. The digital examination revealed a fibroelastic prostate, without pathological findings. The patient did not develop fertility problems throughout his life, being able to have two healthy children.

In the initial evaluation ultrasound, the absence of the left kidney was detected, as well as a left posterolateral multilobed lesion on the location of the seminal vesicle, with cystic areas and echogenic content of approximately 7 × 3.5 cm (Figure 1).

Endoscopic examination reveals an absence of the left ureteral meatus, without other findings.

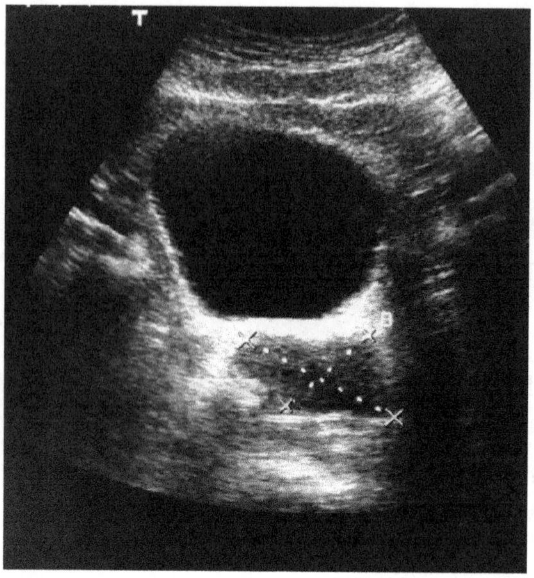

Figure 1: Abdominal ultrasound showing a cystic lesion close to the bladder.

Abdominal-pelvic magnetic resonance imaging (MRI) was performed with acquisition of basal sequences, and after administration of intravenous gadolinium that revealed the absence of parenchyma of the left kidney, a tubular structure in the left lumbar and pelvic region was identified that seemed to correspond to the dilated ureter of up to 12 mm and with probable remnant of the renal pelvis in the most proximal lumbar portion. The ureter empties ectopically into the left seminal vesicle, which is markedly enlarged and multicystic in appearance, measuring approximately 6.9 cm in the oblique longitudinal major axis and 3.5 cm in the anteroposterior axis. Both the ureter and the seminal vesicle show high signal content in both T1 and T2, suggesting hemorrhagic content or a high proteinaceous component, and their walls and septa are thin, without significant contrast enhancement (Figure 2).

The left vas deferens is patent, being more thickened in its part closest to the seminal vesicle. Cystic dilatation of the left ejaculatory duct was observed.

Given the absence of symptoms related to this pathology, observation with periodic ultrasound is decided. The patient continues with his periodic revisions for the bladder tumor, without having any symptoms related to his Zinner syndrome.

3. Discussion

In general, seminal vesicle cysts are identified between the second and third decades of life, during the period of greatest sexual and reproductive activity [2].

There are around 200 published cases in the literature [2], but given the widespread use of imaging tests, it is suspected that there are more cases. A population-based screening study shows that the reported incidence of cystic lesions in the pelvis with agenesis or ipsilateral renal dysplasia is between 0.00035% and 0.0046%. According to several studies, up to 68% of all seminal vesicle cysts are associated with ipsilateral renal agenesis [4].

The especially remarkable characteristics of our case are the findings found in the imaging tests that show the ureteral remnant emptying into the ipsilateral seminal vesicle given the infrequency of this presentation.

Zinner syndrome is considered the male equivalent of the female Mayer-Rokitansky-Kuster-Hauser syndrome [5]. It usually presents as the triad described above, although it can also be associated with other genitourinary disorders such as ureterocele, hypospadias, and testicular, epididymal, or adrenal gland disorders [2]. In the literature, the most frequent symptoms include dysuria, abnormal urinary frequency, prostatitis, perineal or scrotal pain, epididymitis, and painful ejaculation [4].

In our case, the patient remains completely asymptomatic and the diagnosis of Zinner syndrome occurs incidentally in the context of medical monitoring for non-muscle-invasive bladder carcinoma.

Between the fourth and seventh weeks of embryogenesis, the ureter originates as a dorsal bud from the distal mesonephric duct, spreading dorsocranially to find and induce differentiation of the metanephric blastema, which will form the kidney. The mesonephric duct is differentiated in the appendix from the epididymis, paradidymis, epididymis, vas deferens, ejaculatory ducts, seminal vesicle, and hemitrigone. Normal kidney development depends on induction by the ureteric bud and mesonephric duct [6].

If the ureteral bud originates from a more cephalic portion of the mesonephric duct, the delay in absorption of the common distal portion of the mesonephric duct results in delayed absorption, as well as an opening of the ureteral bud in an ectopic location at the trigone level, bladder neck, urethra, or organs derived from the mesonephric duct, such as the ejaculatory duct, the vas deferens, or the seminal vesicle as in the case of our patient [6, 7].

Ultrasound is usually the first imaging test when this condition is suspected, since it is a quick and affordable modality. Thanks to it, we will be able to detect the absence of the renal unit, as well as the presence of a cystic mass in the pelvic

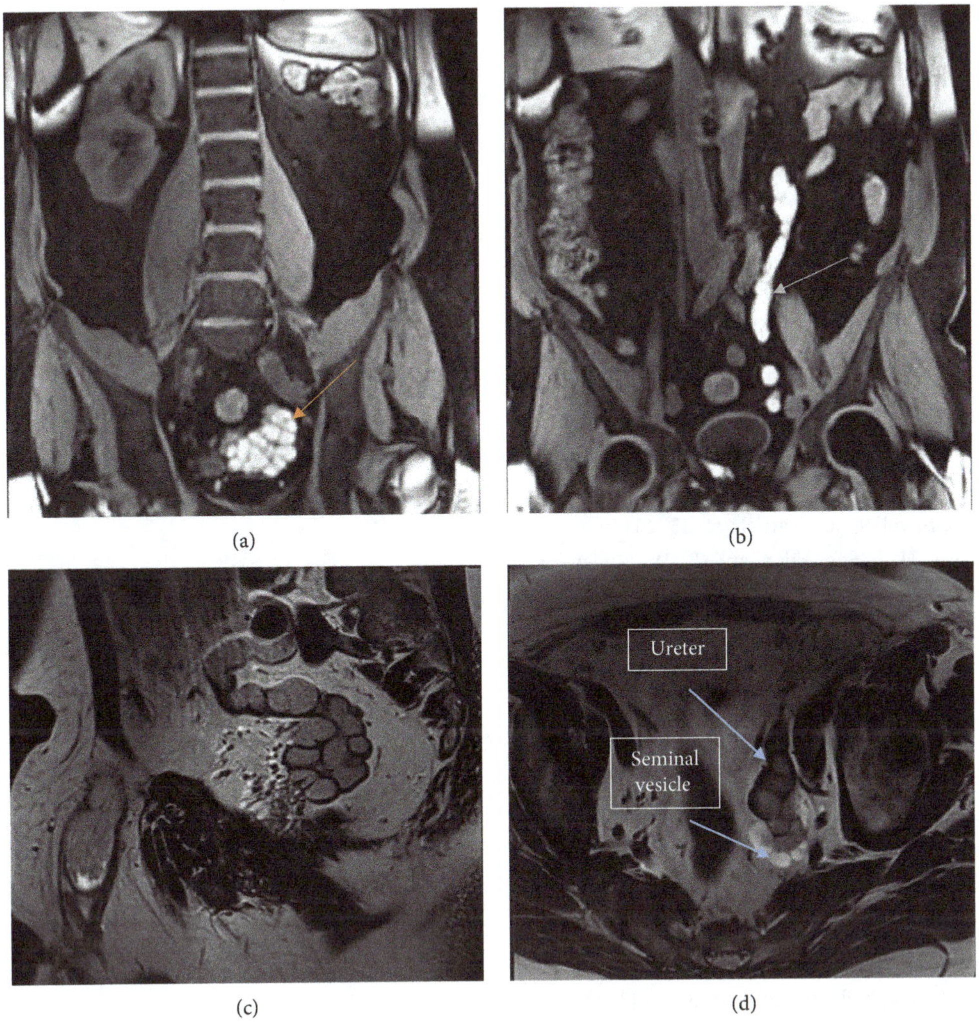

Figure 2: (a) MRI T1 coronal section showed left renal agenesis and dilatation of the left seminal vesicle (red arrow) that shows high signal content, suggesting hemorrhagic content or a high proteinaceous component; (b) tubular structure (green arrow) in the left lumbar and pelvic region that seemed to correspond to the dilated ureter (c). MRI T2 sagittal section reveals the ureter empties ectopically into the left seminal vesicle, which is markedly enlarged and multicystic and (d) shows in the axial the contrast enhancement difference between the ureter and seminal vesicle.

region. Computed tomography (CT) and MRI, especially the latter, are capable of assessing more clearly the lesions and their anatomical characteristics [8].

Differential diagnosis should be made with other entities such as laterally located prostatic cysts, diverticulosis of the vas deferens, ectopic ureterocele, and abscesses. The presence of tumors in seminal vesicle cysts is extremely rare, with two cases of papillary adenocarcinoma reported in the literature. Ultrasound findings are those of an anechoic lesion or with the presence of internal echoes due to bleeding or infection, with a thick and irregular wall, occasionally with calcifications, in a retroprostatic location [3].

The management of this syndrome depends on the symptoms presented by the patient. In asymptomatic or slightly symptomatic cases like ours, observation may be chosen, while patients presenting symptoms will require surgical treatment, either transurethral, transrectal drainage, open surgery, or minimally invasive techniques, the latter being the one that has produced the best results regarding blood loss and hospital stay [9]. Another surgical indication may be infertility [6].

A recently published study has also proposed a new strategy for the analysis of seminal vesicle lesions in the diagnosis and treatment of Zinner syndrome, based on the morphology of the cysts. The study analyzed the size, content, possible calcifications, cyst wall structure, and possible solid lesions in association with cysts [10].

4. Conclusion

Zinner syndrome is a rare entity, with CT and MRI being the diagnostic methods of choice in these patients, given that they allow us a very precise anatomical definition, as well as the diagnosis of other associated malformations.

Surgical treatment is the gold standard in symptomatic patients, while in asymptomatic patients, observation may be chosen.

References

[1] A. Zinner, "Ein fall von intravesikaler samenblasenzyste," *Wiener Medizinische Wochenschrift*, vol. 64, p. 605, 1914.

[2] B. J. Pereira, L. Sousa, P. Azinhais et al., "Zinner's syndrome: an up-to-date review of the literature based on a clinical case," *Andrologia*, vol. 41, no. 5, pp. 322–330, 2009.

[3] L. Livingston and C. R. Larsen, "Seminal vesicle cyst with ipsilateral renal agenesis," *AJR. American Journal of Roentgenology*, vol. 175, no. 1, pp. 177–180, 2000.

[4] B. Hergan, F. A. Fellner, and K. Akbari, "Incidental imaging findings suggesting Zinner syndrome in a young patient with pulmonary embolism: a case report," *Radiology Case Reports*, vol. 15, no. 4, pp. 437–441, 2020.

[5] S. Khanduri, G. Katyal, H. Sharma, A. Goyal, N. Singh, and H. Yadav, "Unique Association of multiple seminal vesicle cysts with contralateral renal agenesis: a rare variant of Zinner syndrome," *Cureus*, vol. 9, no. 7, article e1415, 2017.

[6] C. G. Roehrborn, H. J. Schneider, and E. W. Rugendorff, "Embryological and diagnostic aspects of seminal vesicle cysts associated with upper urinary tract malformation," *The Journal of Urology*, vol. 135, no. 5, pp. 1029–1032, 1986.

[7] S. R. Grimaldo, L. A. F. Chapa, M. J. J. Galán, B. N. I. Ríos, and F. A. Guardiola, "Quistes de vesículas seminales con agenesia renal ipsilateral. Presentación de 3 casos y revisión de la literatura," *Revista Mexicana de Urología*, vol. 68, no. 5, 2008.

[8] S. Mehra, R. Ranjan, and U. C. Garga, "Zinner syndrome–a rare developmental anomaly of the mesonephric duct diagnosed on magnetic resonance imaging," *Radiology Case Reports*, vol. 11, no. 4, pp. 313–317, 2016.

[9] E. Kord, A. Zisman, A. E. Darawsha, N. Dally, P. H. Noh, and A. Neheman, "Minimally invasive approach for treatment of seminal vesicle cyst associated with ipsilateral renal agenesis," *Urologia Internationalis*, vol. 99, no. 3, pp. 338–342, 2017.

[10] Z. Tan, B. Li, L. Zhang et al., "Classifying seminal vesicle cysts in the diagnosis and treatment of Zinner syndrome: a report of six cases and review of available literature," *Andrologia*, vol. 52, no. 1, article e13397, 2020.

23

A Case of Lower-Pole Moiety Ureteral Stenosis Close to Ureteropelvic Junction in an Incomplete Duplicated Collecting System Managed by Retrograde Balloon Dilatation that Needed a 2nd Ureteral Stent to the Upper-Pole

Seiichi Saito

Art Park Urology Hospital & Clinic, Ishiyama-Higashi 3-1-31, Minami-ku, Sapporo 005-0850, Japan

Correspondence should be addressed to Seiichi Saito; apusss@mb.infosnow.ne.jp

Academic Editor: Nicola Zampieri

A 71-year-old woman presented at our institution with the chief complaints of left back pain and fatigue. Radiographic examination revealed left ureteral stenosis close to ureteropelvic junctiòn of the lower-pole with a left incomplete duplicated collecting system. Transurethral retrograde balloon dilatation under general anesthesia was performed, and a ureteral stent was inserted to the lower-pole; however, there was urinary leakage from the upper-pole at the dilated ureteral stenosis lesion, and therefore, another ureteral stent was inserted to the upper-pole just after the first stent insertion. Both stents were removed at 6 weeks and subsequent intravenous pyelography confirmed resolution of the obstruction. The patient has remained asymptomatic during 2 years of follow-up.

1. Introduction

The ureteropelvic junction (UPJ) of the lower-pole, both with a complete and incomplete duplicated system, is a common cause of obstruction. Although minimally invasive treatment like a retrograde endoscopic approach has been reported, most cases are successfully managed [1–4]. I herein report a case with ureteral stenosis close to UPJ of the lower-pole in an incomplete duplicated collecting system managed by retrograde balloon dilatation. However, there was urinary leakage from the upper-pole at the dilated ureteral stenosis lesion, and therefore, another ureteral stent needed to be inserted to the upper-pole.

2. Case Presentation

A 71-year-old woman was referred with dull left back pain and fatigue for 1 year. The patient was evaluated by abdominal computed tomography (CT) and intravenous pyelography (IVP), which revealed incomplete duplication of the left urinary system with lower pole moiety hydronephrosis (Figures 1 and 2). Retrograde pyelography (RP) showed ureteral stenosis close to UPJ with severe hydronephrosis of the lower pole moiety (Figure 3). With the patient in the dorsal lithotomy position under general anesthesia, a 0.038-inch guidewire was inserted into the lower pole of the collecting system, and balloon dilatation (X-Force, 6 mm × 4 cm, Bard Urological Division, C. R. Bard Inc. Covington, GA, 30209, USA) was performed at the narrowed ureteral lesion. Finally, a ureteral stent (InLay Optima, 6Fr × 22 cm, Bard Medical Division, C. R. Bard Inc. Covington, GA, 30209, USA) was inserted to the lower-pole of the collecting system. However, there was urinary leakage with contrast from the upper-pole at the dilated ureteral stenosis lesion, and another ureteral stent (same size and same company) was inserted to the upper-pole of the collecting system (Figures 4 and 5) just after the balloon dilatation. This procedure lasted for 115 minutes, and the patient stayed in the hospital for 5 days. The patient was asymptomatic during the six weeks in which she had two 6 Fr stents in her left ureter. And she was on antibiotics while stenting. Both stents were removed at 6 weeks after operation.

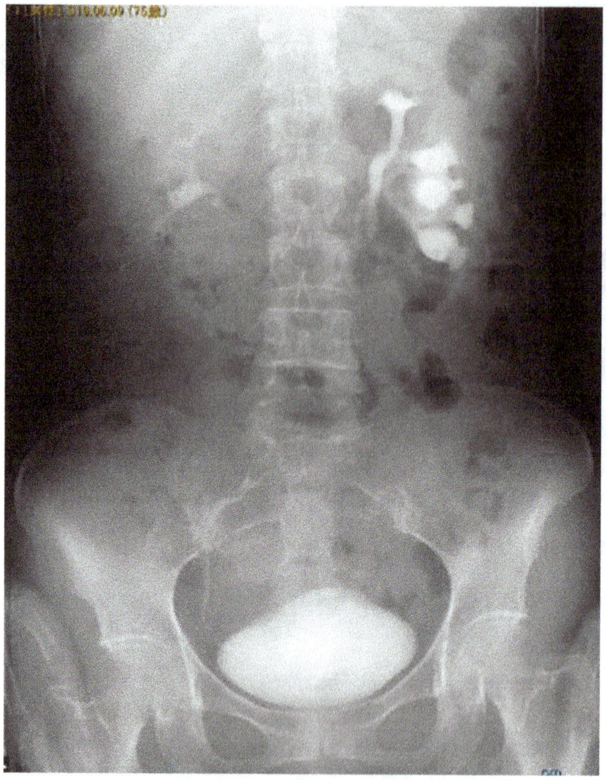

FIGURE 1: IVP shows hydronephrosis of the left lower-pole in the incomplete duplicated collecting system.

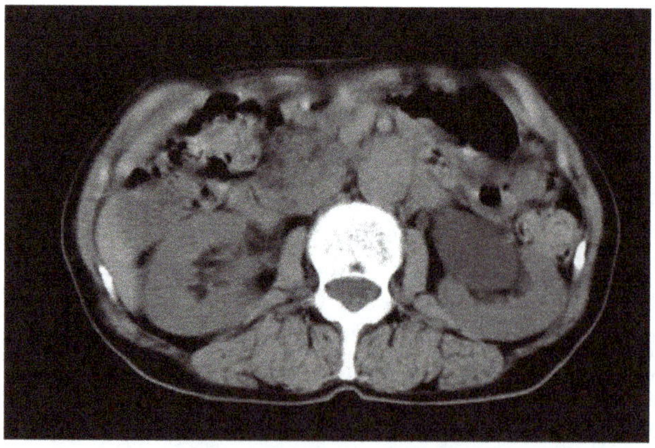

FIGURE 2: CT shows hydronephrosis of the left lower-pole.

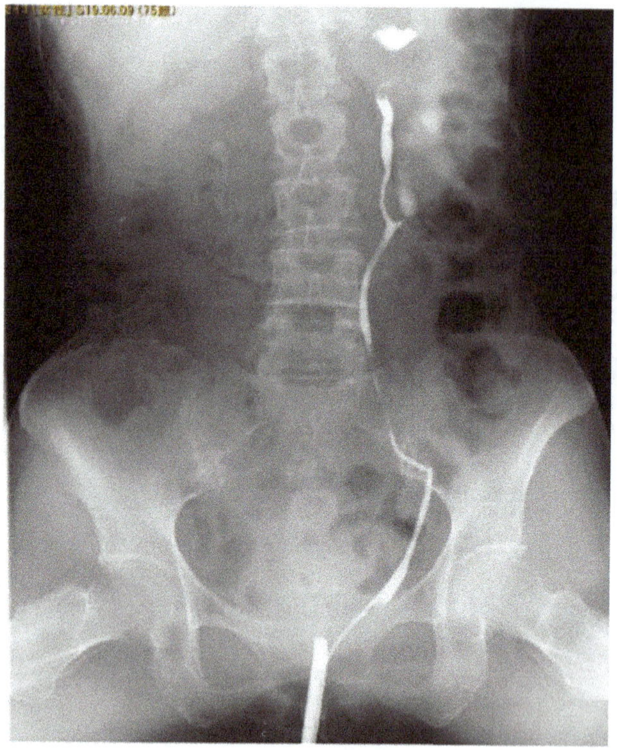

FIGURE 3: RP reveals UPJO of the left lower-pole in the incomplete duplicated system.

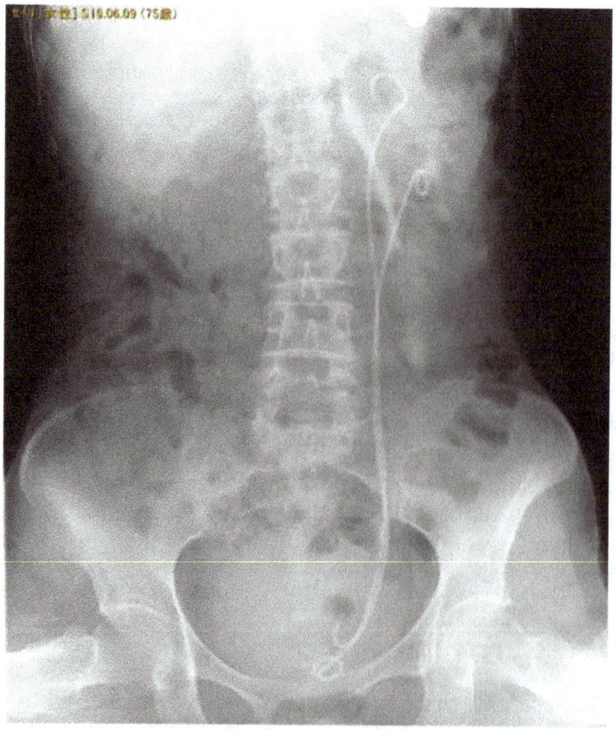

FIGURE 4: Contrast leakage from the upper-pole of the incomplete duplicated collecting system after the inflation of the UPJO, and stents were placed to the upper-pole and lower-pole.

An IVP at 3 months postoperatively showed reduction of the hydronephrosis in the lower-pole moiety (Figure 6), and the patient remained asymptomatic during 2 years of follow-up.

3. Discussion

Duplication of the renal collecting system is the most common upper urinary tract anomaly, occurring in 0.5% of the nonselected population [5]. Of these duplicated systems, approximately 70% are incomplete [6]. Ureteropelvic junction obstruction (UPJO) is the most common cause of pyelocaliectasis, which occurs in approximately 1 in 1500 births

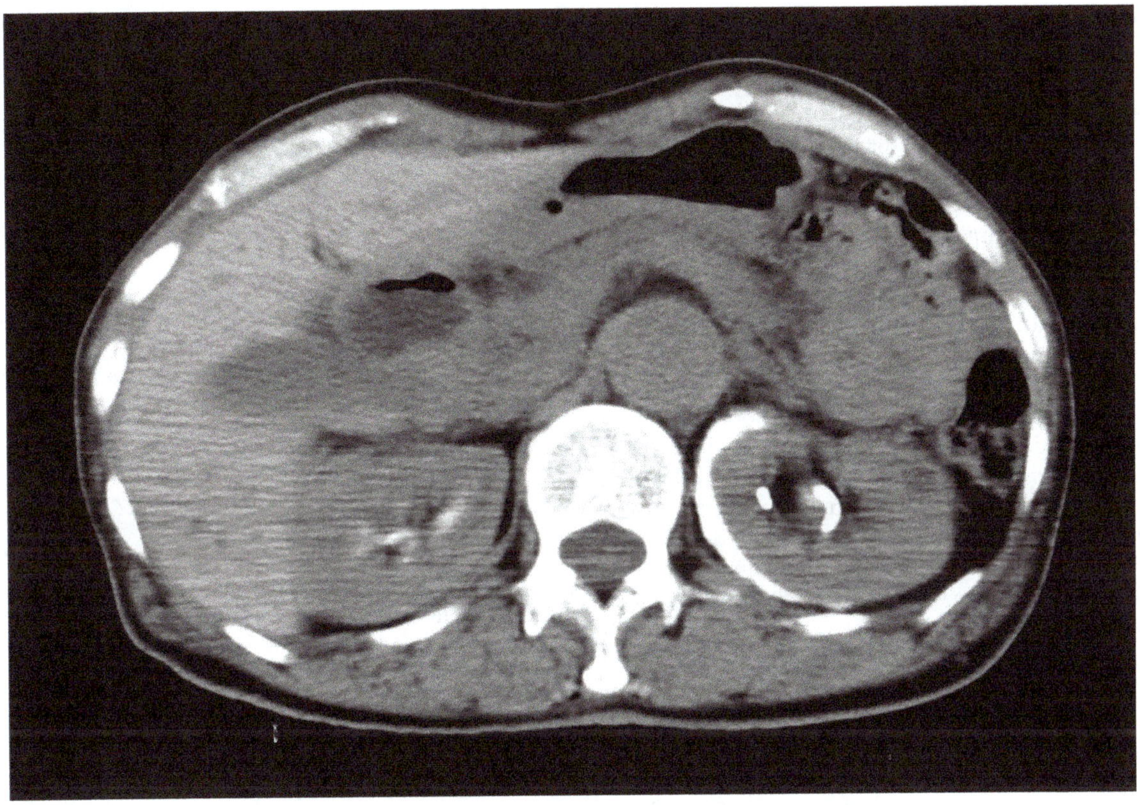

Figure 5: CT shows contrast leakage in the retroperitoneal space.

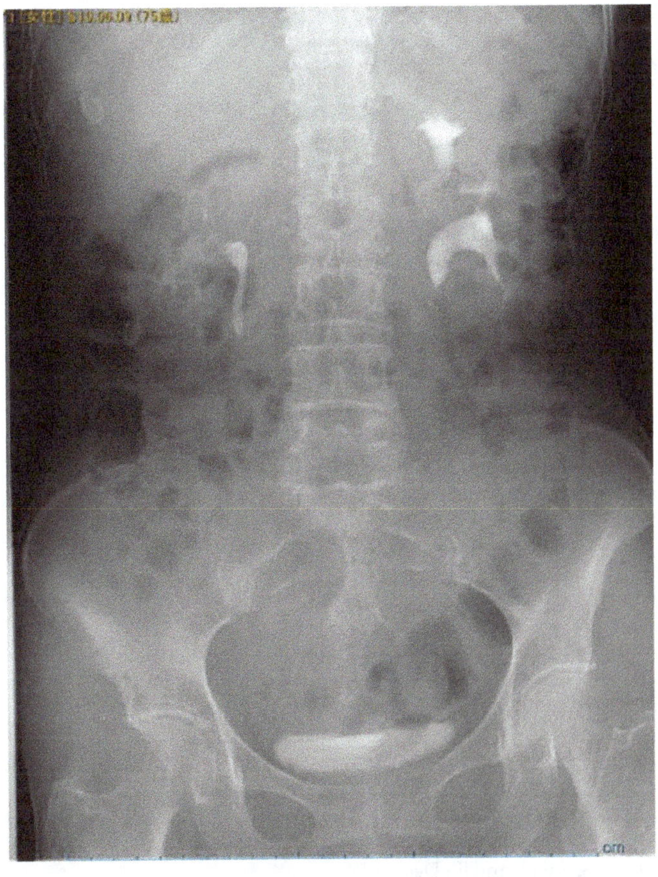

Figure 6: IVP shows the improvement of the hydronephrosis of the left lower-pole 3 months postoperatively.

[7]. In complete and incomplete duplex systems, UPJO of the lower-pole is a common cause of obstruction [2]. This may be explained by the fact that the lower segment is anatomically the analogue of a single renal system, which usually corresponds to about two-thirds of the parenchyma, and at least 2 calyces and a true renal pelvis [2].

Several endoscopic techniques have been developed as alternatives to open surgery, and the endoscopic approach to UPJ has been successful for both antegrade and retrograde procedures, offering the advantages of shorter operative time, less morbidity, reduction of postoperative analgesic requirements, and shorter hospital stay. Retrograde endoscopic procedures thought to be the most minimally invasive, endopyelotomy, laser incision, Acucise, and balloon dilatation have been reported to be performed successfully.

In this case, transurethral retrograde balloon dilatation was performed for the ureteral obstruction close to UPJ of the lower-pole with a left incomplete duplicated collecting system, after which a ureteral stent was inserted to the lower-pole. However, there was urinary leakage at the dilated ureteral stenosis lesion, and therefore, another ureteral stent needed to be inserted to the upper-pole because the ureteral obstruction was close to the junction of upper and lower poles in the incomplete duplicated collecting system; therefore, urinary leakage started from the operated ureteral stricture lesion from the upper-pole. Fortunately, a 2nd ureteral stent could be inserted to the upper-pole just after balloon dilatation and urinary leakage was minimal after operation. Although laparoscopic or open approach might be safer and effective from the beginning in this case, retrograde endoscopic procedures were thought to be the most minimally invasive and should be tried first.

4. Conclusion

When we manage UPJO and/or ureteral stenosis close to UPJ of the lower-pole with an incomplete duplicated system by retrograde balloon dilatation, we should keep in mind the possibility of urinary leakage from the upper-pole and the need for another stent to the upper-pole.

Abbreviations

UPJ: Ureteropelvic junction
UPJO: Ureteropelvic junction obstruction
CT: Computed tomography
IVP: Intravenous pyelography
RP: Retrograde pyelography.

Authors' Contributions

All authors have read and approved the final version of the manuscript.

References

[1] M. Taniguchi, S. Kamei, T. Takeuchi, S. Sakai, and T. Deguchi, "Successful management of lower pole moiety ureteropelvic junction obstruction in a partially duplicated collecting system using retrograde endoureteropyelotomy with the Holmium:YAG laser," *International Journal of Urology*, vol. 12, no. 3, pp. 313–315, 2005.

[2] A. Okamura, A. Komiya, and H. Kitamura, "Retrograde balloon dilatation for the management of upper-pole ureteropelvic junction obstruction in an incomplete duplicated collecting system," *Japanese Journal of Endourolog*, vol. 30, pp. 107–110, 2017.

[3] E. Hwang, Y. H. Kim, S. W. Yang et al., "Successful endourologic management of lower pole moiety ureteropelvic obstruction in a partially duplicated collecting system," *Korean Journal of Urology*, vol. 51, no. 6, pp. 434–437, 2010.

[4] D. Bruno, F. C. Delvecchio, and G. M. Preminger, "Successful management of lower-pole moiety ureteropelvic junction obstruction in a partially duplicated collecting system using minimally invasive retrograde endoscopic techniques," *Journal of Endourology*, vol. 14, no. 9, pp. 727–730, 2000.

[5] C. C. Schulman, "The ureter," in *Pediatric Urology*, B. O'Donnell and S. A. Koff, Eds., pp. 397–418, Butterworths, 1997.

[6] D. B. Joseph, S. B. Bauer, A. H. Colodny, J. Mandell, R. L. Lebowitz, and A. B. Retik, "Lower pole ureteropelvic junction obstruction and incomplete renal duplication," *The Journal of Urology*, vol. 141, no. 4, pp. 896–899, 1989.

[7] S. C. Flashner and L. R. King, "Ureteropelvic junction," in *Clinical Pediatric Urology*, pp. 693–725, WB Saunders, Philadelphia, 3rd edition, 1992.

24

An Unconcealed Reservoir: Case Report of Erosion of Inflatable Penile Implant Reservoir through the Anus

Mark Arthur,[1] **Jonathan Canete**,[2,3] **and Charles Welliver**[1,3]

[1]*Albany Medical College, Department of General Surgery, Division of Urology, Albany, NY, USA*
[2]*Albany Medical College, Department of General Surgery, Section of Colon and Rectal Surgery, Albany, NY, USA*
[3]*Albany Stratton Veterans Affairs Medical Center, Albany, NY, USA*

Correspondence should be addressed to Mark Arthur; arthurm@amc.edu

Academic Editor: Mohamed A. Ghoneim

Inflatable penile prosthesis (IPP) involves placement of the fluid reservoir into an abdominal or pelvic location. While the space of Retzius (SOR) was the preferred site for many years, the change from open to robotic prostatectomy made this space less desirable due to the violation of the peritoneum with the robotic approach. Other factors like previous abdominal or pelvic surgeries (particularly inguinal hernia repair with mesh) may also require a change in location of the reservoir during IPP placement. In this report, we discuss a previously undescribed result of alternative reservoir placement (ARP) with erosion of the reservoir through the colon and out of the anus in a man with multiple previous abdominal surgeries. Management of this clinical problem is also discussed.

1. Introduction

Inflatable penile prosthetics (IPP) are a surgical treatment of erectile dysfunction (ED) often reserved for medically refractory cases. The typical IPP consists of 3 parts: inflatable cylinders within the penis, a scrotal pump, and a fluid reservoir which is placed in the abdomen or pelvis.

Traditionally, the fluid reservoir was placed within the space of Retzius (SOR) for IPP. With the change to robotically assisted laparoscopic prostatectomy (RALP) and resulting concerns about the safety of the SOR after the violation of the peritoneum that occurs with RALP, alternative reservoir placement (ARP) sites have grown in popularity [1]. The abdominal wall space avoids the SOR but has its own unique set of complications [2–4].

In this case, we present a unique device herniation and resulting patient management. In this case, a patient's reservoir eroded through the colon and ultimately out of his anus.

2. Case Presentation

A 56-year-old male patient presented to the emergency department after passing two dark brown, loose stools followed by the feeling of something protruding from his anus. The protrusion was observed to be the reservoir for his IPP (Figures 1 and 2).

The patient's past medical history includes an IPP (AMS CX 700, Boston Scientific, Marlborough, Massachusetts) placed through a penoscrotal approach three years prior to presentation at our emergency department. The reservoir was placed via abdominal incision due to previous bilateral inguinal hernia repair with mesh. The reservoir was placed below the rectus muscles on the right side after entering through the fascia. A month prior to his presentation at our institution, he had a laparoscopic appendectomy complicated with postoperative ileus. At the time of clinical presentation in the emergency department, his white blood cell count was not elevated and he was afebrile. His scrotum was mildly erythematous, but otherwise, his IPP was not concerning for clinical infection.

He was initially treated with intravenous antibiotics and scheduled for surgery the next day. His IPP was found to still be functional before surgery (Figure 3). During surgery, urology removed the IPP and colorectal surgery performed a diagnostic laparoscopy that did not identify an intraperitoneal

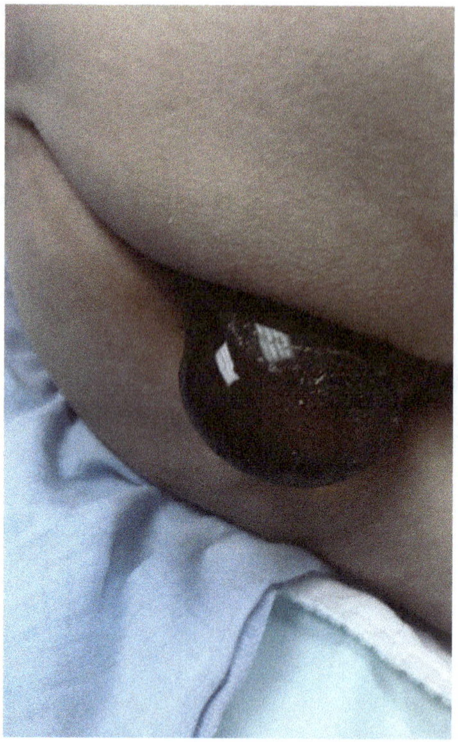

FIGURE 1: Posterior view of reservoir protrusion through the anus.

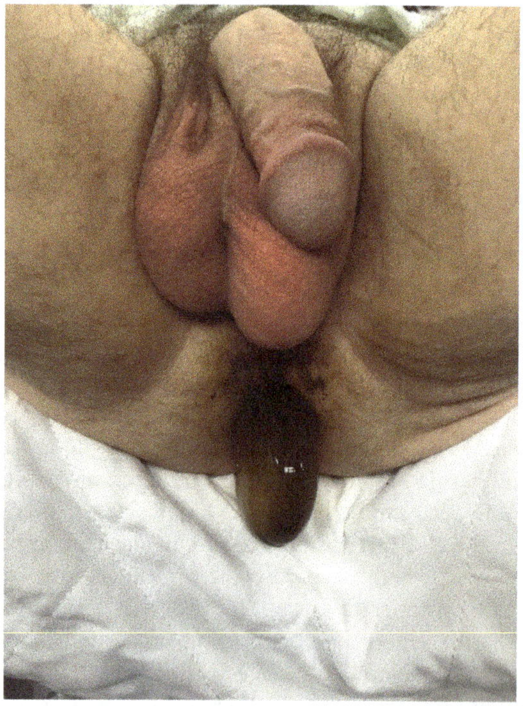

FIGURE 2: Inferior view of reservoir protrusion through the anus.

component of the penile implant. Loop sigmoid colostomy was then created. Anorectal examination using an anoscope could not identify laceration or other injury to the colon even to a distance 10 cm proximal to the anal verge. After IPP removal and washout, a malleable implant was placed through the penoscrotal incision.

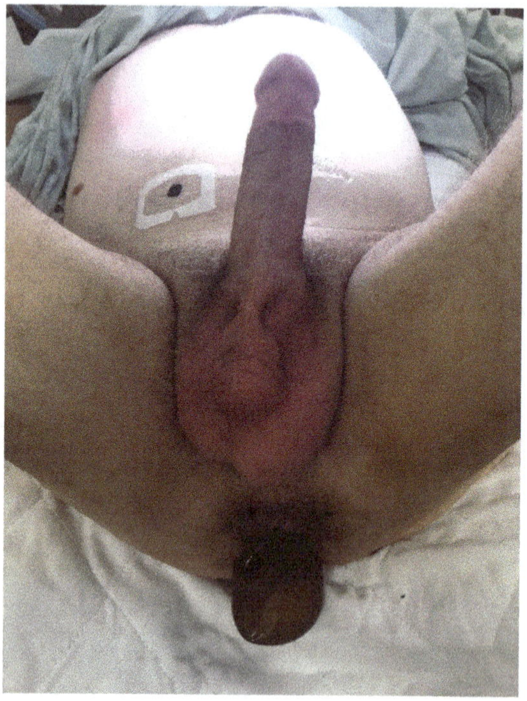

FIGURE 3: Protrusion of a deflated reservoir through the anus demonstrating maintained function of implant device.

At urology follow-up, the malleable implant was without signs of infection. At six-week surgical follow-up with colorectal surgery, a gastrografin enema was performed to evaluate the integrity of the rectum, and a small linear streak of contrast was seen emanating from the anterior aspect of the rectum. Spontaneous resolution was anticipated, and the patient was advised to keep the loop colostomy. At the next follow-up two months later, another gastrografin enema was performed and leakage from the rectum was not observed at which point the colostomy was reversed, and normal bowel function resumed.

3. Discussion

Historically, placement of the reservoir during IPP was through the inguinal canal into the SOR. However, ARP is gaining popularity as this approach does not risk damaging retropubic structures and can be done safely in patients with prior pelvic surgeries (principally RALP) [1, 2]. In this case, ARP was required as the SOR was inaccessible due to previous bilateral hernia repair with mesh. Unfortunately, ARP and the subsequent surgeries led to a previously undescribed finding of the reservoir protruding from the anus.

The advent and resulting increase in the use of RALP, with its violation of the peritoneum to access the pelvis, changed how implanters approach placement of the reservoir. ARP does allow for implants to avoid the SOR but is not without its own unique set of complications. As most penile implants are placed via penoscrotal incision [5], the placement into either the SOR or the ARP is done blindly. In an interesting study looking at reservoir insertion through the penoscrotal approach into a projected high submuscular space, 80% were found in the ideal spot anterior to the transversalis muscle. However, reservoirs were also found in the retroperitoneal (10%), preperitoneal (5%), and intraperitoneal spaces (5%) [6]. In a multicenter study looking at the need for surgical revisions of IPP reservoirs, statistically similar rates were seen between ARP and SOR placement (2.0 vs 1.3%, $p = 0.44$) with reservoir fluid leakage the most common reason for device revision [2].

While our complication of the reservoir protruding from the anus has not been previously described, erosion into visceral strictures including the bowel is not unique. A comprehensive review and case series done by Levine et al. in 2012 found 8 cases with reservoir herniation into the bowel, 6 into the small intestine, and 2 into the large intestine [7]. All 8 individuals had prior pelvic or abdominal surgeries. Other older reports have also described bowel erosion even during the time of standard SOR reservoir placement [8, 9].

The nonemergent way this clinical problem was managed is also notable. While the implant was obviously infected due to the bowel-related erosion and exposure of the reservoir, the patient presented without life threatening or urgent signs of infection. In this case, intravenous antibiotics were started to decrease any surrounding soft tissue infection around the device with surgical treatment the next day. Malleable implant was then placed which has a high success rate even with clinically infected implants [10].

4. Conclusion

Previous abdominal surgery is clearly a risk factor for visceral erosion of IPP reservoirs but may be managed with antibiotics and delayed malleable implant placement in patients without concerning clinical signs of infection.

Disclosure

Albany Medical College had no influence on the research, authorship, and/or publication of this article.

Acknowledgments

The authors received financial support for the APC from Albany Medical College.

References

[1] D. S. Stember, B. B. Garber, and P. E. Perito, "Outcomes of abdominal wall reservoir placement in inflatable penile prosthesis implantation: a safe and efficacious alternative to the space of Retzius," *The Journal of Sexual Medicine*, vol. 11, no. 2, pp. 605–612, 2014.

[2] J. C. Hernández, L. Trost, T. S. Kohler et al., "Emerging complications following alternative reservoir placement during inflatable penile prosthesis placement: a 5-year multi-institutional experience," *The Journal of Urology*, vol. 201, no. 3, pp. 581–586, 2019.

[3] J. Clavell-Hernández, A. Shah, and R. Wang, "Non-infectious reservoir-related complications during and after penile prosthesis placement," *Sexual Medicine Reviews*, vol. 7, no. 3, pp. 521–529, 2019.

[4] M. S. Gross, D. S. Stember, B. B. Garber, and P. E. Perito, "A retrospective analysis of risk factors for IPP reservoir entry into the peritoneum after abdominal wall placement," *International Journal of Impotence Research*, vol. 29, no. 5, pp. 215–218, 2017.

[5] W. Bass, B. O'Connor, C. Welliver et al., "Worldwide trends in penile implantation surgery: data from over 63,000 implants," *Translational Andrology and Urology*, vol. 9, no. 1, pp. 31–37, 2020.

[6] M. J. Ziegelmann, B. R. Viers, D. J. Lomas, M. R. Westerman, and L. W. Trost, "Ectopic penile prosthesis reservoir placement: an anatomic cadaver model of the high submuscular technique," *The Journal of Sexual Medicine*, vol. 13, no. 9, pp. 1425–1431, 2016.

[7] L. A. Levine and M. P. Hoeh, "Review of penile prosthetic reservoir: complications and presentation of a modified reservoir placement technique," *The Journal of Sexual Medicine*, vol. 9, no. 11, pp. 2759–2769, 2012.

[8] I. Singh and C. J. Godec, "Asynchronous erosion of inflatable penile prosthesis into small and large bowel," *The Journal of Urology*, vol. 147, 3, Part 1, pp. 709-710, 1992.

[9] G. E. Leach, C. E. Shapiro, R. Hadley, and S. Raz, "Erosion of inflatable penile prosthesis reservoir into bladder and bowel," *The Journal of Urology*, vol. 131, no. 6, pp. 1177-1178, 1984.

[10] M. S. Gross, E. A. Phillips, A. Balen et al., "The malleable implant salvage technique: infection outcomes after Mulcahy salvage procedure and replacement of infected inflatable penile prosthesis with malleable prosthesis," *The Journal of Urology*, vol. 195, no. 3, pp. 694–698, 2016.

25

Torsion of an Epididymal Cyst: A Rare Finding on Scrotal Exploration for Acute Scrotum

A. M. Omar Mohamed Ozaal,[1] B. Pragalathan,[1] S. Lavanya,[1] and S. T. Sarma[2]

[1]*General Surgery, University Surgical Unit, Teaching Hospital Jaffna, Sri Lanka*
[2]*University Surgical Unit, Teaching Hospital Jaffna, Sri Lanka*

Correspondence should be addressed to A. M. Omar Mohamed Ozaal; ozaalnew@gmail.com

Academic Editor: Tun-Chieh Chen

Torsion of epididymal cyst (EC) is an exceedingly rare cause of acute scrotum in both children and adults. We add our case as the ninth case to literature which was an 8-year-old child presented with features of acute scrotum with history of EC on conservative management. Doppler sonography showed perfused normal bilateral testes and a 4.1 × 1.7 cm septate cystic lesion of right epididymis. On scrotal exploration, we found a haemorrhagic cystic lesion attached to the upper pole of right testis and twisted for 540 degrees with normal testis and appendage. Cyst was excised, and histopathology revealed a haemorrhagic EC. Our case was peculiar due to, presenting as acute scrotum in a child of 1-10 years age group who was conservatively managed for right-sided EC and presence of 540 degrees torsion.

1. Introduction

Acute scrotum can be considered as a urological equivalent of acute abdomen in general surgery. There are myriad of causes for acute scrotum ranging from torsion of testes or appendages, traumatic injuries, infections and inflammatory conditions of testes. Several conditions will require scrotal exploration, and patients should be assessed clinically along with imaging studies as it is time sensitive.

Epididymal cyst (EC) is a benign lesion in children and ranges from 5% to 20% in the literature in contrast to adults where it is common [1]. They are of unknown aetiology, common in testicular maldescent, and managed conservatively with spontaneous regression in most instances [2]. Torsion of EC is rare and a scarce finding on scrotal exploration for acute scrotum. There were eight paediatric cases reported in the literature (Table 1), and among them, seven cases were all adolescents, and one was an infant [1, 3–5]. Our patient is an 8-year-old child and the first case of EC torsion in this age group to be reported and added as the ninth case to the literature.

2. Case Presentation

An 8-year-old boy was admitted to our casualty ward with persistent scrotal pain of 2 days duration associated with nausea and one episode of vomiting. He was treated by local general practitioner with analgesics the day prior and denied preceding trauma to scrotum. But he was investigated for right hemi-scrotal pain without any history of trauma 2 months back in a peripheral hospital. He was diagnosed to have a right-sided EC and opted for conservative management.

On examination, right hemi-scrotal tenderness and high riding right testis were found. Left hemi-scrotal palpation, abdominal examination, and hernial orifices were unremarkable. Urgent sonography with Doppler showed a septate cystic lesion of right epididymis, sized 4.1 cm × 1.7 cm (Figure 1) along with bilateral normally echogenic and perfused testes.

Scrotal exploration under general anaesthesia was performed which revealed oedematous tunica vaginalis, age appropriately sized right testis, normal testicular appendage, and 4 cm × 2 cm sized dark haemorrhagic cystic lesion. The

Table 1: List of cases in literature with brief description.

Case no.	Authors	Brief description
1st case	RI. Kaye et al., 1990	Left-sided 360° torsed EC in a 13-year-old boy
2nd case	N. Liolios et al., 1997	Left-sided 360° torsed EC in a 6-month-old male
3rd case	E. Yılmaz et al., 2004	Left-sided 720° torsed EC in a 13-year-old boy with history of scrotal trauma
4th case	V. Erikçi et al., 2013	Left-sided 720° torsed EC in an 11-year-old boy on conservative management for EC with no history of scrotal trauma
5th case	Y. Akın et al., 2014	Bilateral simple ECs in a 14-year-old boy with no history of scrotal trauma
6th case	M. Ameli et al., 2015	Left-sided 720° torsed EC in a 14-year-old boy with history of scrotal trauma
7th case	C. Bleve et al., 2018	Right-sided 720° torsed EC in a 16-year-old boy with no history of scrotal trauma
8th case	M. Messina et al., 2019	Left-sided twisted EC in a 13-year-old boy with no history of scrotal trauma
This case		Right-sided 540° torsed EC in an 8-year-old child with no history of scrotal trauma who was on conservative management for EC.

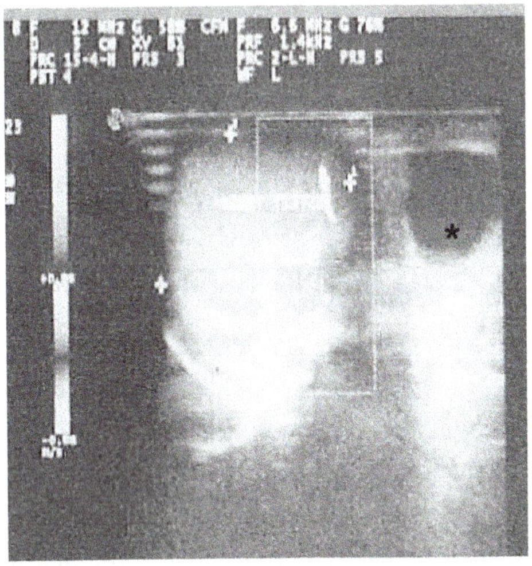

Figure 1: Ultrasound image of right testis with epididymal cyst* (on acute presentation).

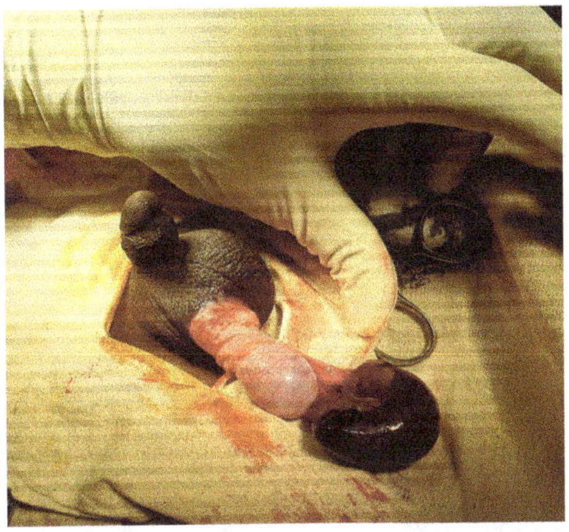

Figure 2: Twisted right Epididymal cyst with normal testis.

lesion appeared to be attached to the upper pole of right testis and was twisted for 540 degrees (Figure 2).

Cyst was untwisted (Figure 3) and excised, and the testis was fixed. Histopathological assessment revealed haemorrhagic EC (Figure 4). Patient was discharged the next day following unremarkable recovery, with analgesics and oral antibiotics.

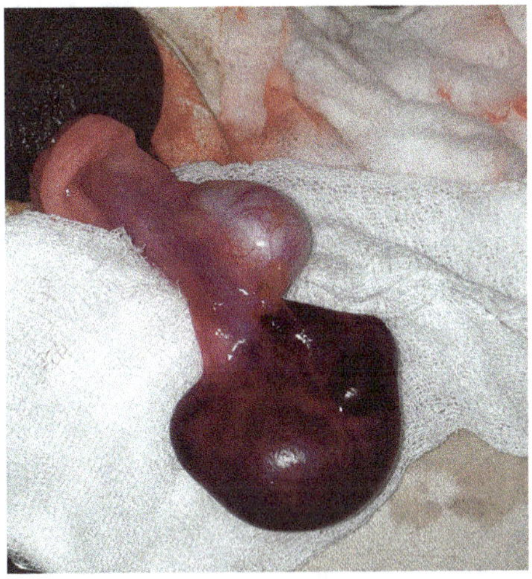

Figure 3: Untwisted hemorrhagic right Epididymal cyst.

3. Discussion

Epididymal cysts occur in 94.9% of boys older than 10 years, and 71.2% of them are older than 14 years [2]. In our case, the patient was 8 years old and presented with features of an acute scrotum. At the time of admission to ward, neither history of previous ultrasound evidence of a right-sided EC was provided by the patient and guardian nor the previous medical records were available with the patient.

Our line of management was towards torsion of testis derived from the acuteness of presentation with swollen and high ridden testis. Even though Doppler sonography showed a perfused right testis, the patient had persistent scrotal pain with few bouts of vomiting. This prompted us to go ahead with scrotal exploration. Torsion of an EC was not considered into the differential diagnosis due to its rarity over a torsion of testicular appendage.

Intraoperative finding of a twisted haemorrhagic cystic lesion arising from the epididymal location of the right testis attached to its upper pole, confirmed the diagnosis of a torsed

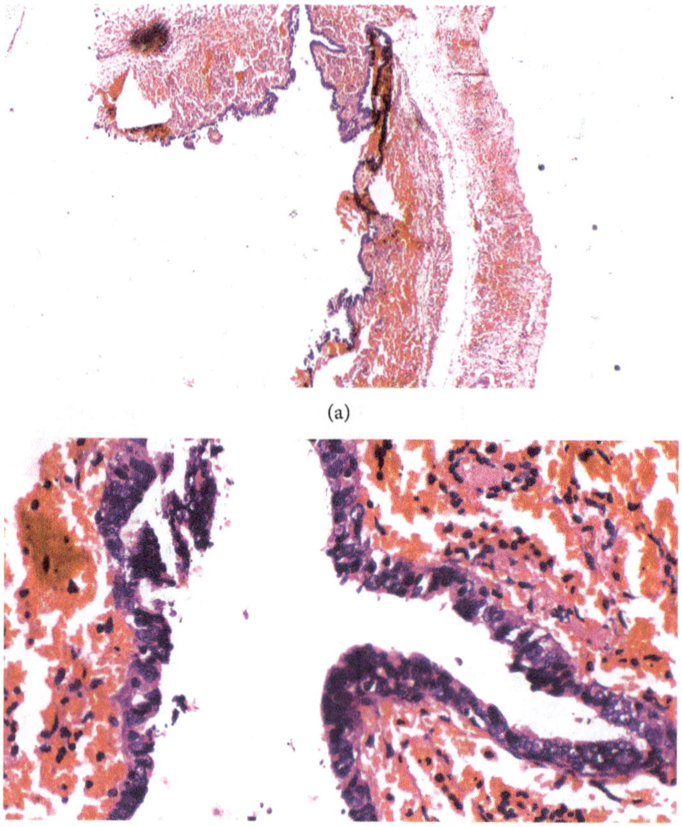

(a)

(b)

Figure 4: (a) Low and (b) high power views of the epididymal cyst wall with columnar epithelium showing congestion and haemorrhage.

EC and led us to carry out excision. The twist was 540 degrees, whereas in the literature, it ranged from 360 to 720 degrees [1, 3–5]. In line with majority of the literature, there was no associated prior scrotal trauma.

Particularity of our case was due to being the first case of torsed EC in a child of 1-10 years age group and being torsed for 540 degrees. It is the second case of a right-sided EC and has an acute presentation in previously diagnosed case of an EC. Bleve et al. [3] reported the first case of torsed right sided EC and the remaining seven cases in the literature (Table 1) are left sided lesions.

Erikci et al. [1] also have reported a case of EC torsion in an 11-year-old boy who was put on conservative management for an EC [1]. Presentation with features of acute scrotum such as pain and swelling was similar among all reported cases [1, 3–5]. Management of an EC is usually conservative as 60% of the cases regress on its own more importantly if less than 3 cm in size [2].

4. Learning Points

In conclusion, in line with literature, it is acceptable to perform elective surgery in children for ECs more than 10 mm in size, which are symptomatic, and which are persistent in nature [2].

In cases of ECs opted for conservative management, patients and guardians should be advised on symptoms of acute scrotum and when to seek immediate medical help.

We emphasize the importance of adequate background history taking from the patient as well as the guardian. And it can help to consider a torsed EC as a differential diagnosis in acute scrotum, even though it is rare but important in cases with past history of an EC.

Consent

Informed written consent was obtained from the guardian for publication of this case report and the image. A copy of it is available for review in our unit.

References

[1] V. Erikçi, M. Hosgör, M. Yildiz et al., "Torsion of an epididymal cyst: a case report and review of the literature," *The Turkish Journal of Pediatrics*, vol. 55, no. 6, pp. 659–661, 2013.

[2] J. Niedzielski, M. Miodek, and M. Krakós, "Epididymal cysts in childhood-conservative or surgical approach?," *Polski Przeglad Chirurgiczny*, vol. 84, no. 8, pp. 406–410, 2012.

[3] C. Bleve, M. L. Conighi, V. Bucci, L. Costa, and S. F. Chiarenza, "Torsion of huge epididymal cyst in a 16-year-old boy: case report and review of the literature," *La Pediatria Medica e Chirurgica*, vol. 40, pp. 20–22, 2018.

[4] M. Messina, G. Fusi, F. Ferrara et al., "A rare cause of acute scrotum in a child: torsion of an epididymal cyst. Case report

and review of the literature," *La Pediatria medica e chirurgica: Medical and surgical pediatrics*, vol. 41, no. 1, 2019.

[5] M. Ameli, S. Boroumand-Noughabi, and L. Gholami-Mahtaj, "A 14-year-old boy with torsion of the epididymal cyst," *Case Reports in Urology*, vol. 2015, Article ID 731987, 3 pages, 2015.

26

Utilizing Colpocleisis to Repair a Vesicovaginal Fistula in a Cervical Cancer Patient with History of Pelvic Radiation: A Case Report and Literature Review

Ahmad Dahman,[1] Daniel McClelland,[2] Stanley Zaslau,[2,3] Valerie Galvan Turner,[3] Omar Duenas,[3] and Robert Shapiro[2,3]

[1] *West Virginia University School of Medicine, Morgantown, WV 26506, USA*
[2] *Department of Urology, West Virginia University School of Medicine, Morgantown, WV 26506, USA*
[3] *Department of Obstetrics & Gynecology, West Virginia University School of Medicine, Morgantown, WV 26506, USA*

Correspondence should be addressed to Robert Shapiro; rshapiro@hsc.wvu.edu

Academic Editor: Sigurdur Gudjonsson

Background. Vesicovaginal fistula is a rare and distressing urological condition. It is especially prevalent in developing countries with the predominant etiology secondary to obstructed labor. Radiation therapy in female patients with cervical cancer is a risk factor for vesicovaginal fistula formation in the United States. *Case Presentation.* A 53-year-old woman with a history of cervical cancer and radiation presented with continuous urinary incontinence. Following diagnostic vaginoscopy, a 1 cm vesicovaginal fistula was diagnosed at the vaginal apex. The patient elected for surgical repair. She subsequently underwent successful transvaginal fistula closure using colpocleisis to optimally address the systemic factors of poor wound healing associated with irradiated tissue. Because of the adjacent tissue having been compromised by pelvic radiation, we opted to use a biologic graft made of human cadaveric pericardial tissue (CPT) instead of a native tissue flap to provide additional support for the fistula repair. *Conclusion.* A transvaginal approach for surgical repair of vesicovaginal fistula can be successful in patients with a prior history of pelvic radiation. Transvaginal colpocleisis is a viable option to augment vesicovaginal fistula repair for patients with significant comorbidities when sexual intercourse is no longer desired.

1. Introduction

Vesicovaginal fistula (VVF) is a distressing gynecologic complication that occurs when an abnormal connection forms between the bladder and the vagina [1]. While rare in the United States, it is still a prevalent issue for women in developing countries with studies projecting upwards of three million women living with unrepaired VVFs [1]. The most common etiology of VVF is obstructed labor, accounting for around 90% of fistulas in women of developing countries [1]. Other risk factors include adjacent malignancy, radiation, and repetitive pelvic operations. Classically, a patient presents with continuous urine leakage from her vagina. If radiation is a contributing factor, this presentation may be delayed by years. Diagnosis is clinical with a relevant history and physical examination but can be confirmed with instillation of methylene blue into the bladder and further characterized with specific imaging studies.

The mainstay of treatment is surgery with the option to approach vaginally or abdominally [2]. The vaginal approach minimizes blood loss, hospital stay, and pain [2]. In the following, we report a case of a 54-year-old woman with a challenging VVF resulting from stage four cervical cancer and history of brachytherapy to the vagina. The fistula was successfully treated with transvaginal colpocleisis.

2. Case Presentation

A 53-year-old woman first presented to our clinic as a referral for evaluation of urinary incontinence. She had a complex history, including stage four cervical cancer nine years prior that had invaded the bladder and been treated with combination brachytherapy, external beam radiation, and chemotherapy. Her urinary incontinence complaint traced back seven months and was characterized as a complete loss of bladder control. Speculum examination revealed the pooling of urine in the vaginal vault with a high suspicion for VVF. The patient did not have evidence of recurrent cervical cancer. Two weeks later, she underwent rigid cystourethroscopy with bilateral ureteral catheterization, bilateral retrograde pyelography, and vaginoscopy. The procedure showed a fistula tract on the anterior vaginal wall extending medially into the bladder just posterior to the trigone (Figure 1). No evidence of upper tract obstruction was seen on retrograde pyelography. No vaginal stricture was present preventing access to the fistula. The fistula tract was biopsied and revealed no evidence for recurrence of her cervix cancer.

Due to her prior history of pelvic radiation and morbid obesity with a BMI of 54.95 kg/m^2, a vaginal approach was opted for to limit postoperative complications associated with poor wound healing. We began by inserting a 22 French rigid cystoscope with a 30-degree lens into the bladder through the urethra. Bilateral ureteral orifices were in normal position, and the large fistula tract was noted to be supratrigonal, away from the ureteral orifices. We then placed a 0.035 straight sensor wire into the left ureteral orifice up to the kidney. A 5-French Pollack catheter was passed over this wire and the procedure was repeated on the right side, providing identification of the ureters for the remainder of the procedure. Vaginoscopy was then performed, and a 0.035 straight sensor wire was passed through the fistula opening. We returned to the bladder with the cystoscope, where we grasped the distal end of the sensor wire. A 10-French silicone catheter was placed over this using a modified Seldinger technique with 10 mL in the balloon to identify the fistula tract. The setup was completed and we moved forward with the fistula repair (Figure 2).

We began by placing 3-0 Vicryl sutures on the superior and inferior aspects of the labia majora to provide more retraction. A lone star retractor was placed with skin hooks deeper in the vagina to maximize exposure. Following exposure, vasopressin solution was injected circumferentially around the fistula and posterior vaginal wall to provide hemostasis and hydrodissection. Using a 15-blade scalpel, the anterior vagina was incised circumferentially around the fistulous tract. In the same plane, the vagina was dissected away from surrounding tissue with Metzenbaum scissors. This maneuver was repeated on the posterior aspect of the vagina. After the vaginal flaps were elevated sufficiently, we continued dissection proximally to the fistula. Once around the tract, we used 3-0 Vicryl sutures on a UR6 needle to close the mucosal edges over the fistula tract. A moderate fill test of the bladder revealed no leak. A biologic graft made of CPT was prepped with a soak time of 30 minutes and cut into 2 × 2 cm squares. With the 3-0 Vicryl on a UR6, we placed the dermis in a quilted fashion overlying the repair (Figure 3). Once properly placed, we began sewing the rectovaginal fascia to the pubovesical fascia with 3-0 Vicryl on a UR6 in a tension-free fashion to obliterate the vaginal opening. We concluded by trimming and closing the vaginal mucosa, thereby finishing the colpocleisis to provide the extra layer of support (Figure 4). A final moderate fill test was performed, which ensured no leak.

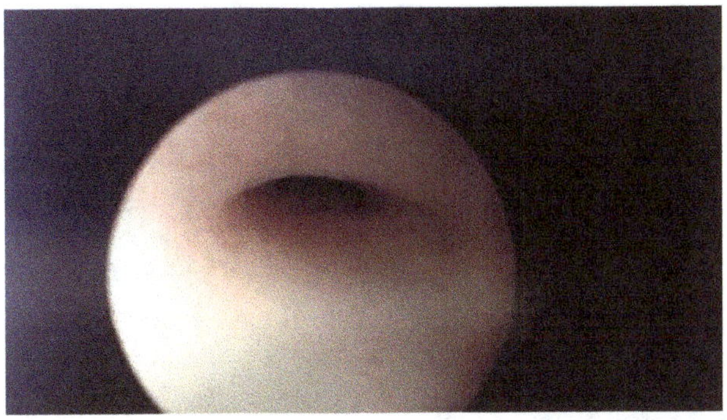

FIGURE 1: Fistula tract visualized by rigid cystourethroscopy in the urinary bladder.

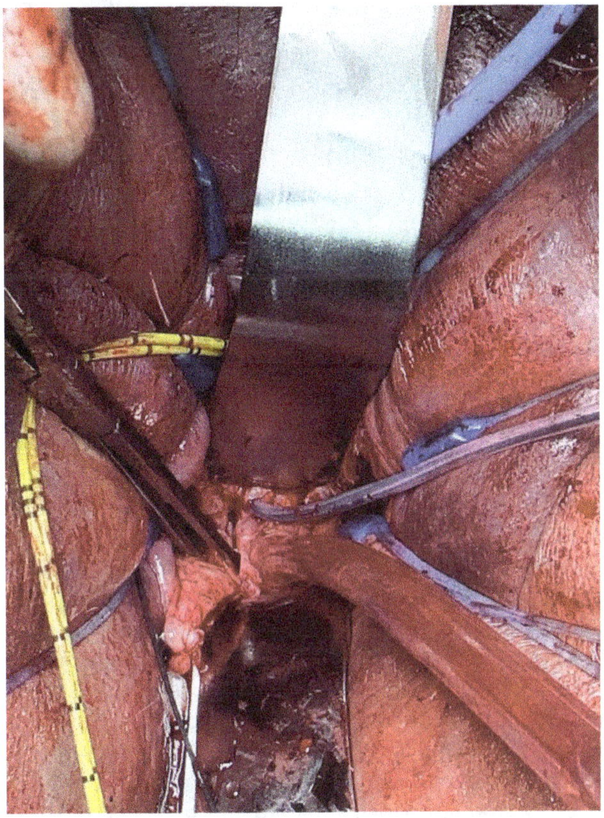

FIGURE 2: Ureteral catheters (yellow) retracted away from the operative field. A 10F Foley catheter was shown exiting the fistula tract along the anterior vaginal wall just inferior to the metal retractor.

The patient presented two weeks postoperatively with a negative cystogram. The patient was seen at six months from surgery and continues to be completely dry.

3. Discussion

Surgical management of vesicovaginal fistulas includes multiple approaches either abdominally or vaginally. The specific

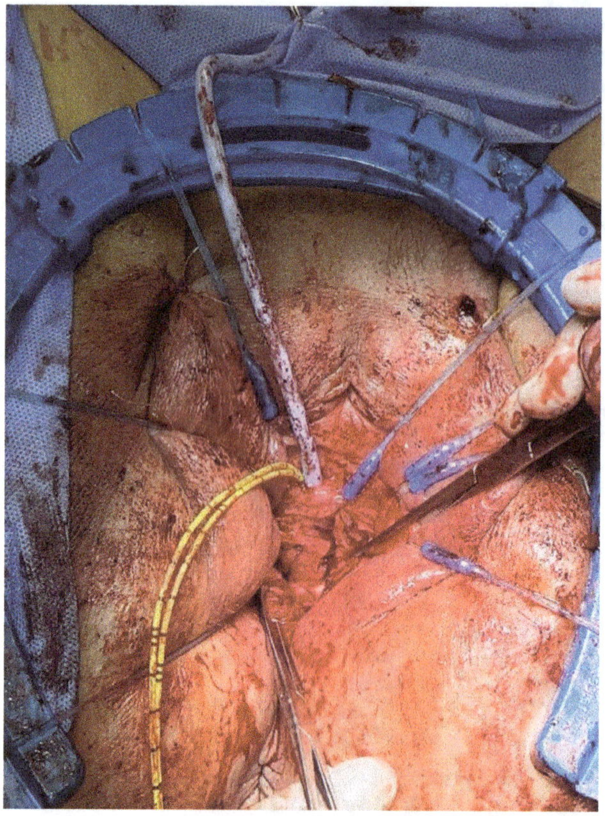

Figure 3: Biologic graft made of human cadaveric dermis placed over the fistula tract using allis clamps.

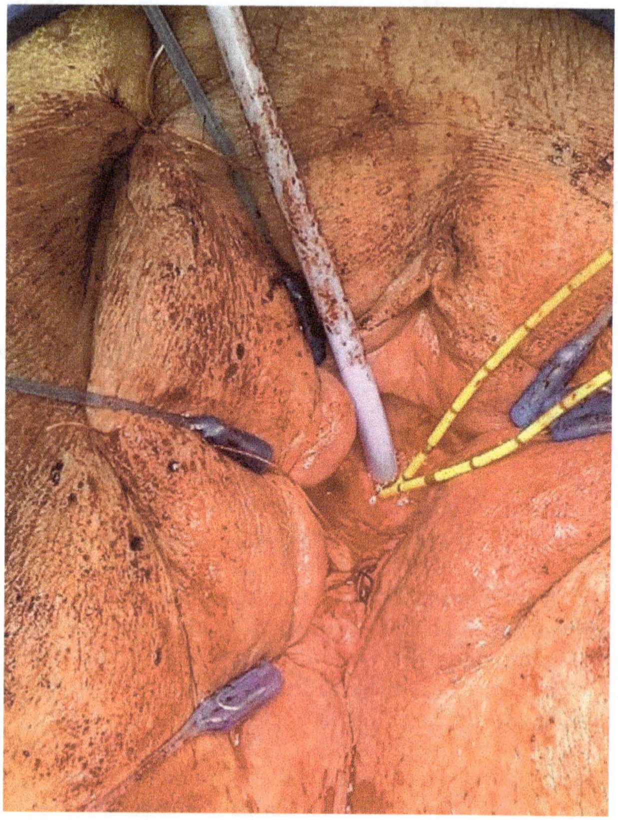

Figure 4: Completed fistula repair using colpocleisis to obliterate the vaginal opening.

characteristics of each patient help direct the optimal approach. In the case of a patient with significant radiation history, such as ours, access to the vagina may be limited on account of stricture formation. The reported incidence of radiation-induced vaginal stricture among patients with cervical cancer is highly variable ranging from 1% to 88% [3]. This is likely on account of the wide variation in patient, tumor, and treatment factors. In our case, no vaginal stricture was present, and the fistula was easily accessible through the vagina. The vaginal approach may be advantageous over the abdominal approach for wound healing and recovery time, especially amongst patients that are morbidly obese.

Although little research exists regarding the physiologic mechanisms of vaginal wound healing, there are some known observations that may potentially make this an optimal approach for healing compared to the abdominal route. First, the vagina is highly vascularized [4], and because the wound-healing process is mediated by inflammation and neovascularization [5], this feature may account for improved wound healing compared to the abdominal route. Certain growth factors, such as platelet-derived growth factor [6], transforming growth factor [7], and fibroblast growth factor [8], have been shown to play a role in the wound-healing process. In theory, greater concentrations of these factors in the vagina versus the abdomen may improve wound healing.

In a traditional fistula repair, a flap can be used for tissue interposition as an adjunct to improve healing. Various interposition flaps have been described in the literature. These include omentum, peritoneum, labial, and gracilis muscle flaps [9–11]. When operating transvaginally, the Martius flap can be used. The Martius flap is derived from the labial fat pad [11]. The flap is tunneled under the labia minora to the site of fistula repair [11]. Because of this patient's prior history of malignancy and pelvic radiation, the tissue integrity of the labia was likely compromised. Therefore, we opted to use a biologic graft made of CPT instead of a native tissue flap to provide additional support for the fistula repair. Our case is unique with the usage of CPT to augment the closure and thereby reduce the risk of fistula recurrence.

A paucity of studies exists on biologic grafts used in the setting of vesicovaginal fistulas. Caja et al. reported on the use of CPT interposition to decrease the risk of vesicovaginal fistula formation [12]. Due to the low cost, ease of handling, and less immunogenicity, CPT may be used to help prevent fistula formation [13]. Literature from colon and rectal surgery reports good success with utilizing porcine submucosa to close fistula tracts of the anus [14].

Traditionally, colpocleisis was used to treat advanced pelvic organ prolapse in patients that no longer wished to be sexually active [15]. In 1942, Latzko reported a technique (derived from Simon's procedure), whereby vault vesicovaginal fistulas were treated through a purely vaginal approach. It consists of a vault colpocleisis without any attempt at the dissection of the fistulous tract [16]. A review of literature revealed a retrospective study done that examined the success of the procedure [17]. Over a 15-year period from 1991 to 2005, the procedure was done to repair 11 VVFs. The mean size of the fistula was 12 mm and all eleven fistulas healed. No intraoperative complications occurred and only one postoperative lower urinary tract infection resulted. The mean hospital stay was 6 days. In select patients, the approach is a safe and effective option.

The radiated surrounding tissue and morbid obesity were some of the specific challenges unique to our patient. Unlike the Latzko procedure, we completely dissected the fistulous tract and sutured it closed without tension. Fully dissecting the fistula tract is somewhat controversial. Cruikshank [18] and Raz [19] reported a 100% success rate in their respective series of 11 and 65 patients without fistulous tract dissection. Because of the impaired blood supply of the surrounding irradiated tissue, we decided to fully dissect the fistula tract to optimize healing. Following the operation, the patient was discharged home on the same day and avoided any hospital stay. The major disadvantage of the technique is it has to be patient-specific as they will no longer be able to be sexually active in the future. In patients who no longer desire to be sexually active, this is a viable and safe approach to repair fistulas in challenging patients with significant medical comorbidities.

4. Conclusion

Vesicovaginal fistula is a rare clinical entity that is associated with high morbidity for many women. A thorough history and physical examination can help guide diagnosis, which can be confirmed using imaging such as vaginoscopy. Surgical correction is the mainstay of management and can be approached from different routes. While exposure can be more difficult, a transvaginal approach offers benefits regarding hospital stay and recovery. If the patient has additional comorbidities, as in our case with radiation and morbid obesity, wound healing appears to be an additional benefit to the transvaginal approach. Colpocleisis is a useful surgical technique to assist in closure and wound healing if the patient no longer desires to be sexually active. Such an approach provides a safe, less invasive option with the goal of decreasing morbidity.

Authors' Contributions

Ahmad Daman, Daniel McClelland, Stanley Zaslau, Valerie Galvan Turner, Omar Duenas, and Robert Shapiro carried out conception and design, acquisition, analysis, interpretation of data, and drafting. They reviewed the paper and gave final approval.

References

[1] M. Stamatakos, C. Sargedi, T. Stasinou, and K. Kontzoglou, "Vesicovaginal fistula: diagnosis and management," *The Indian Journal of Surgery*, vol. 76, no. 2, pp. 131–136, 2014.

[2] H. H. Woo, D. J. Rosario, and C. R. Chapple, "The treatment of vesicovaginal fistulae," *European Urology*, vol. 29, no. 1, pp. 1–9, 2017.

[3] P. Hartman and A. W. Diddle, "Vaginal stenosis following irradiation therapy for carcinoma of the cervix uteri," *Cancer*, vol. 30, no. 2, pp. 426–429, 1972.

[4] L. C. Junqueira, L. C. J. Vagina, and J. Carneiro, Eds., "Basic histology: text and atlas," in *Chapter 23: The Female Reproductive System*, pp. 493–496, McGraw-Hill Companies, New York, 10th ed edition, 2003.

[5] M. R. Hausman and B. D. Rinker, "Intractable wounds and infections: the role of impaired vascularity and advanced surgical methods for treatment," *American Journal of Surgery*, vol. 187, no. 5, pp. S44–S55, 2004.

[6] Z. Gao, T. Sasaoka, T. Fujimori et al., "Deletion of the PDGFR-beta gene affects key fibroblast functions important for wound healing," *The Journal of Biological Chemistry*, vol. 280, no. 10, pp. 9375–9389, 2005.

[7] E. B. Tredget, J. Demare, G. Chandran, E. E. Tredget, L. Yang, and A. Ghahary, "Transforming growth factor-beta and its effect on reepithelialization of partial-thickness ear wounds in transgenic mice," *Wound repair and regeneration*, vol. 13, no. 1, pp. 61–67, 2005.

[8] H. Chuma, H. Mizuta, S. Kudo, K. Takagi, and Y. Hiraki, "One day exposure to FGF-2 was sufficient for the regenerative repair of full- thickness defects of articular cartilage in rabbits," *OSTEOARTHRITIS CARTILAGE*, vol. 12, no. 10, pp. 834–842, 2004.

[9] V. Singh, R. J. Sinha, S. Mehrotra, S. N. Sankhwar, and S. Bhatt, "Repair of vesicovaginal fistula by the transabdominal route: outcome at a north Indian tertiary hospital," *International Urogynecology Journal*, vol. 23, no. 4, pp. 411–416, 2012.

[10] S. Raz, K. J. Bregg, V. W. Nitti, and E. Sussman, "Transvaginal repair of vesicovaginal fistula using a peritoneal flap," *The Journal of Urology*, vol. 150, no. 1, pp. 56–59, 1993.

[11] T. E. Elkins, J. O. DeLancey, and E. J. McGuire, "The use of modified Martius graft as an adjunctive technique in vesicovaginal and rectovaginal fistula repair," *Obstetrics and Gynecology*, vol. 75, no. 4, pp. 727–733, 1990.

[12] M. Caja, M. Lamonde, J. Barnard, S. Zaslau, and R. E. Shapiro, "Use of cadaveric pericardial tissue in the surgical treatment of neurogenic bladder," *Case Reports in Urology*, vol. 2019, Article ID 6182397, 4 pages, 2019.

[13] J. Hosseini, S. Hosseini, M. A. Hosseini, and Y. Rezaei, "Pericardium in reconstructive urologic surgeries: a systematic review and meta-analysis," *Urologia Internationalis*, vol. 102, no. 2, pp. 131–144, 2019.

[14] E. Bubbers and K. Cologne, "Management of complex anal fistulas," *Clinics in Colon and Rectal Surgery*, vol. 29, no. 1, pp. 43–49, 2016.

[15] S. Abbasy and K. Kenton, "Obliterative procedures for pelvic organ prolapse," *Clinical Obstetrics and Gynecology*, vol. 53, no. 1, pp. 86–98, 2010.

[16] W. Latzko, "Postoperative vesicovaginal fistulas: genesis and therapy," *American Journal of Surgery*, vol. 58, no. 2, pp. 211–228, 1942.

[17] Y. Ansquer, G. Mellier, P. Santulli et al., "Latzko operation for vault vesicovaginal fistula," *Acta Obstetricia et Gynecologica Scandinavica*, vol. 85, no. 10, pp. 1248–1251, 2006.

[18] S. H. Cruishank, "Early closure of post-hysterectomy vesicovaginal fistulas," *Southern Medical Journal*, vol. 81, no. 12, pp. 1525–1528, 1988.

[19] S. Raz, *Female urology*, no. article 3730377, 1893WB SaundersPhiladelphiapp, 1893.

27

Pathogenesis, Diagnosis and Management of Splenogonadal Fusion: A Literature Review

Youssef Kadouri,[1] Damien Carnicelli,[2] Hachem El Sayegh,[1] Lounis Benslimane,[1] and Yassine Nouini[1]

[1]*Faculty of Medicine and Pharmacy of Rabat Morocco, Ibn Sina Hospital, Department of Urology A, Mohammed V University, Morocco*
[2]*Department of Urology and Andrology, Center Hospitalier Métropole Savoie, Chambery, France*

Correspondence should be addressed to Youssef Kadouri; youcef.kadouri@gmail.com

Academic Editor: Apul Goel

Introduction. Splenogonadal fusion is a rare congenital anomaly, defined by the presence of ectopic splenic tissue caused by an abnormal connection between the spleen and the gonad or mesonephrotic derivatives during the embryonic period. *Materials and Methods.* By reporting an observational case and performing a review of the literature according to the CARE guidelines (using the PubMed database and guidelines from urology, general surgery, and pediatric learned societies), we present the embryological genesis of the splenogonadal fusion, the associated anatomical anomalies, and the diagnostic procedure. *Observation.* We report the case of a patient aged 45, with no notable history, reporting left testicular pain. A small nodule on the upper pole of the left testicular was clinically palpable. Tumor markers were normal, and scrotal ultrasound depicted a hypoechoic hypervascular nodule measuring 8 * 6 * 8 mm. After validation in a multidisciplinary oncology consultation meeting and opinion from a uro-andrologist expert, the patient underwent an inguinal lumpectomy with an extemporaneous examination which did not objectify any signs of malignancy. Ultimately, it is a normal spleen tissue in the testicular ectopic position. *Discussion.* Splenogonadal fusion corresponds to a rare congenital malformation; less than 200 cases have been published in the literature, most often affecting boys, with a sex ratio of 15/1. Two types are described, depending on the continuity of the link between the orthotopic spleen and the gonad: the continuous and discontinuous forms. In a third of the cases, there are associated congenital malformations and particularly in the continuous forms (44 to 50% of the cases): anomalies of the limbs, micrognathia, microgyria, and hepatic and digestive abnormalities. Cryptorchidism is associated with the continuous form in 31% of cases. The preoperative diagnosis remains difficult because of its morphological and clinical characteristics suggesting a tumor process.

1. Introduction

Splenogonadal fusion (SGF) is a rare congenital malformation, defined by the presence of ectopic splenic tissue caused by an abnormal connection between the spleen and the gonad or mesonephrotic derivatives during the embryonic period. Described for the first time in 1883 by Farthouat et al. [1] The age of the patients is less than 10 years in half of the cases reported, and 82% of the cases occur in young men under the age of 30. [2] The sex ratio is 15/1 [3]. It is often associated with other congenital anomalies and poses a problem of differential diagnosis with testicular tumors.

2. Materials and Methods

By reporting an observational case and performing a review of the literature according to the CARE guidelines (using the PubMed database and guidelines from urology, general surgery, and pediatric learned societies), we present the embryological genesis of the splenogonadal fusion, associated anatomical anomalies, and the diagnostic procedure. We used the following key word associations in French and English: "splenogonadal fusion" (Fusion splénogonadique) AND "congenital anomalies" (Anomalies congénitales), "splenogonadal fusion" AND "cryptorchidism" (Cryptorchidie), "splenogonadal fusion" AND

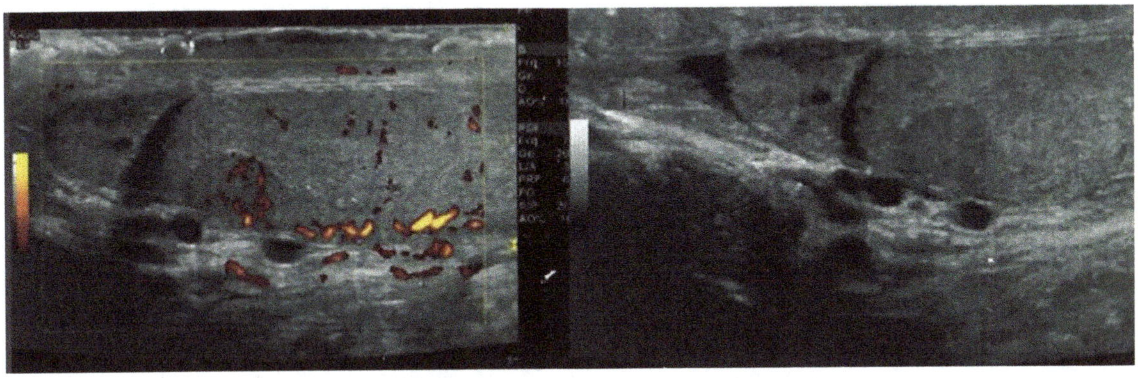

FIGURE 1: Scrotal ultrasound showing hypervascular hypoechogene testicular module measuring 8 * 6 * 8 mm.

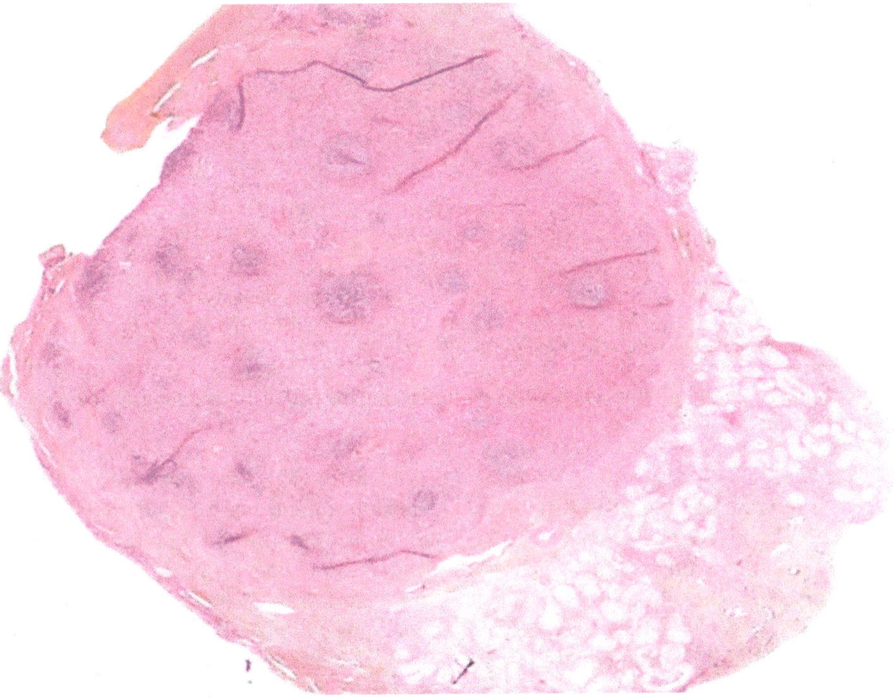

FIGURE 2: Microscopic examination: normal splenic tissue consisting of congestive red pulp and numerous mature lymphoid foci forming the white pulp, limited by a fibrous capsule.

"testicular masses ", " splenogonadal fusion" AND "limb defect syndrom".

Only reviews published in English or French were analyzed. The reviews were selected on the basis of their level of evidence and their relevance.

3. Observation

We report the case of a 45-year-old patient, with no significant history, reporting left testicular pain for 5 years. A small solid nodule at the upper pole of the left testicular was clinically palpable. Scrotal ultrasound described a hypoechoic hypervascular nodule measuring 8 * 6 * 8 mm (Figure 1).

As a testicular tumor is strongly suspected, an assay for testicular tumor markers was requested: alpha-fetoprotein, human chorionic gonadotropin (hCG), and lactate dehydrogenase (LDH) were found to be normal.

Although the presentation of this file presents the key diagnostic elements of testicular cancer (hypoechogenic solid mass palpable intrascrotal with doppler hypervascularization), signs make this diagnosis suspect: the chronic pain felt by the patient, especially after intense physical exercise and negative tumor markers. After validation in a multidisciplinary consultation meeting and a uro-andrologist expert, the patient underwent an inguinal lumpectomy with an extemporaneous examination which did not objectify any signs of malignancy. Ultimately, the anatomopathological analysis concluded with normal splenic tissue in the testicular ectopic position (Figure 2).

4. Discussion

SGF is a rare benign congenital malformation, reported in detail by Carragher [4] in 1889, although Boestrom had

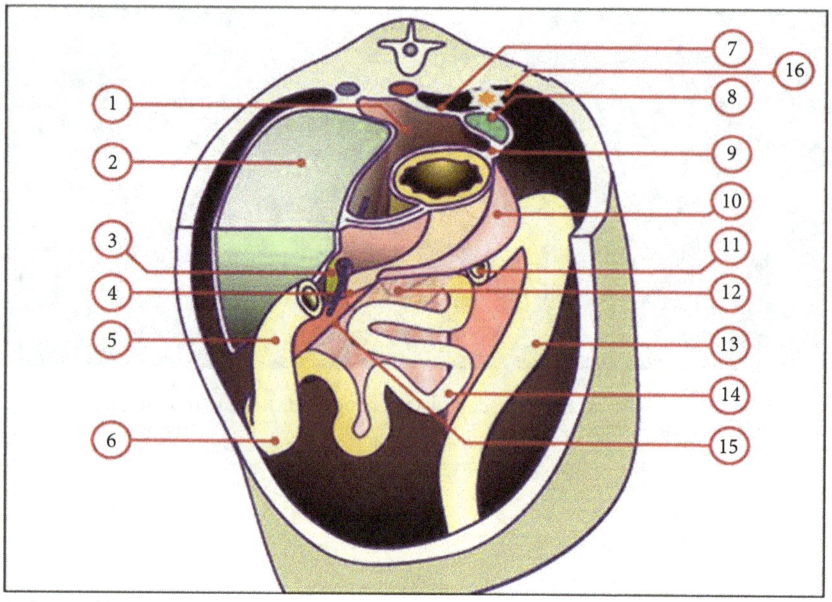

1 Omental bursa
2 Liver
3 Gall bladder
4 Duodenum
5 Right colon
6 Caecum
7 Splenorenal ligament
8 Spleen
9 Gastrosplenic ligament
10 Big omentum
11 Transverse colon
12 Mesentery
13 Descending colon
14 Intestinal convolution
15 Radix mesenterii
16 Genital crest

✶ Aggression between the spleen and the genital crest

FIGURE 3: Horizontal section at the height of the stomach and spleen explaining the SGF genesis after gastric rotation and the splenic draft of the genital crest between the 5th and 8th weeks of gestation.

described this anomaly in 1883. It was Sneath [5]. who published the first case of splenogonadic fusion in the American literature in 1913. Until 1917, all the reported cases were discovered fortuitously during autopsy studies, and thus, less than 200 cases were published in the literature [6]. This anomaly concerns almost exclusively the male sex; only 8 cases have been reported in women, [7] although this incidence is probably underestimated due to the inaccessibility of the ovaries to clinical examination. SGF mainly affects the left gonad between the fifth and sixth weeks of gestation (98% of cases) before the start of gonadal descent [8]. Note that a single case has been published in animals, more specifically in horses [9].

Putschar and Manion [10] describe two types of splenogonadal fusion: the continuous form characterized by the presence of a cord between the orthotopic spleen and the gonad and the discontinuous form which has no connection to the main spleen and the splenic tissue ectopic, directly fused to the testicular albuginea. Previous studies indicate that the frequency of the two types is equal [9], but other studies suggest that the frequency of the discontinuous type of SGF was lower than that of the continuous type [11, 12].

In the continuous form, the main spleen is connected to the gonad by an entirely fibrous cord or includes islets of splenic tissue, or even entirely composed of splenic tissue. [13] Most often, this cord comes from the upper pole of the spleen and ends at the upper pole of the gonad.

Congenital malformations occurring in the continuous form of SGF are 5 times more frequent than in the discontinuous form [12]. Cryptorchidism and inguinal hernias are the most frequently associated malformations. In 1980, Cortes et al. [14] examined 111 cases of splenogonadic fusion of which 31% had cryptorchidism (59% bilateral, 26% right intra-abdominal, and 65% left intra-abdominal). In case of continuous FSG, about 50% are accompanied by other congenital malformations, the most common of which are limb malformations: ectromelia, peromelia, amelia, phocomelia [15, 16], and micrognathia. [17] Other malformations are more exceptional: cardiac anomalies, [18] microgastronomy, [16] cleft palate, hypospadias, sexual ambiguities, varicocele, and spina bifida. [19] The association of splenogonadal fusion with major malformations of the limbs and mandible defines the splenogonadal fusion limb defect syndrome (SGFLD) of which 30 cases have been published in the literature; the SGFLD is marked by a perinatal mortality rate ranging from 40 to 50%. [1] Bonneau et al. [20] examined 29 cases of SGFLD, of which 24 cases (82.7%) were continuous, while 70% were associated with micrognathia.

The discontinuous forms are quite different since there are generally no associated malformations. The gonad is fused with a supernumerary spleen with no connection to the main spleen. The splenic tissue can be simply adherent to the elements of the cord or can be enveloped by the albugine tunic of the testicle, but it can also be separated from it; in this form, the testicle is often ectopic [21, 22], sometimes dysgenic, explaining possible degeneration [21].

Our case was of the discontinuous type, as no link between the main spleen and the testicle was objectified,

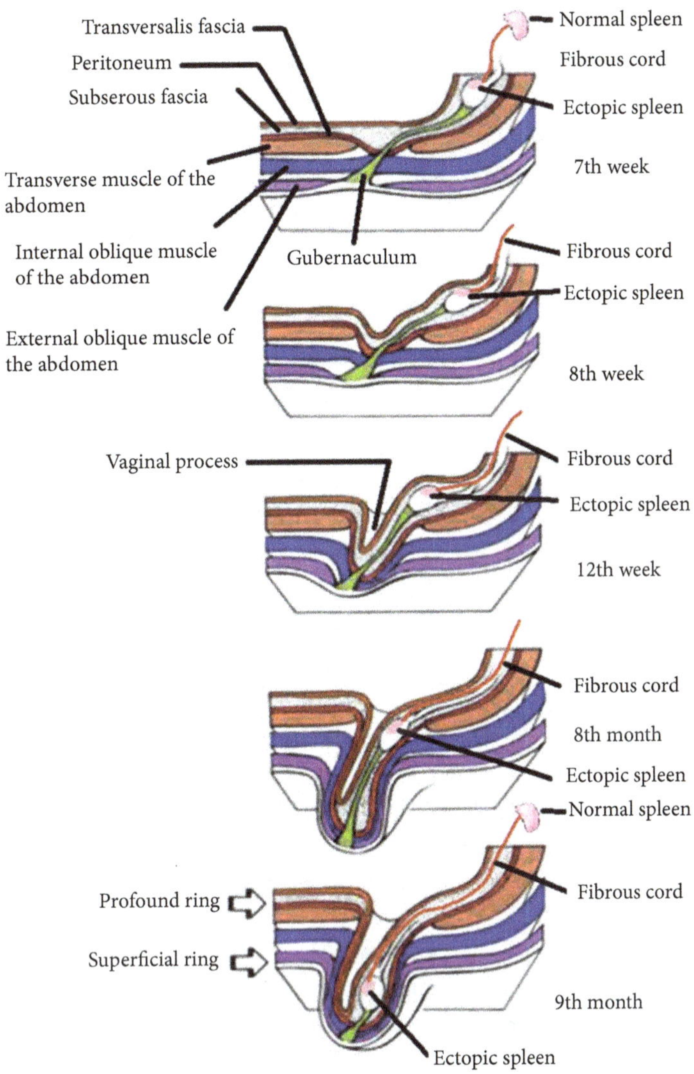

FIGURE 4: Diagram explaining the genesis of the continuous form of the SGF during the gonadal descent.

TABLE 1: Comparison between the continuous and discontinuous form of the SGF.

	SGF continuous type	SGF discontinuous type
Definition	There is a cord between the main spleen and the gonad	Lack of connection between the main spleen and the gonad or ectopic splenic tissue
Frequency	56%	44%
Associated malformations	Common: cryptorchidism	Uncommon
Imaging (ultrasound, CT, MRI)	Visualization of the connecting cord between the main spleen and the gonad	No link between the main spleen and the gonad
Tc-99 m scintigraphy	Similar fixation of the radioactive tracer in the main spleen and suspect mass	Similar fixation of the radioactive tracer in the main spleen and suspect mass

either by ultrasound or during surgical exploration, and the patient was free from any associated clinically evident malformation and the clinical examination did not objectify limb or mandible malformations, which agrees with the data in the literature.

The exact pathogenesis of splenogonadic fusion is not yet clear, but it is generally believed to occur before gonadal descent, between the fifth and sixth weeks of pregnancy. During embryogenesis and precisely from the fifth week of gestation, the stomach is moved to the left of the median plane and turns around its axis, this gastric rotation brings together the two spleen and gonad tissues, an event occurring during this period can cause fusion of the surface of the developing genital ridge and the splenic outline (Figure 3), which accounts

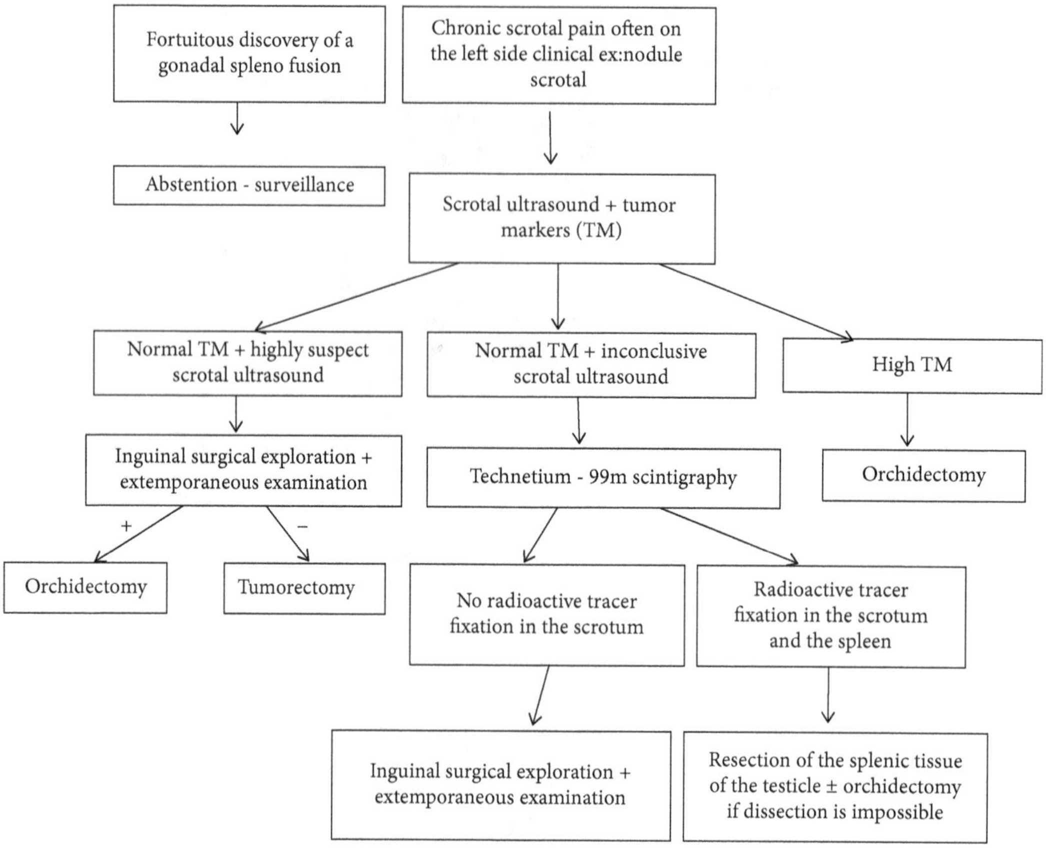

FIGURE 5: Decision tree in front of a chronic testicular nodule.

for the frequency of left localization of splenogonadal fusions, although cases of fusion of splenic tissue with the right testicle have been described. Some authors also evoke the possibility of migration of spleen cells by retroperitoneal route under the effect of an unknown teratogenic agent, [23] or of an hereditary participation in an autosomal recessive form. [24] The subsequent descent of the gonad between the 8th and the 10th week leads to a simultaneous descent of part of the spleen (Figure 4), so that the spleen tissue can appear in any place of the gonadal descent path, even in the inguinal canal or in the scrotum to arrive at the continuous form of SGF [12, 19]. These embryological hypotheses allow us to underline the importance of the classification proposed by Guarin et al., [15] distinguishing two types of SGF with quite different consequences (Table 1).

The clinical presentation of SGF is not specific, and the diagnosis is often accidentally made during surgery for inguinal hernia and/or cryptorchidism, which are the two most frequently associated anomalies or on histological examination after an orchidectomy for tumor. The discontinuous form usually presents as a hard scrotal nodule, imitating a testicular tumor, often asymptomatic, unless the patient develops a disease with splenic involvement (leukemia, mononucleosis, malaria, and salmonellosis [14]), because the splenic ectopic tissue is also affected, causing symptoms of increased volume and pain. Its association with germ tumors has been described in a few cases with the particularity that these patients had ipsilateral cryptorchidism. Other cases have been discovered in front of intestinal obstruction caused by the intraperitoneal cord [25], traumatic rupture of the ectopic spleen, or an association with an intra-abdominal seminoma. However, some rare cases have also been diagnosed preoperatively by ultrasound, computed tomography, or magnetic resonance imaging, [26, 27] most were of the continuous type, demonstrating a tubular structure fused with the testes. Splenic scintigraphy using technetium-99 m (99mTc) is a valid option once splenogonadic fusion is suspected. The binding of the radioactive tracer in the spleen and testicular mass is similar, confirming the ectopic splenic origin of this mass. [28]

Given this clinical diversity and diagnostic difficulty, we propose a diagnostic algorithm for each chronic testicular nodule (Figure 5).

The treatment of splenogonadic fusion is controversial, even if it is an almost always mild pathology. For some authors, surgery is compulsory in order to confirm the diagnosis and exclude the infrequent association with a testicular neoplasm [11]. The association with a testicular tumor has only been described in four cases [10]. There is no obvious causality between the splenogonadic fusion and the malignant transformation. The rare cases observed were probably prone to developing testicular neoplasm due to cryptorchidism [29]. If surgery is performed, orchidectomy is generally not indicated, splenic tissue can usually be easily dissected from gonadal structures and the testicle can be kept. [4, 30] For other authors, abstention can be discussed if the anomaly is recognized preoperatively and if it does not manifest clinically. [31]

5. Conclusion

Splenogonadal fusion is a rare benign congenital disease with diagnostic difficulties due to the absence of typical clinical symptoms. Better knowledge of this disease will prevent a misdiagnosis of testicular tumors and the need for an unnecessary orchidectomy. We offer a decision tree for a better management of this pathology.

Data Availability

By reporting an observational case and performing a review of the literature according to the PRISMA recommendations (using the PubMed database and guidelines from urology, general surgery and pediatrics learned societies), we present the embryological genesis of the splenogonadal fusion, associated anatomical anomalies, and the diagnostic procedure. We used the following key word associations in French and English: "splenogonadal fusion" (Fusion splénogonadique) AND "congenital anomalies" (Anomalies congénitales), "splenogonadal fusion" AND "cryptorchidism" (Cryptorchidie), "splenogonadal fusion" AND "testicular masses ", "splenogonadal fusion" AND "limb defect syndrom"

Consent

Informed consent was obtained from all individual participants included in the study.

Authors' Contributions

All authors have contributed to this work and have read and approved the final version of the manuscript.

References

[1] P. Farthouat, S. Faucompret, P. Debourdeau, T. Cruel, and Y. Breda, "Unusual testicular tumor: an ectopic spleen," *Annales de chirurgie*, vol. 126, no. 1, pp. 67–69, 2001.

[2] A. B. M. Khairat and A. M. Ismail, "Splenogonadal fusion: case presentation and literature review," *Journal of Pediatric Surgery*, vol. 40, no. 8, pp. 1357–1360, 2005.

[3] P. J. Moore, E. P. Hawkins, C. A. Galliani, and M. L. Guerry-Force, "Splenogonadal fusion with limb deficiency and micrognathia," *Southern Medical Journal*, vol. 90, no. 11, pp. 1152–1155, 1997.

[4] A. M. Carragher, "One hundred years of splenogonadal fusion," *Urology*, vol. 35, no. 6, pp. 471–475, 1990.

[5] W. A. Sneath, "An apparent third testicle consisting of a scrotal spleen," *Journal of Anatomy and Physiology*, vol. 47, Part 3, pp. 340–342, 1913.

[6] J. A. S. B. Jayasundara, V. H. Vithana, and A. K. Lamahewage, "A case of continuous-type splenogonadal fusion," *Singapore Medical Journal*, vol. 54, no. 6, pp. e123–e124, 2013.

[7] M. F. Meneses and M. L. Ostrowski, "Female splenic-gonadal fusion of the discontinuous type," *Human Pathology*, vol. 20, no. 5, pp. 486–488, 1989.

[8] A. S. Gouw, J. D. Elema, M. T. Bink-Boelkens, H. J. de Jongh, and L. P. ten Kate, "The spectrum of splenogonadal fusion. Case report and review of 84 reported cases," *European Journal of Pediatrics*, vol. 144, no. 4, pp. 316–323, 1985.

[9] D. E. Noakes and R. A. White, "Splenic-gonadal fusion in the horse," *The Veterinary Record*, vol. 98, no. 19, pp. 382-383, 1976.

[10] W. G. Putschar and W. C. Manion, "Splenicgonadal fusion," *The American Journal of Pathology*, vol. 32, no. 1, pp. 15–33, 1956.

[11] R. I. Lopes, M. T. . Medeiros, M. A. Arap, M. Cocuzza, M. Srougi, and J. Hallak, "Splenogonadal fusion and testicular cancer: case report and review of the literature," *Einstein (Sao Paulo)*, vol. 10, no. 1, pp. 92–95, 2012.

[12] O. Bosnalı, İ. Cici, S. Moralıoğlu, and A. Cerrah-Celayir, "Continuous-type splenogonadal fusion: report of a rare case," *The Turkish Journal of Pediatrics*, vol. 56, no. 6, pp. 680–683, 2014.

[13] G. Lungarella, L. Fonzi, A. De Martino, and M. Giacchi, "A rare case of continuous type spleno-gonadal fusion," *Annales d'anatomie pathologique*, vol. 25, no. 3, pp. 217–230, 1980.

[14] D. Cortes, J. M. Thorup, and J. Visfeldt, "The pathogenesis of cryptorchidism and splenogonadal fusion: a new hypothesis," *British Journal of Urology*, vol. 77, no. 2, pp. 285–290, 1996.

[15] U. Guarin, Z. Dimitrieva, and S. J. Ashley, "Splenogonadal fusion-a rare congenital anomaly demonstrated by 99Tc-sulfur colloid imaging: case report," *Journal of nuclear medicine: official publication, Society of Nuclear Medicine*, vol. 16, pp. 922–924, 1975.

[16] G. A. Mandell, S. Heyman, A. Alavi, and M. M. Ziegler, "A case of microgastria in association with splenic-gonadal fusion," *Pediatric Radiology*, vol. 13, no. 2, pp. 95–98, 1983.

[17] S. Tsingoglou and A. W. Wilkinson, "Splenogonadal fusion," *The British Journal of Surgery*, vol. 63, no. 4, pp. 297-298, 1976.

[18] K. F. Loomis, G. W. Moore, and G. M. Hutchins, "Unusual cardiac malformations in splenogonadal fusion-peromelia syndrome: relationship to normal development," *Teratology*, vol. 25, no. 1, pp. 1-9, 1982.

[19] P. J. Le Roux and R. M. Heddle, "Splenogonadal fusion: is the accepted classification system accurate?," *BJU International*, vol. 85, no. 1, pp. 114-115, 2000.

[20] D. Bonneau, J. Roume, M. Gonzalez et al., "Splenogonadal fusion limb defect syndrome: report of five new cases and review," *American Journal of Medical Genetics*, vol. 86, no. 4, pp. 347–358, 1999.

[21] W. S. Falkowski and M. F. Carter, "Splenogonadal fusion associated with an anaplastic seminoma," *The Journal of Urology*, vol. 124, no. 4, pp. 562–564, 1980.

[22] A. E. Finkbeiner, P. A. DeRidder, and S. E. Ryden, "Splenic-gonadal fusion and adrenal cortical rest associated with bilateral cryptorchism," *Urology*, vol. 10, no. 4, pp. 337–340, 1977.

[23] R. L. Cirillo, B. D. Coley, L. A. Binkovitz, and R. V. Jayanthi, "Sonographic findings in splenogonadal fusion," *Pediatric Radiology*, vol. 29, no. 1, pp. 73–75, 1999.

[24] K. C. Balaji, A. A. Caldamone, R. Rabinowitz, J. Ortenberg, and D. A. Diamond, "Splenogonadal fusion," *The Journal of Urology*, vol. 156, no. 2S, pp. 854–856, 1996.

[25] J. R. Hines and P. R. Eggum, "Splenic-gonadal fusion causing bowel obstruction," *Archives of Surgery*, vol. 1960, no. 83, pp. 887–889, 1961.

[26] D. R. Varma, G. R. Sirineni, M. V. Rao, K. M. Pottala, and B. V. P. Mallipudi, "Sonographic and CT features of splenogonadal fusion," *Pediatric Radiology*, vol. 37, no. 9, pp. 916–919, 2007.

[27] W. C. Croxford, K. L. M. Pfistermuller, F. Scott, and A. J. Pope, "Splenogonadal fusion presenting clinically and radiologically as a seminoma," *Urology case reports*, vol. 3, no. 6, pp. 204-205, 2015.

[28] S. Ando, T. Shimazui, K. Hattori, T. Yamamoto, K. Kuriyagawa, and H. Akaza, "Splenogonadal fusion: case report and review of published works," *International Journal of Urology*, vol. 13, no. 12, pp. 1539–1541, 2006.

[29] P. Sountoulides, F. Neri, R. Bellocci, L. Schips, and L. Cindolo, "Splenogonadal fusion mimicking a testis tumor," *Journal of Postgraduate Medicine*, vol. 60, no. 2, pp. 202–204, 2014.

[30] G. Verga and G. B. Parigi, "Splenic gonadal fusion: a plea for conservative surgery," *Urology*, vol. 35, no. 1, p. 99, 1990.

[31] M. I. Karaman and E. T. Gonzales, "Splenogonadal fusion: report of 2 cases and review of the literature," *The Journal of Urology*, vol. 155, no. 1, pp. 309–311, 1996.

28

Idiopathic Scrotal Calcinosis: A Case Report and Review of Postoperative Outcomes

Mathew Yamoah Kyei,[1] **Robert Djagbletey**,[2] **Afua Darkwa Abrahams**,[3] **and James Edward Mensah**[4]

[1]*Department of Surgery and Urology, University of Ghana Medical School, P.O. Box 4236, Accra, Ghana*
[2]*Department of Anaesthesia, University of Ghana Medical School, P.O. Box 4236, Accra, Ghana*
[3]*Department of Pathology, University of Ghana Medical School, P.O. Box 4236, Accra, Ghana*
[4]*Department of Surgery and Urology, University of Ghana Medical School, P.O. Box 4236, Accra, Ghana*

Correspondence should be addressed to Mathew Yamoah Kyei; matkyei@yahoo.com

Academic Editor: Yankai Xia

Idiopathic scrotal calcinosis is a rare condition, characterized by the idiopathic deposition of calcium in the scrotal dermis leading to the formation of a single nodule or multiple nodules of different sizes. Surgical excision of the nodules reduces symptoms and improves cosmesis. We present a case of idiopathic scrotal calcinosis that had an en bloc excision of scrotal skin nodules and primary closure of the scrotal skin. Handling each hemiscrotum as a separate entity and preserving the median raphe with its uninvolved skin improved the cosmesis. Reported outcomes of surgery were satisfactory with no postoperative complications. At 30 months of follow-up, the residual scrotal skin had regained its laxity and the scrotum its normal configuration. There is the risk of recurrence of the calcific nodules post excision, but these may be smaller in size and with regained scrotal configuration that could be amenable to excision with further preservation of the native scrotal skin.

1. Introduction

Idiopathic scrotal calcinosis is a rare condition characterized by the idiopathic deposition of calcium in the scrotal dermis leading to the formation of a single nodule or multiple nodules of different sizes. Historically, it was first reported by Lewinski in 1883 and named as idiopathic scrotal calcinosis by Shapiro in 1970 [1]. It is benign and common in the third decade of life.

Patients usually present because of concern about cosmesis and itching which adversely affect their quality of life. Other reported presentations include pain, superimposed infection, and exudation of chalky substances [2].

There is no underlying metabolic disorder with normal serum calcium, phosphate, and parathyroid hormone levels [3].

Imaging studies such as CT scans will show calcifications in the scrotal wall [4] but are usually not needed as diagnosis is mainly clinical and confirmed with histology of excised nodules.

Surgery is the treatment approach, and it is to reduce symptoms and improve cosmesis [5]. This involves en bloc excision of the scrotal wall containing the nodules with/or selected excision of each nodule [2]. The aim is to excise all nodules while leaving enough scrotal skin to allow for primary closure or scrotoplasty using the native scrotal skin.

We present a case of idiopathic scrotal calcinosis that had an en bloc excision of scrotal skin nodules and primary closure of the scrotal skin. Handling each hemiscrotum as a separate entity and preserving the median raphe with its uninvolved skin improved the cosmesis. The residual scrotal skin regained its laxity with the scrotum assuming its normal

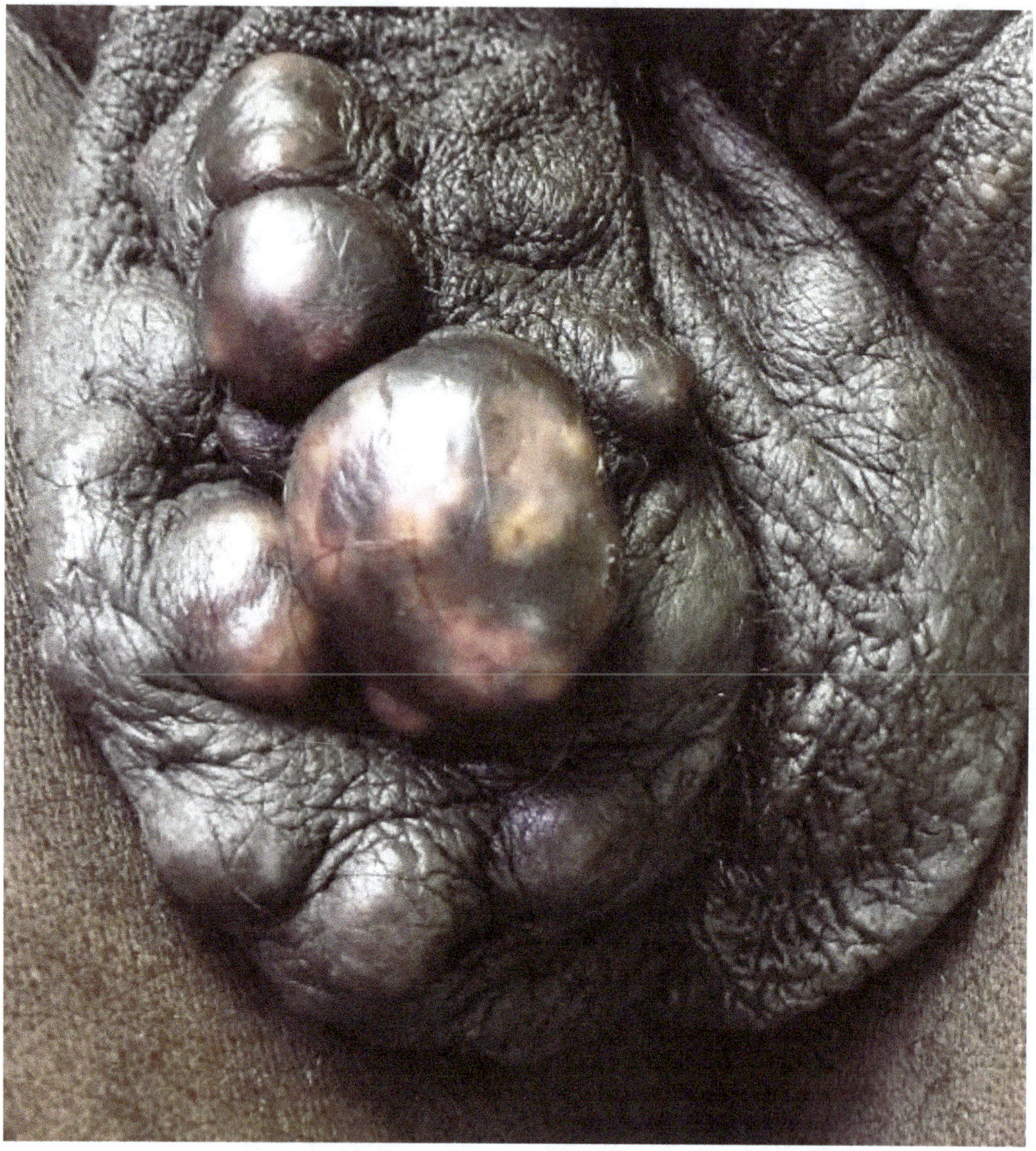

FIGURE 1: Showing the scrotum with multiple intradermal nodules of different sizes.

configuration at 30 months of follow-up. The patient gave consent for publication of this case report.

We also reviewed the postoperative outcomes after surgical intervention for idiopathic scrotal calcinosis.

2. Case Presentation

A 32-year-old married man presented in December 2017 with slow-growing multiple nodules on the scrotum of 5-year duration.

He self-reported because of cosmesis and occasional mild itch. He indicated he had been applying talcum powder to the scrotum for many years aiming to reduce sweating in the area. There was no history of trauma or infection of the scrotum. He also had no systemic or metabolic disease.

On examination, the scrotum had multiple, nontender, hypopigmented, firm nodules of different sizes that were intradermal. The largest was about 25 mm in size. It was bilateral but much larger nodules on the right hemiscrotum. The testes were normal, and there was no inguinal lymphadenopathy (Figure 1).

His serum calcium, phosphate, and parathyroid hormone levels were normal.

An important differential considered was multiple epidermal cysts of the scrotum.

The patient consented for an excision biopsy of the scrotal nodules.

The procedure was done under spinal anaesthesia using 2.5 mls of 0.5% hyperbaric bupivacaine through the L4-L5 interspace with a gauge 26 Whitacre needle.

The patient was positioned supine, and the site was cleaned with povidone-iodine and draped. The scrotum was inspected, and all nodules were noted considering each hemiscrotum as a unit. On careful inspection, the skin over the

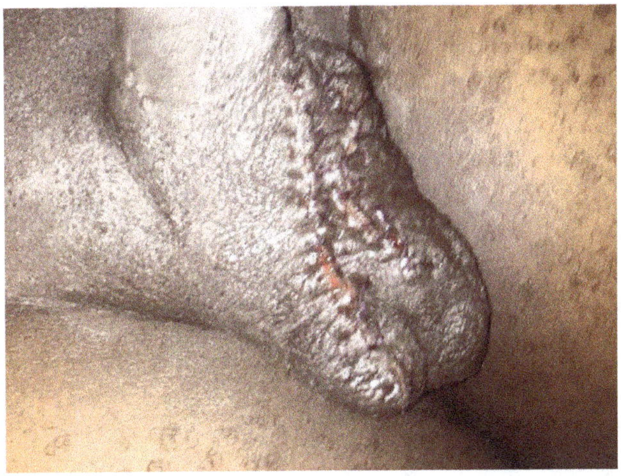

FIGURE 2: Scrotum four days post scrotoplasty with preserved skin over the median raphe.

median raphe was noted not having any nodules. A decision was made to preserve it.

A wide local excision of the involved scrotal skin was made removing the nodules en block while taking each hemiscrotum as a unit. This required a semielliptical incision on the lateral aspects and a vertical paramedian raphe incision on the medial aspects. Dissecting was just below the dermis so as not to disrupt the dartoic muscle layer which was spared.

The wound was then closed with vicryl 2-0 using an interrupted technique (Figure 2).

The histology of the excised specimen showed dense fibrosis of the dermis with foci of calcifications surrounded by multinucleated giant cells of the foreign body type. The overlying epidermis was normal confirming the diagnosis of scrotal calcinosis (Figures 3(a)–3(c)).

Thirty months post excision at follow-up, the natural laxity and configuration of the scrotum had returned and the patient was satisfied with the outcome. A recurrence of a single nodule (5 mm) on the right hemiscrotum was however observed, but it was of no bother to the patient and he therefore declined excision (Figures 4(a) and 4(b)).

3. Discussion

Idiopathic scrotal calcinosis is a rare condition with debated aetiology. While no underlying aetiology has been widely accepted, some researchers have indicated that the cause could be attributed to dystrophic deposition of calcium in an existing epidermal cyst, eccrine epithelial cyst, or degenerated dartoic muscle [5, 6]. Most patients present for cosmetic reasons as well as itching as seen in this patient [2]. The patient at 32 years had had the initial nodules when he was 27 years old supporting the observation that it tends to occur in the third decade.

The examination findings of multiple firm, intradermal, nontender nodules of different sizes and brownish in colour (hypopigmented in a dark skin) are the typical examination findings [2]. There is usually no associated inguinal lymphadenopathy as was observed in this case supporting the benign nature of the condition.

The absence of an underlying abnormality in calcium metabolism in idiopathic scrotal calcinosis [3] was also observed as the serum calcium, phosphate, and parathyroid hormones of the patient were normal.

Surgical excision for histology, limited to the involved scrotal skin but ensuring removal of all nodules, confirms the diagnosis and also treats the condition. The surgery so offered also provides the needed cosmesis. The procedure is usually performed under local or spinal anaesthesia [5, 7]. In this current case, the procedure was done under spinal anaesthesia. The use of spinal anaesthesia allows time for the performance of more complex reconstruction that may take a longer duration to accomplish. Careful inspection of the scrotum taking into consideration the number of nodules present and the extent of involvement of the scrotum allows one to plan the excision process. This could be excising each nodule separately using elliptical incisions or en bloc as a wide local excision or combination of both techniques [2, 5, 7]. The aim is to preserve adequate scrotal skin for the reconstruction and so maintain the scrotal function.

While the median raphe is preserved if the nodules involved only one hemiscrotum, it tended to be part of the en bloc excision when both ventral hemiscrota are involved [5, 8]. In this case, we performed a wide local excision of the scrotal skin with the involved nodules en bloc considering each hemiscrotum as a unit. This allowed for the preservation of the skin over the median raphe. The decision to preserve the median raphe with its overlying skin was done because it was not involved and the incision used was able to allow for the complete removal of the nodules. An involved median raphe skin if observed needs to be excised to allow for complete removal of the nodules so as to prevent recurrence. Hedhli et al. recently published their report where they excised the lesion on either side of the median raphe and centered their scrotal reconstruction on the scrotal median raphe to provide a scrotal lift shape [9].

The suture used in this case was vicryl 2-0 (absorbable suture) which worked well with no complications. Other reports have preferentially used nonabsorbable sutures such as 3-0 prolene for the reconstruction [7].

This presentation showed that the preservation of the median raphe of the scrotum with its skin, if not involved, enhances the outcome in terms of cosmesis. There was also the regain of the scrotal laxity and configuration over time.

The finding in this case as reported by others is that of calcium deposition in the dermis with associated granulomatous reaction [9]. There was a giant cell reaction in this case reported as observed in other reports [5].

Though there is a debate about the probability of recurrence of the calcific nodules after excision, this case demonstrated a single recurrence at two and half years (30 months) of follow-up supporting views of risk of recurrence after excision [10]. However, the recurred nodule with its size (5 mm) in relation to the regained laxity and configuration of the scrotum could allow for a second excision if so desired with further preservation of the scrotal skin and cosmesis.

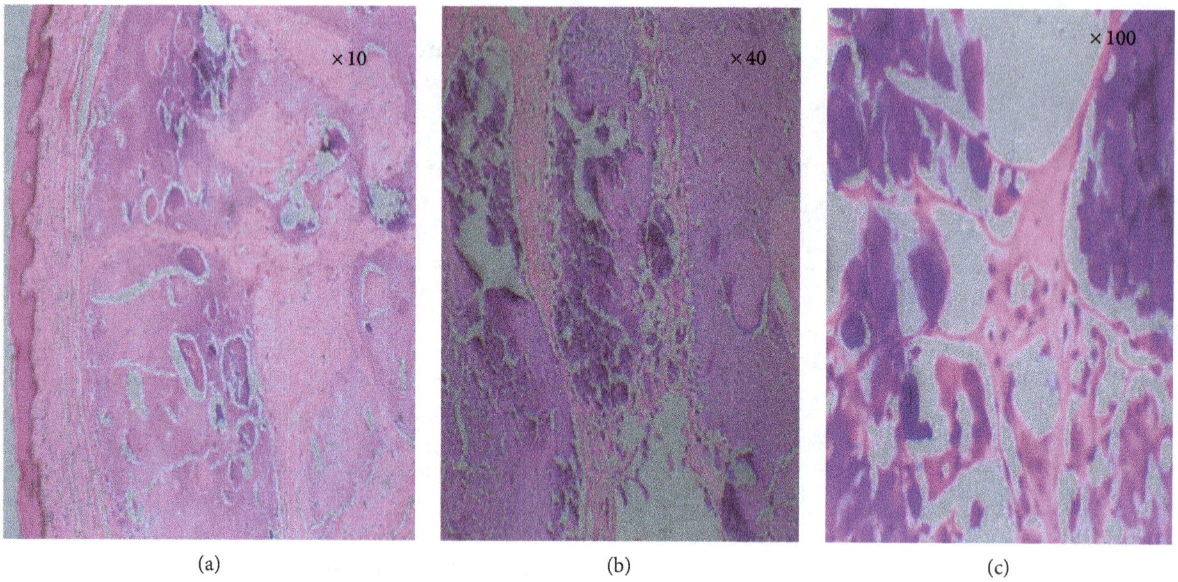

FIGURE 3: Histology of excised tissue showing (a) intact overlying epidermis with calcium deposits in the dermis (×10), (b) calcium deposits in the dermis (×40), and (c) inflammatory reaction around the deposits (×100).

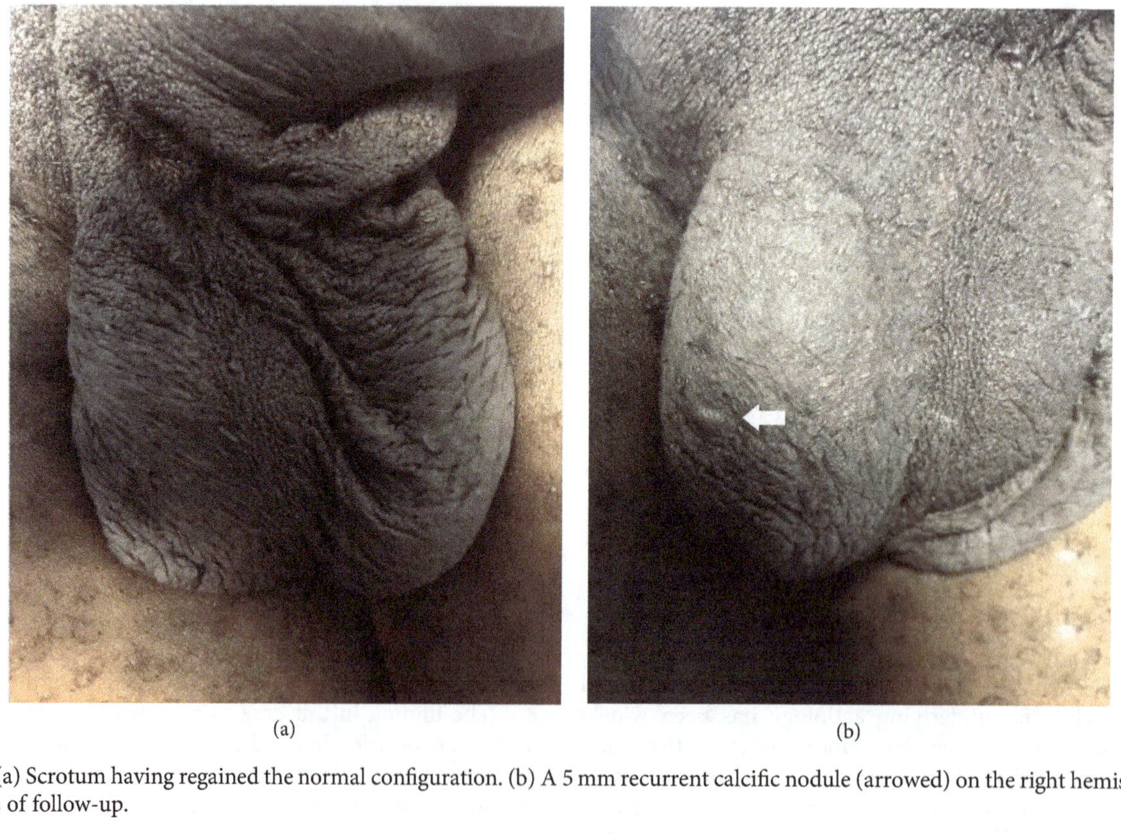

FIGURE 4: (a) Scrotum having regained the normal configuration. (b) A 5 mm recurrent calcific nodule (arrowed) on the right hemiscrotum at 30 months of follow-up.

Most authors reported no postoperative complications and satisfactory or good cosmetic outcomes after surgical excision and primary closure.

Pompeo et al. (multiple nodules) reported no recurrence at 3 months of follow-up [2]. Both Khallouk et al. (multiple nodules) and Tsai et al. (single nodule) reported no recurrence at 12 months of follow-up [5, 12]. A single recurrent nodule of size 5 mm was seen in our case at 30 months of follow-up.

4. Conclusion

Surgery is the mainstay of treatment of idiopathic scrotal calcinosis with an overall good cosmetic outcome. Preserving the median raphe with its uninvolved skin improved the aesthetics after surgery. The residual scrotal skin regained its laxity with the scrotum assuming its normal configuration at follow-up. There is the risk of recurrence of the calcific nodules, but these may be small in relation to the regained configuration of the scrotum and thus could be amenable to excision with further preservation of the native scrotal skin.

Acknowledgments

This study was funded by the authors.

References

[1] A. M. Baruchin, F. W. B. Preis, M. Cavallini, and D. Ben-Dor, "Idiopathic calcinosis of the scrotum: report of five cases and review of the literature," *European Journal of Plastic Surgery*, vol. 21, no. 6, pp. 282–285, 1998.

[2] A. Pompeo, W. R. Molina, G. D. Pohlman, D. Sehrt, and F. J. Kim, "Idiopathic scrotal calcinosis: a rare entity and a review of the literature," *Canadian Urological Association Journal*, vol. 7, no. 5-6, pp. E439–E441, 2013.

[3] A. G. Saad and G. S. Zaatari, "Scrotal calcinosis: is it idiopathic?," *Urology*, vol. 57, no. 2, p. 365, 2001.

[4] T. Grenader and L. Shavit, "Scrotal calcinosis," *The New England Journal of Medicine*, vol. 365, no. 7, p. 647, 2011.

[5] A. Khallouk, O. El Yazami, S. Mellas, M. F. Tazi, J. el Fassi, and M. H. Farih, "Idiopathic scrotal calcinosis: a non-elucidated pathogenesis and its surgical treatment," *Revista de Urología*, vol. 13, pp. 95–97, 2011.

[6] D. T. King, S. Brosman, F. M. Hirose, and L. M. Gillespie, "Idiopathic calcinosis of scrotum," *Urology*, vol. 14, pp. 92–94, 1979.

[7] A. O. Akinboro, D. A. Onilede, Babatunde TO, S. O. Oiwoh, O. A. Suleiman, and O. P. Olabode, "Idiopathic scrotal calcinosis: report of 2 cases, and review of pathogenesis and factors that determine patients' acceptance of surgical treatment," *Clinical, Cosmetic and Investigational Dermatology*, vol. 11, pp. 333–337, 2018.

[8] U. M. Tela and M. B. Ibrahim, "Scrotal calcinosis: a case report and review of pathogenesis and surgical management," *Case Reports in Urology*, vol. 2012, Article ID 475246, 3 pages, 2012.

[9] H. Hedhli, A. Hermi, M. Raboudi et al., "Idiopathic scrotal calcinosis: a new case report," *Urology Case Reports*, vol. 32, article 101225, 2020.

[10] D. H. Song, K. H. Lee, and W. H. Kang, "Idiopathic calcinosis of the scrotum: histopathologic observations of fifty-one nodules," *Journal of the American Academy of Dermatology*, vol. 19, no. 6, pp. 1095–1101, 1988.

[11] D. P. Ruiz-Genao, L. Ríos-Buceta, L. Herrero, J. Fraga, M. Aragüés, and A. García-Díez, "Massive scrotal calcinosis," *Dermatologic Surgery*, vol. 28, p. 745, 2002.

[12] Y.-S. Tsai, T.-S. Tzai, J. S.-N. Lin, and Y.-C. Tong, "Scrotal calcinosis presenting with prostatitis-like symptoms," *Urology*, vol. 59, no. 1, p. 138, 2002.

29

Management of an Infected Vesicourachal Diverticulum in a 42-Year-Old Woman

Maria Erodotou,[1] **Maria Isaia**,[1] **Georgios Fragkiadakis**,[1] **Theocharis Tontikidis**,[2] **Kosmas Tyriakidis**,[2] **Spyridon Palaiologos**,[2] **and Nikolaos Nikolaou**[1]

[1]*General Surgery Department, Larnaca General Hospital, Larnaca, Cyprus*
[2]*Urology Department, Larnaca General Hospital, Larnaca, Cyprus*

Correspondence should be addressed to Maria Erodotou; ma_riaax@hotmail.com

Academic Editor: Giorgio Carmignani

Urachal remnant anomalies are uncommon in adults and can be confused with a variety of clinical conditions when symptomatic or infected. Vesicourachal diverticulum is the rarest type, accounting for approximately 3% to 5% of congenital urachal anomalies. We report the case of a 42-year-old female patient, who presented to the emergency department with lower abdominal pain and a palpable abdominal mass. An infected vesicourachal diverticulum was diagnosed after imaging studies and was initially treated with intravenous antibiotic therapy and drainage of the urachal diverticulum to the urinary bladder through a JJ stent. Finally, the patient underwent open surgical excision of the urachal remnant. The postoperative course was uneventful, and the histopathological examination confirmed the diagnosis of vesicourachal diverticulum. We recommend drainage of an infected vesicourachal diverticulum through the bladder by JJ stent placement inside its lumen during cystoscopy, as an alternative to percutaneous drainage reported in the literature.

1. Introduction

Urachal remnant anomalies are rare in adulthood, with a reported incidence of 1 : 5000 in adults, and a higher prevalence in men than women with a ratio 2 : 1 [1, 2]. The urachus is an embryologic remnant of the cloaca and the allantois [1], and incomplete obliteration of its lumen results in four different types of urachal anomalies [1, 2]. Vesicourachal diverticulum, where there is a persistence of the vesical portion of the urachus, is the most uncommon, accounting for approximately 3% to 5% of congenital urachal anomalies [3]. It is generally asymptomatic and discovered incidentally at imaging studies [1, 3]. Infection is the most common complication of urachal remnants and may present with nonspecific abdominal or pelvic symptoms. When urachal diverticula become symptomatic or infected, surgical management is indicated [1, 3].

2. Case Presentation

A 42-year-old woman presented to the emergency department complaining of progressively deteriorating lower abdominal pain of 2 days duration. Her past medical history was unremarkable, and hysterectomy and appendectomy were reported from her surgical history. On physical examination, diffuse tenderness in the lower abdomen and a palpable midline suprapubic mass were found. An incarcerated incisional hernia was suspected initially. Her vital signs were stable. Laboratory tests revealed leucocytosis of 13.5×10^9/L with 77.2% neutrophil predominance and a high C-reactive protein of 93.4 mg/L. Urine analysis was normal and urine culture showed no bacterial growth. Abdominal ultrasonography (US) revealed a cystic lesion extending from the umbilicus to the bladder dome, measuring 7.8×3.5 cm, and free fluid in the pouch of Douglas. Computed Tomography

(CT) revealed a cystic lesion with peripheral enhancement arising from the bladder dome and extending to the umbilical region, leading to a suspected diagnosis of an infected urachal diverticulum (Figures 1 and 2). A cystography was additionally performed which also revealed findings compatible with an infected urachal diverticulum (Figure 3). The initial treatment included empirical intravenous broad-spectrum antibiotic therapy with ciprofloxacin 400 mg twice daily. Cystoscopy revealed the orifice of the infected vesicourachal diverticulum, which was narrow with purulent content, so a JJ stent was placed through for drainage. Three months later, the patient underwent a scheduled open surgical excision of the urachal remnant including a cuff of normal bladder, through an infraumbilical vertical midline incision (Figures 4–6). The postoperative course was uneventful, and the patient was discharged on the 9th postoperative day with the urinary catheter in place. On a follow-up visit at two weeks, the catheter was removed, and the patient remained asymptomatic. The histopathological examination confirmed the diagnosis of vesicourachal diverticulum.

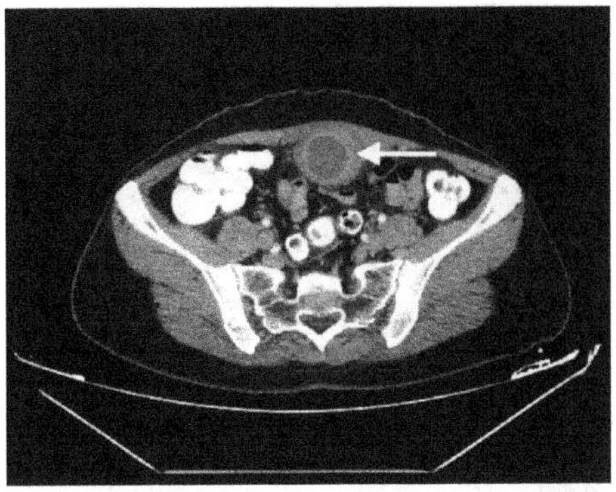

FIGURE 1: Contrast-enhanced computed tomographic image showing a cystic lesion with peripheral enhancement (arrow), thus excluding the initial diagnosis of an incarcerated hernia.

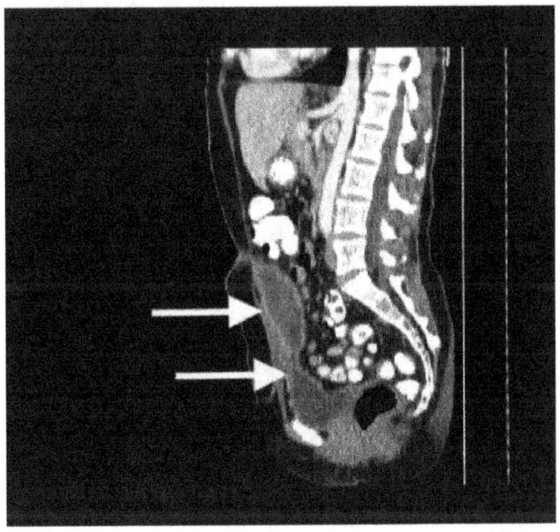

FIGURE 2: Contrast-enhanced computed tomography (sagittal plane) showing the cystic lesion (arrow-above) arising from the bladder dome (arrow–below) and extending to the umbilical region, leading to a suspected diagnosis of an infected vesicourachal diverticulum.

3. Discussion

The urachus, or median umbilical ligament, is a midline ductal remnant of the allantois and the cloaca that connects the anterosuperior bladder to the umbilicus. This fibrous remnant is located extraperitoneally in the space of Retzius (or retropubic space), between the transverse fascia anteriorly and the parietal peritoneum posteriorly. It varies from 3 to 10 cm in length, and it commonly has an approximate diameter of 8 to 10 mm [1–3]. Histologically, the urachus is composed of three layers, an inner layer lined with transitional epithelium in 70% of cases and with columnar epithelium in 30%, a middle submucosal layer of connective tissue, and an outermost muscular layer in continuum with the detrusor muscle. However, urachal remnants without an epithelial lining have also been described [1, 3, 4].

The urachus involutes before birth and remains as a connective tissue band, the median umbilical ligament. Incomplete obliteration of the urachus results in four types of congenital anomalies such as patent urachus (50%) in which a communication between the bladder and the umbilicus exist, umbilical-urachal sinus (15%) in which the urachus opens into the umbilicus and drainage from the umbilicus can be present, vesicourachal diverticulum (3-5%) in which the urachus has a wide patent opening into the bladder, and urachal cyst (30%) in which the urachus encompasses a cyst-like lesion within its length [3, 5]. Patent urachus is purely congenital, while the other types may close normally after birth but reopen in association with conditions that are often categorized as acquired diseases. These include infection and neoplasm [3]. With the widespread use of imaging, more asymptomatic cases are identified, and according to a more recent study, urachal cysts are the most common type, accounting for 69% [1].

Urachal remnants may remain asymptomatic, but when complicated by infection they may be confused with other abdominal or pelvic diseases at clinical examination or with malignant tumors at imaging, due to nonspecific symptoms [1, 3]. Vesicourachal diverticula are generally asymptomatic, as they usually have a large opening and drain well into the bladder, decreasing the possibility of complications [1]. However, a small opening can lead to debris collection or intraurachal stone formation from intermittent occlusion of the lumen, resulting in the clinical presentation of urinary tract infections, palpable mass, or acute abdominal pain if ruptured [6]. An increased prevalence of carcinoma after puberty is also reported in association with vesicourachal diverticula [3]. In the present case, cystoscopy revealed a small opening of the diverticulum to the bladder, which was blocked leading to infection. This was also demonstrated by the CT cystography where no contrast material was diffused inside the diverticulum lumen.

The urachus is located in a clinically silent area, so the clinical signs in case of infection or neoplasm may be nonspecific, delayed, or absent [5]. Patients with infection may present with abdominal pain with tenderness and palpable mass, as in the present case, fever, erythema, purulent urinary discharge, and dysuria or as an acute abdomen [1, 5]. Laboratory tests may show signs of inflammation such as elevated sedimentation rate or leukocytosis. On urine

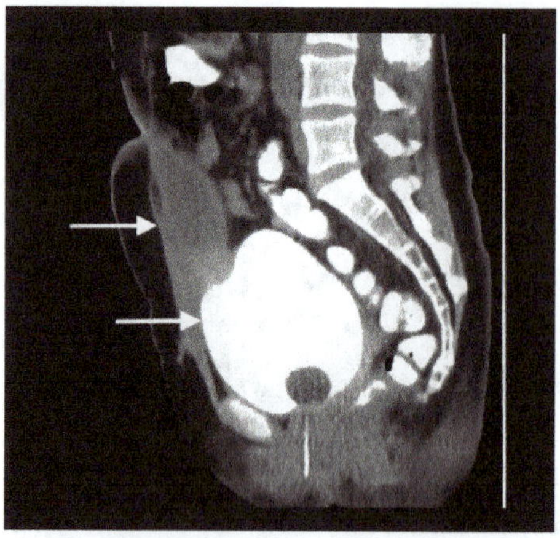

Figure 3: Cystography showing the bladder filled with contrast (arrow-below) without diffusion of the contrast inside the vesicourachal diverticulum (arrow-above), probably due to infection and a small opening of its lumen.

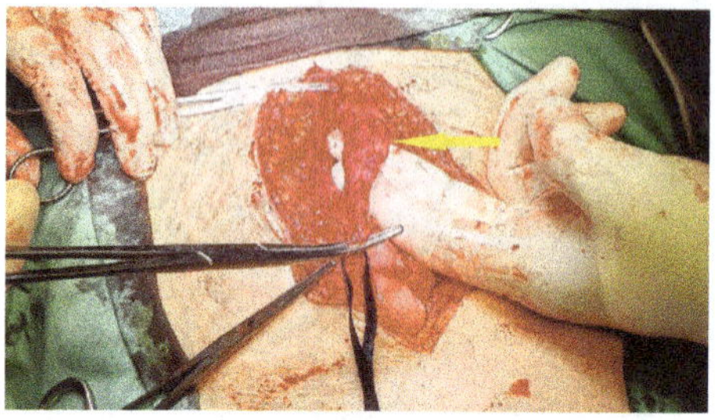

Figure 4: Intraoperative image during the dissection of the urachal remnant (arrow).

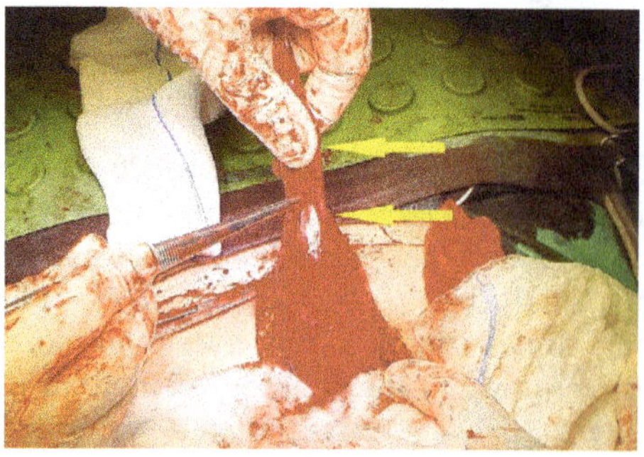

Figure 5: Intraoperative image showing the vesicourachal diverticulum (arrow-above) arising from the anterosuperior margin of the bladder (arrow-below).

analysis, bacteriuria and pyuria are absent in more than 80% and urine culture is negative [5], as in the present case. Consequently, infected urachal remnants can be confused with a wide spectrum of diseases, such as complicated Meckel's diverticulum, acute prostatitis, acute appendicitis, ovarian torsion, endometriosis, recurrent urinary tract infections, abdominal colicky pain of unknown origin, or incarcerated hernia [1, 5]. In a reported case, presentation and physical examination suggested an incarcerated umbilical hernia as the predominant pathology, before imaging studies revealed

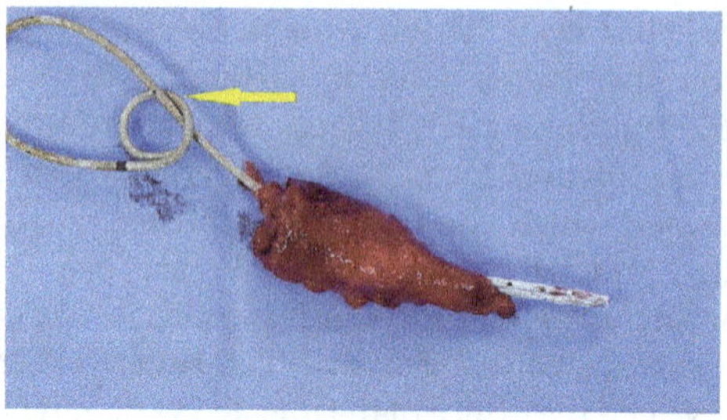

Figure 6: Surgical specimen of the resected vesicourachal diverticulum with a bladder cuff and the JJ stent in place (arrow).

an infected urachal cyst [7]. Similarly, in the present case, an incarcerated incisional hernia was suspected initially.

Abdominal US, CT scan, MRI, cystography, sinography, and cystoscopy can help with the differential diagnosis and they can show the relationship of the infected urachal anomaly with the surrounding tissue and adjacent organs [1]. Imaging findings such as complex echogenicity at US and heterogenous attenuation with variable contrast enhancement at CT scan make it difficult to differentiate an infected urachal remnant from urachal carcinoma. *In* most of the cases, percutaneous needle biopsy or fluid aspiration may be necessary for the diagnosis and therapeutic planning [3]. However, the presence of hematuria, palpable suprapubic mass, and calcifications on CT (70% of cases) is diagnostic for urachal carcinoma [1, 4]. Urachal carcinomas are rare accounting for less than 1% of bladder cancers [1] and are typically silent because of their extraperitoneal location, with a poor prognosis due to late presentation and advanced disease with local invasion [1, 3].

The initial management of infected urachal anomalies should include broad–spectrum antibiotic therapy, combined with percutaneous or surgical drainage. Total surgical excision should be performed after the infection has cleared [1]. This two-stage approach is considered by most as the treatment of choice [2, 5]. It emphasizes infection resolution before surgical intervention as superior, for reducing the risk of postoperative complications, like wound infection or urine leak, as well as reducing hospital stay [7]. However, the primary excision of the urachal remnant before the inflammation subsides has also been reported, and it can be considered safe in cases of isolated urachal cyst infection [5, 7]. The two-stage approach may be more appropriate in the management of cases complicated by bladder fistula, large abscesses, and sepsis [7]. The present case was considered as complicated because of the communication with the bladder, therefore antibiotic therapy and drainage were implemented as a first step. However, we did not perform percutaneous or surgical drainage as described in the literature [1, 5]. The infected vesicourachal diverticulum was drained through the bladder, by placing a JJ stent inside its lumen during cystoscopy. To our knowledge, nothing similar is described in the literature. We consider the placement of a JJ stent as a simple, safe, and effective technique for the drainage of an infected vesicourachal diverticulum with a narrow opening to the bladder.

The recommended surgical approach for all the types of urachal anomalies is complete excision of the urachal remnant, in order to avoid the 30% risk of infection recurrence and the potential of malignant transformation later in life [1]. Anomalies that extend to the bladder, like patent urachus and vesicourachal diverticulum, additionally require resection of a cuff of normal bladder. This radical excision requires removing the urachus and each medial umbilical ligament, along with the adjacent peritoneum from the umbilicus to the bladder dome [1, 5]. In the traditional open surgical technique, an infraumbilical transverse or vertical midline incision is used [1, 5]. Laparoscopic surgery is a safe and effective technique, alternative to open surgery in the management of urachal remnants, with the advantages of minimal invasiveness [2, 5]. Robotic-assisted approach has also been reported [8].

4. Conclusion

Vesicourachal diverticulum is the most uncommon type of urachal remnant anomalies. Although rarely detected and even more rarely presenting with symptoms of infection, it should be considered in the differential diagnosis of cases with abdominal pain. Because of nonspecific symptoms at presentation, imaging studies like ultrasound, computed tomography, and cystoscopy are essential for final diagnosis. The initial management of infected urachal diverticula should include antibiotic therapy combined with adequate drainage. We would like to add drainage through the bladder by JJ stent placement inside the diverticulum as an alternative to percutaneous drainage reported in the literature. The total excision of the urachal remnant, including resection of a cuff of normal bladder, consists of the final treatment, in order to prevent infection recurrence or future malignancy.

References

[1] C. Parada Villavicencio, S. Z. Adam, P. Nikolaidis, V. Yaghmai, and F. H. Miller, "Imaging of the urachus: anomalies, complications, and mimics," *Radiographics*, vol. 36, no. 7, pp. 2049–2063, 2016.

[2] S. Passoni, A. Guerra, and M. Marengo, "Laparoscopic treatment of an infected urachalcyst and diverticulum in a young adult: presentation of a case and review of the literature," *International Journal of Surgery Case Reports*, vol. 49, pp. 87–90, 2018.

[3] J. S. Yu, K. W. Kim, H. J. Lee, Y. J. Lee, C. S. Yoon, and M. J. Kim, "Urachal remnant diseases: spectrum of CT and US findings," *Radiographics*, vol. 21, no. 2, pp. 451–461, 2001.

[4] A. Nimmonrat, W. Na-ChiangMai, and M. Muttarak, "Urachal abnormalities: clinical and imaging features," *Singapore Medical Journal*, vol. 49, no. 11, pp. 930–935, 2008.

[5] F. Tazi, M. Ahsaini, A. Khalouk et al., "Abscess of urachal remnants presenting with acute abdomen: a case series," *Journal of Medical Case Reports*, vol. 6, no. 1, 2012.

[6] J. B. Lewis, J. W. Morse, M. F. Eyolfson, and S. L. Schwartz, "Spontaneous rupture of a vesicourachal diverticulum manifesting as acute abdominal pain," *Academic Emergency Medicine*, vol. 3, no. 12, pp. 1140–1143, 1996.

[7] A. Elkbuli, K. Kinslow, J. D. Ehrhardt Jr., S. Hai, M. McKenney, and D. Boneva, "Surgical management for an infected urachal cyst in an adult: case report and literature review," *International Journal of Surgery Case Reports*, vol. 57, pp. 130–133, 2019.

[8] P. Frazzini Padilla and S. Kwon, "Robotic-assisted excision of a urachal diverticulum," *Journal of Minimally Invasive Gynecology*, vol. 25, no. 2, p. 328, 2018.

30

A Case of Left Retroexternal Iliac Artery Megaureter Associated with Additional Renal and Vascular Congenital Anomalies

Amin A. Karadaghy, Matthew T. Bell, Daniel T. Daly, and Yun Tan

Center for Anatomical Science and Education, Department of Surgery, Saint Louis University School of Medicine, Saint Louis, MO 63104, USA

Correspondence should be addressed to Daniel T. Daly; daniel.daly@health.slu.edu

Academic Editor: Tun-Chieh Chen

Introduction. A number of rare anatomical anomalies, including retroexternal iliac ureter, extrarenal calyces (ERCs), and vascular anomalies, were observed in a 96-year-old female cadaver during a routine dissection. *Description.* A markedly dilated left extrarenal pelvis (ERP) with a diameter of 3.15 cm was noticed. Three major calyces were found outside of the normal-sized left kidney. The abdominal aorta (AA), instead of normal bifurcation, branched to the right common, left external, and left internal iliac arteries. The median sacral artery was a direct branch from the right common iliac artery. No hydronephrosis was observed on the affected side, and no urinary tract anomalies were observed on the right side. *Significance.* The retroiliac megaureter is a rare congenital anomaly, with fewer than 25 cases reported to date. Additionally, the ERCs are amongst the rarest anomalies of the renal collecting system. Further, the current case is one of few reported cases where the particular branching pattern of the AA was observed. The combination of such anatomical anomalies is rare, and the relationship between them is unclear. Common clinical manifestations of retroiliac ureters are the results of ureteric obstruction, hydronephrosis, and secondary infection. Precise knowledge of anomalies of the kidney and urinary tract can help radiologists and surgeons make a definitive diagnosis and prevent inadvertent injury during surgery.

1. Introduction

Congenital abnormalities of the kidney and urinary tract (CAKUT) encapsulates a wide range of structural abnormalities that arise during the development of the kidneys and urinary tract. CAKUT represents 20% of all birth defects and is a major cause of pediatric end-stage renal disease [1]. Known risk factors for CAKUT include intrauterine exposures, such as exposure to ACE inhibitors, and family history [2].

One well-described form of CAKUT is megaureter, defined simply as a ureter with a larger than normal diameter with or without involvement of the renal pelvis. A normal ureter is ~25-30 cm in length from the renal pelvis to the bladder and ~3-5 mm in diameter along its length. Megaureters are divided into four categories: obstructive, refluxing, refluxing with obstruction, and nonrefluxing/nonobstructing [3]. These four categories are further subdivided into two subcategories: primary (vesicoureteral junction dysfunction) or secondary (bladder obstruction) [4]. The decision to begin treatment is multifactorial and depends on symptomology, severity, and underlying conditions [5].

Secondary obstructive megaureter is most commonly due to obstruction at the level of the bladder by posterior urethral valves [6, 7]. This occurs most commonly on the left side and in males due to a remnant of embryological membranes [5, 8].

Much less commonly, secondary obstructive megaureter can be due to a retroiliac ureter wherein the ureter passes deep to the iliac artery. There have been a very small number (24) of documented retroiliac ureter cases reviewed to date [9]. Obstructive megaureter is associated with several anatomic variations including retro-common iliac artery (CIA) with lack of internal iliac artery (IIA), retro-IIA, and circumiliac ureter [7, 10, 11].

In the current report, we describe a novel case of left retro-external iliac artery (EIA) megaureter. This case includes other renal and vascular anomalies, specifically the absence of a left CIA, the presence of ERC, and a unique AA branching pattern. Because this case was found postmortem, it permitted detailed exploration and measurement.

This case is of interest for its rarity and clinical implications. The importance of understanding vascular anatomical variations is highlighted in a case of development of the left lower limb ischemia following a routine nephrectomy due to an aberrant EIA originating from the left renal artery [12]. This case emphasizes the importance of how knowledge of anatomical variations can help clinicians exercise caution in a clinical setting.

2. Case Presentation

A 96-year-old female body was received through the Saint Louis University Gift of Body Program of the Center for Anatomical Science and Education (CASE) with the signed informed consent from the donor. The CASE gift body program abides by all rules set forth by the Uniform Anatomical Gift Act (UAGA). Information obtained through the CASE program did not specify a cause of death but did mention a history of Alzheimer's disease, COPD, and atrial fibrillation in this donor. During dissection in 2018, it was observed that the donor was status post hysterectomy and status post ventral hernia repair with mesh.

During routine dissection, a markedly dilated left ureter was noticed and further explored (Figure 1). The left renal pelvis was located outside of the kidney sitting medially, inferiorly, and slightly posteriorly from the kidney. The path of the ureter curved slightly posteriorly and medially before turning laterally. The ureter then turned sharply medially and anteriorly before continuing over the psoas major muscle. The ureter was most dilated as it passed anteriorly to the left psoas minor muscle, where its diameter measured at 1.70 cm. The ureter then passed posterior to the EIA and anterior to the IIA, about 0.50 cm away from the bifurcation of the AA.

Upon further dissection, it was found that what was initially identified as the left CIA was in fact the left EIA. The donor had three terminal arterial branches off the AA: the right CIA, left IIA, and left EIA. The left IIA branched off the posterior side of the AA. As a result, the median sacral artery was shifted and was observed branching off the right CIA (Figure 2). After passing beneath the left EIA, the left ureter returned to a normal size (0.45 cm) and position following a normal path to the bladder (Figure 3).

The three major calyces of the left kidney were found to join together outside of the kidney (Figure 4(a)). All arteries and veins of the left kidney were normal, and no evidence of hydronephrosis was observed (Figure 4(b)). Constriction of the ureteropelvic junction (UPJ) was noted, though this slight constriction did not result in any gross renal pathology (Figure 4(c)).

Finally, the subject exhibited extensive surgical sutures, likely from the hysterectomy, along the lateral paravertebral muscles as well as near the left IIA, inferolateral to the ureter.

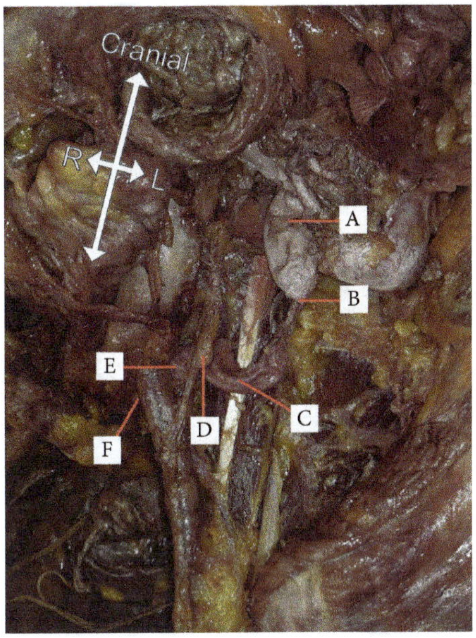

Figure 1: Dissected path of left ureter from the kidney to the iliac arteries. (A) The beginning of the renal pelvis (diameter: 3.15 cm), (B) the end of the renal pelvis (diameter: 0.88 cm), (C) passing over psoas minor (diameter: 1.70 cm), (D) passing under ovarian artery/vein, (E) passing under external iliac artery (diameter: 1.65 cm), and (F) emerging medial to external iliac artery (diameter: 0.45 cm).

3. Discussion

The only review found in the literature on retroiliac ureter described 24 cases, many of which were associated with various genitourinary anomalies including those of ectopic vas deferens, horseshoe kidney, and imperforate anus [13]. The current case appears to be the first reported with the constellation of various anomalies including a left retro-EIA ureter with ERC and absent left CIA with a unique AA branching pattern. The importance of the present report is several fold.

First, this case highlights yet another form of secondary obstructive megaureter wherein the aberrant ureter is obstructed between the IIA and EIA and thus may be called retro-EIA megaureter. Similar cases of retro-IIA, retro-CIA, and circumiliac artery ureter have been previously described [7, 10, 11]. More commonly, secondary obstructive megaureter is caused by aneurysm of the iliac arteries, arteriovenous malformation, and persistent umbilical artery [14–20]. These common causes of obstructive megaureter were not observed in the cadaveric body under study, rather the obstruction was due to the ureter coursing posterior to the EIA.

Second, the observed branching pattern of the AA seems to be very unique. As noted above, the current cadaveric body lacks a left CIA and the left IIA was observed branching directly off the posterior side of the AA with the left EIA arising directly from the lateral side of the AA. Generally, cases of vascular anomalies in the iliac and femoral vessels are rare [21]. One study reported the case of the unilateral lack of iliac arteries, with a network of collateral arteries supplying the normal vascular territory [21]. Similar cases include absence

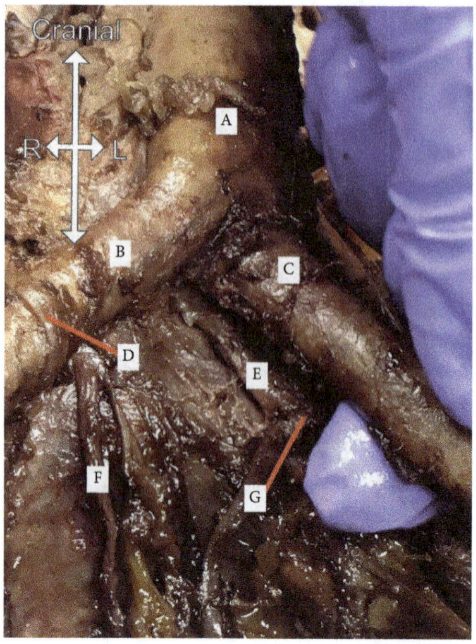

Figure 2: Terminal branches of the abdominal aorta and paths of ureters. (A) Abdominal aorta, (B) right common iliac artery, (C) left external iliac artery, (D) right ureter passes over common iliac artery, (E) let internal iliac artery, (F) median sacral artery branches off the right common iliac artery, and (G) the left ureter passes between the left internal iliac artery and external iliac artery.

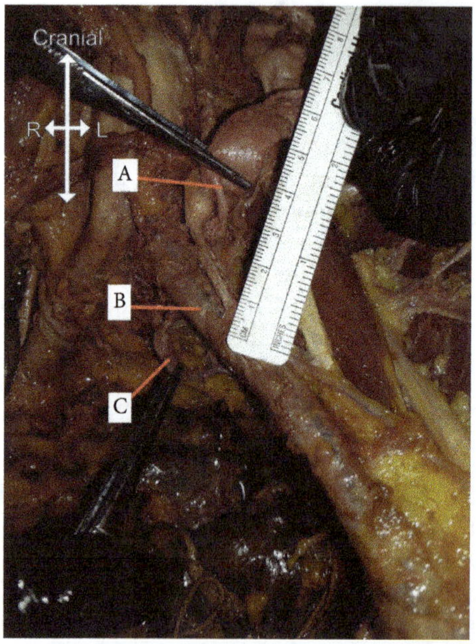

Figure 3: Ureter passes beneath the left external iliac artery and emerges distally with a normal diameter. (A) Proximal, preobstruction end of ureter, (B) the point of obstruction under the left external iliac artery, and (C) distal, postobstruction end of the ureter.

of CIA and IIA with an aberrant EIA arising from the renal artery, absence of right CIA with aberrant left IIA, and absence of bilateral CIA and left IIA with prominent collateral vasculature [12, 22, 23]. A very similar iliac artery branching pattern to this case has been described but included absent bilateral, rather than unilateral, CIAs [24]. Variations in terminal branches of iliac and femoral arteries have been described more thoroughly, with several classification systems used to categorize variations in iliac artery branches [25].

Third, this case is notable for its associated urinary tract anomalies, namely dilated ERP, ERC, and UPJ stenosis, all present with a conspicuous absence of hydronephrosis. ERP is an anatomical variant that appears just outside the renal sinus and can be confused with hydronephrosis, especially on renal ultrasound, but can be distinguished by its lack of dilated calyces, parenchymal thinning, hydroureter, or enlarged kidney [26]. ERP is estimated to be seen in up to 10% of the population and is asymptomatic in most cases. Extrarenal calyces (ERCs) are among the rarest anomalies of the renal collecting system, with only 20 cases reported to date [19]. The ERC association with UPJ obstruction is described only rarely in the literature [27]. The etiology of ERC is unclear and is most commonly associated with ectopic kidney, which is usually the result of variation in degrees of embryological kidney nonrotation [19]. The clinical presentation of ERC includes flank pain and recurrent UTIs usually as a result of stasis, calculi, and infection [19, 28]. It has been diagnosed incidentally during cadaveric dissection or investigation of hydronephrosis [19, 27]. As described by one paper, treatment is not always necessary but includes either a classic pyeloplasty, resection of the pelvis, and an ureterocalicostomy with fusion of the calyces, or a single-stage nephroureterectomy [27]. Interestingly, no other genitourinary anomalies were present in this body. The bladder and urethra were examined and no abnormalities regarding size or positioning were noted.

Fourth, this case is notable because it provides important information regarding embryologic aspects. The ureter originates from the ureteric bud, an evagination of the mesonephric (Wolffian) duct that forms during the fourth or fifth week of gestation. Through repeated rounds of elongation and branching, the buds eventually mature into the bilateral ureters [29]. Starting in the sixth or seventh week of gestation, the developing kidney migrates rostrally, passing anterior to the iliac vessels which develop as branches off the umbilical artery. Abnormalities in this migration are generally considered to be a cause of secondary obstructive megaureter arising from an aberrant ureter [7]. Therefore, it would be reasonable to suggest that the aortic abnormalities represent the primary aberration and not the ureteric migration. For the same reason, a similar condition previously called retrocaval ureter was redefined as the preureteral vena cava [30]. The genetic programming underlying ureteric bud positioning and migration has been implicated in the development of retroiliac ureter and extensively studied [29, 31–34].

Fifth, this case is also important because it could modify the respective prenatal screening to make it more accurate and informative. CAKUT is a major cause of chronic kidney disease in children, often resulting in end-stage renal disease thereby requiring a kidney transplant [35]. CAKUT and its associated abnormalities are often detected during prenatal ultrasound examination, which is recommended by the American College of Obstetricians and Gynecologists to be

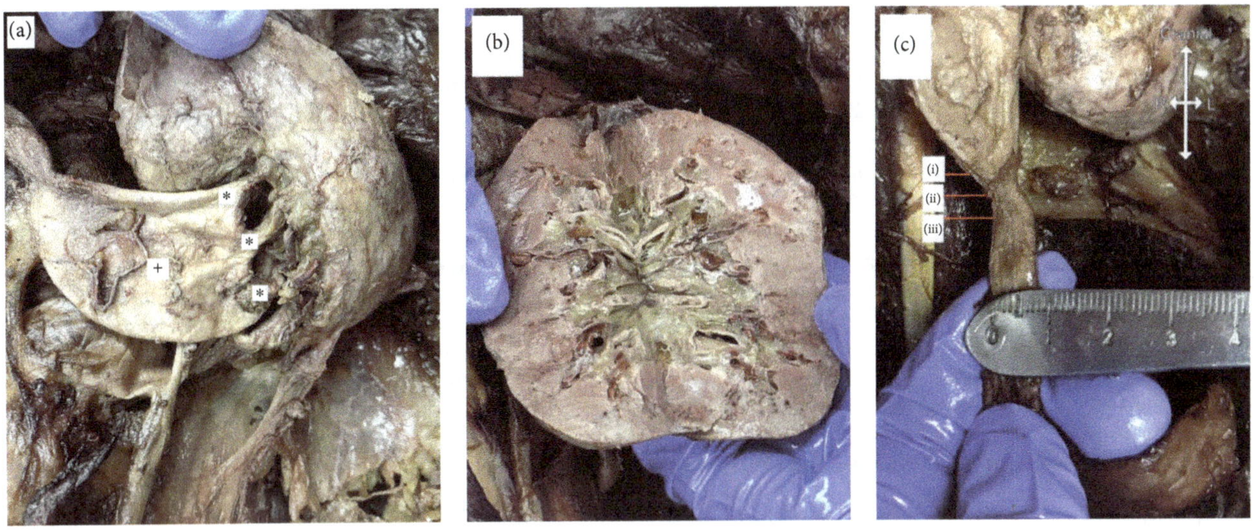

(a) (b) (c)

FIGURE 4: (a) A posterior view of the affected (left) kidney showing three major calyces (asterisks) joining outside of the kidney and a dilated renal pelvis (plus sign). (b) A view inside the affected (left) kidney showing normal-sized minor calyces and pyramids without evidence of hydronephrosis. (c) Also notable was a slight, yet still noticeable, stenosis of the ureteropelvic junction: (i) pre-ureteropelvic junction (diameter: 0.88 cm), (ii) ureteropelvic junction (diameter: 0.50 cm), (iii) post-ureteropelvic junction (diameter 0.75 cm).

performed at least once during pregnancy. One retrospective study of congenital malformations showed that 73% of cases of congenital hydronephrosis were diagnosed prenatally [8]. In countries where prenatal ultrasound examination is rare, postnatal ultrasound in children with UTI, or those at higher risk, could also detect congenital abnormalities [36, 37]. According to other publications, the incidence of prenatally diagnosed megaureter is not currently known and may be due to the fact that detection of a dilated ureter by ultrasound prenatally is a difficult endeavor [8].

Finally, this case has a high clinical value. Indeed, surgical treatment of retroiliac ureter is most commonly done by transposition of the ureter around the obstruction. Other documented treatments include iliac artery diversion, nephroureterectomy, and transureteroureterostomy [13]. Knowledge of the anatomical variants was highlighted by a report where an anomalous EIA arising from the renal artery was unexpectedly compromised during a nephrectomy [12].

4. Conclusion

This postmortem case of a novel retroexternal iliac artery megaureter with absent left common iliac artery and presence of extrarenal calyces is of interest for both its rarity and clinical significance. The embryological etiology of this particular genitourinary and vascular variant is unclear at this time. However, this variant does pose clinical significance for the medical and surgical community. Common clinical manifestations of retroiliac ureters are usually the result of obstruction and secondary infection though, to our knowledge, this patient was not experiencing any of those. Furthermore, identifying the location and orientation of anatomical details of the abdominal aorta and iliac vasculature as well as ureteral anomalies is essential for performing various pelvic surgeries ranging from uterine fibroid removal to hernia repair. Failure to consider these potential variations can lead to preventable morbidity and mortality during surgery.

Disclosure

These data were presented in part at the annual American Association of Clinical Anatomists meeting (Abstracts Presented at the 36th Annual Meeting of the American Association of Clinical Anatomists, 11th–15th June 2019 at Tulsa, Oklahoma, Clin Anat, doi:10.1002/ca.23451).

Acknowledgments

This study was supported by the Center for Anatomical Science and Education, Saint Louis University School of Medicine. The authors thank Evan Qu and Mia Jenkins for their help with the initial dissection as well as to Andrey Frolov for his help with manuscript preparation.

References

[1] S. Sanna-Cherchi, P. Ravani, V. Corbani et al., "Renal outcome in patients with congenital anomalies of the kidney and urinary tract," *Kidney International*, vol. 76, no. 5, pp. 528–533, 2009.

[2] W. O. Cooper, S. Hernandez-Diaz, P. G. Arbogast et al., "Major congenital malformations after first-trimester exposure to ACE inhibitors," *The New England Journal of Medicine*, vol. 354, no. 23, pp. 2443–2451, 2006.

[3] E. D. Smith, "Report of working party to establish an international nomenclature for the large ureter," *Birth Defects Original Article Series*, vol. 13, no. 5, pp. 3–8, 1977.

[4] L. R. King, "Megaloureter: definition, diagnosis and management," *The Journal of Urology*, vol. 123, no. 2, pp. 222-223, 1980.

[5] S. J. Hodges, D. Werle, G. McLorie, and A. Atala, "Megaureter," *The Scientific World JOURNAL*, vol. 10, Article ID 530925, 10 pages, 2010.

[6] C. Manzoni, "Megaureter," *Rays*, vol. 27, no. 2, pp. 83–85, 2002.

[7] R. L. Mehl, "Retro-iliac artery ureter," *The Journal of Urology*, vol. 102, no. 1, pp. 27–29, 1969.

[8] M. K. Farrugia, R. Hitchcock, A. Radford et al., "British Association of Paediatric Urologists consensus statement on the management of the primary obstructive megaureter," *Journal of Pediatric Urology*, vol. 10, no. 1, pp. 26–33, 2014.

[9] H. Prasad, V. Karthikeyan, M. Shivalingaiah, and C. Ratkal, "Retroiliac ureter presenting as right upper ureteric obstruction – report of a rare case," *International Journal of Research in Medical Sciences*, vol. 3, no. 8, pp. 2143-2144, 2015.

[10] K. Taibah, P. D. Roney, D. E. McKay, and J. L. Wellington, "Retro-internal iliac artery ureter," *Urology*, vol. 30, no. 2, pp. 159–161, 1987.

[11] A. M. Tawfik and M. H. Younis, "Computed tomography imaging appearance of a unique variant of retroiliac ureter," *Urology*, vol. 88, pp. e7–e9, 2016.

[12] G. D. Oduro, L. H. Cope, and I. M. Rogers, "Case report: lower limb arterial blood supply arising from the renal artery with congenital absence of the ipsilateral iliac arteries," *Clinical Radiology*, vol. 45, no. 3, pp. 215–217, 1992.

[13] D. H. Nguyen, N. Koleilat, and R. Gonzalez, "Retroiliac ureter in a male newborn with multiple genitourinary anomalies: case report and review of the literature," *The Journal of Urology*, vol. 141, no. 6, pp. 1400–1403, 1989.

[14] R. Safran, R. Sklenicka, and H. Kay, "Iliac artery aneurysm: a common cause of ureteral obstruction," *The Journal of Urology*, vol. 113, no. 5, pp. 605–609, 1975.

[15] A. Kaynan, V. Rosenberg, and P. Szuchmacher, "Ureteral obstruction secondary to iliac artery aneurysms," *Mount Sinai Journal of Medicine*, vol. 45, no. 3, pp. 334–341, 1978.

[16] S. Maeda, K. Ogura, Y. Arai, H. Takeuchi, O. Yoshida, and K. Mori, "Ureteral obstruction caused by aneurysm of iliac artery," *Hinyokika kiyo. Acta Urologica Japonica*, vol. 39, no. 11, pp. 1047–1049, 1993.

[17] K. Mineta, M. Nomura, N. Fujimoto, K. Takahashi, and T. Matsumoto, "Ureteral obstruction due to retroperitoneal fibrosis secondary to a solitary internal iliac aneurysm," *International Journal of Urology*, vol. 11, no. 11, pp. 1024–1027, 2004.

[18] S. K. Sharma, A. K. Goswami, G. P. Sharma, G. C. Malakondiah, and S. K. Khanna, "Congenital iliac arteriovenous malformation: a cause of massive hematuria and ureteral obstruction," *The Journal of Urology*, vol. 139, no. 2, pp. 355-356, 1988.

[19] T. Gupta, S. K. Goyal, A. Aggarwal, D. Sahni, and A. K. Mandal, "Extrarenal calyces: a rare renal congenital anomaly," *Surgical and Radiologic Anatomy*, vol. 37, no. 4, pp. 407–410, 2015.

[20] M. Krishna, S. Theodore, P. K. Varma, and K. S. Neelakandhan, "Spontaneous iliac arteriovenous fistula: recognition and management," *The Journal of Cardiovascular Surgery*, vol. 46, no. 182, pp. 181-182, 2005.

[21] D. A. Dabydeen, A. Shabashov, and K. Shaffer, "Congenital absence of the right common iliac artery," *Radiology Case Reports*, vol. 3, no. 1, 2008.

[22] J. Llauger, J. M. Sabaté, E. Guardia, and J. Escudero, "Congenital absence of the right common iliac artery: CT and angiographic demonstration," *European Journal of Radiology*, vol. 21, no. 2, pp. 128–130, 1995.

[23] C. S. Green and M. A. Helmy, "Novel, congenital iliac arterial anatomy: absent common iliac arteries and left internal iliac artery," *Radiology Case Reports*, vol. 9, no. 3, 2014.

[24] A. O. Mansfield and J. M. Howard, "Absence of both common iliac arteries. A case report," *The Anatomical Record*, vol. 150, no. 4, pp. 363-364, 1964.

[25] H. Mohammadbaigi, M. Darvishi, and A. Moayeri, "Variations of anterior and posterior division of internal iliac artery: a systematic review and clinical implications," *Biomedical Research and Therapy*, vol. 6, no. 5, pp. 3189–3206, 2019.

[26] A. Koratala and D. Bhattacharya, "Extrarenal pelvis mimicking hydronephrosis: a case for caution," *Clinical Case Reports*, vol. 5, no. 10, pp. 1720-1721, 2017.

[27] B. V. Raghunath, B. M. Narendra, B. C. Gowrishankar, and S. Ramesh, "Extrarenal calyces associated with pelviureteric junction obstruction: a case report of a rare anomaly," *Journal of Indian Association of Pediatric Surgeons*, vol. 17, no. 3, pp. 124-125, 2012.

[28] P. Garg, R. Godara, and R. K. Karwasra, "Extrarenal calyces: a rarity," *Urologia Internationalis*, vol. 71, no. 3, pp. 331-332, 2003.

[29] T. Bohnenpoll and A. Kispert, "Ureter growth and differentiation," *Seminars in Cell & Developmental Biology*, vol. 36, pp. 21–30, 2014.

[30] A. Lesma, A. Bocciardi, and P. Rigatti, "Circumcaval ureter: embryology," *European Urology Supplements*, vol. 5, no. 5, pp. 444–448, 2006.

[31] J. Blake and N. D. Rosenblum, "Renal branching morphogenesis: morphogenetic and signaling mechanisms," *Seminars in Cell & Developmental Biology*, vol. 36, pp. 2–12, 2014.

[32] H. M. Rasouly and W. Lu, "Lower urinary tract development and disease," *Wiley Interdisciplinary Reviews. Systems Biology and Medicine*, vol. 5, no. 3, pp. 307–342, 2013.

[33] V. Capone, W. Morello, F. Taroni, and G. Montini, "Genetics of congenital anomalies of the kidney and urinary tract: the current state of play," *International Journal of Molecular Sciences*, vol. 18, no. 4, 2017.

[34] I. V. Yosypiv, "Congenital anomalies of the kidney and urinary tract: a genetic disorder?," *International Journal of Nephrology*, vol. 2012, Article ID 909083, 2012.

[35] J. Harambat, K. J. van Stralen, J. J. Kim, and E. J. Tizard, "Epidemiology of chronic kidney disease in children," *Pediatric Nephrology*, vol. 27, no. 3, pp. 363–373, 2012.

[36] Y. Gong, Y. Zhang, Q. Shen et al., "Early detection of congenital anomalies of the kidney and urinary tract: cross-sectional results of a community-based screening and referral study in China," *BMJ Open*, vol. 8, no. 5, article e020634, 2018.

[37] P. Vachvanichsanong, P. Dissaneewate, and E. McNeil, "What did we find from imaging studies in childhood urinary tract infection and which studies are mandatory?," *Urology*, vol. 111, pp. 176–182, 2018.

31

Multiple Urethral Hemangiomas Associated with Urethral Stricture: An Uncommon Aetiology for Urethral Bleeding

Raquel Varea-Malo,[1] Félix Campos-Juanatey,[2] José Antonio Portillo Martín,[3] and Luisana Castillo Carvajal[4]

[1] *Urology Department, Marqués de Valdecilla University Hospital, Santander, Spain*
[2] *Urology Department, Marqués de Valdecilla University Hospital, Institute of Investigation Marqués de Valdecilla (IDIVAL), Santander, Spain*
[3] *Urology Department, Marqués de Valdecilla University Hospital, University of Cantabria, Santander, Spain*
[4] *University Foundation of Health Sciences, San Jose Hospital, Bogotá, Colombia*

Correspondence should be addressed to Raquel Varea-Malo; raquelvareamalo@gmail.com

Academic Editor: Fumitaka Koga

Urethral haemangiomas are rare benign vascular tumours. They usually cause painless urethral bleeding and haematospermia. Urethroscopy is the preferred diagnostic tool, while complementary radiologic studies could describe the extension of the tumour. Treatment should be tailored to each case, considering size, location, and number of lesions. We present a case of a male patient diagnosed with urethral haemangiomas following painless spontaneous urethral bleeding associated with voiding symptoms.

1. Introduction

Urethral bleeding aetiology is diverse (traumas, infections, prostatic origin,. . .), even though vascular malformations are a rare cause. The urethral haemangioma is an uncommon vascular tumour [1] with benign constitution, usually presenting as isolated episodes of urethral bleeding and haematospermia [2]. The preferred diagnostic method is urethrocystoscopy, with identification of haemangiomas typical appearance and with ability to describe size, location, and number of lesions. Due to different clinical presentations, they would require to customize its treatment [3, 4].

Our purpose is to present a case of urethral haemangiomas found in a male. The clinical presentation and diagnostic tests are described. We performed a revision of the existing literature regarding this entity and its treatment.

2. Case Report

A 61-year-old man was admitted with acute painless urethral bleeding associated with lower urinary tract symptoms (LUTS), mainly voiding obstruction. He had past medical history of hypertension (HT) and dyslipidemia. When asked about urological backgrounds, the patient described two episodes of acute strong urethral bleeding 20 years ago. Likewise, he underwent surgical primary suture of bleeding areas when haemangiomas of the glans penis were first diagnosed.

Physical examination confirmed several haemangiomas in the glandular urethra, located at submeatal level. Those were only visible by gently spreading the external urethral meatus (Figure 1). In addition, we found scrotal haemangiomas and prominent varicose veins in both legs. Digital rectal examination revealed a nonsuspicious medium-sized adenomatous prostate and uroflowmetry showed no value due to a low voiding volume. A short proximal bulbar urethral stricture was diagnosed through a retrograde urethrogram and voiding cystourethrogram (RUG + VCUG). During RUG, contrast extravasation to the peribulbar veins was evident (Figure 2). Urethroscopy confirmed the stricture ring close to the external urinary sphincter.

After discussion with the patient, an internal urethrotomy under direct vision was the preferred treatment. During this procedure, glans haemangiomas and small haemangiomas

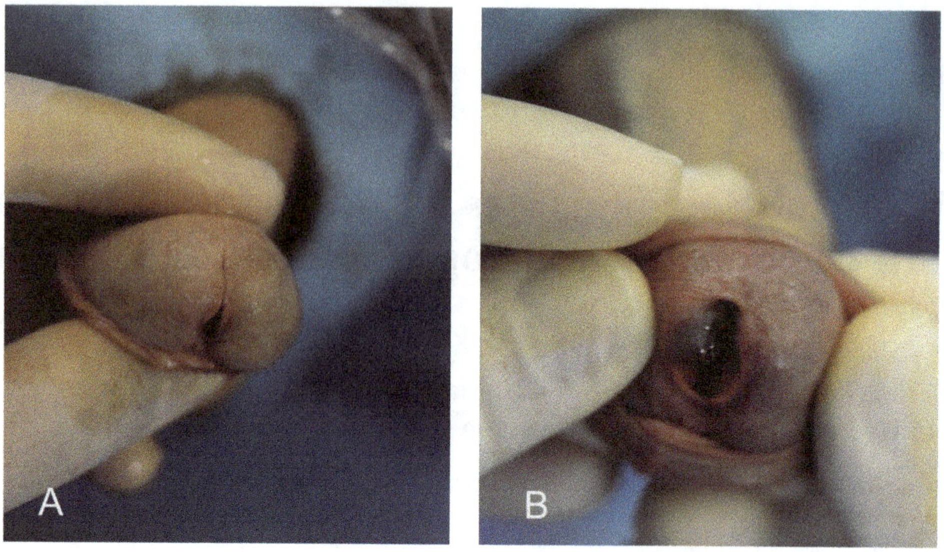

(a) (b)

Figure 1: External aspect of glans. (a) External vision, without appreciating hemangioma. (b) Open external urethral meatus, with protrusion of vascular lesion.

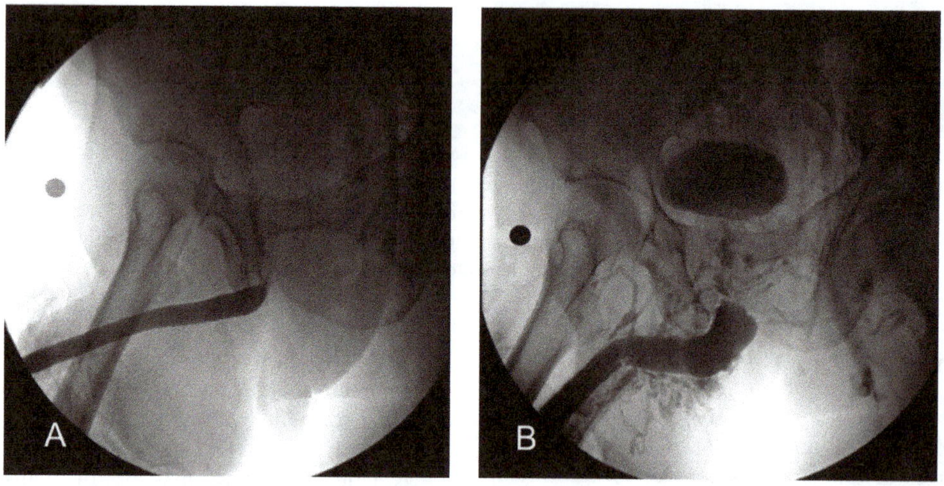

(a) (b)

Figure 2: Retrograde urethrogram and voiding cystourethrogram. (a) Proximal bulbar urethral stricture. (b) Contrast extravasation to peribulbar veins.

in prostatic urethra were identified (Figure 3), unrelated to urethral stricture area. The latter were only visible after opening the strictured segment, but since they did not cause any further bleeding, conservative management was applied. The urethrotomy did not present any haemorrhagic incident, and the catheter was removed on the fifth day after the procedure without any subsequent complications. Follow-up flowmetry evidenced Qmax=12.9 mL/sec, Qmed=5.3 mL/sec with 180 mL of voided volume.

Considering endoscopic findings, a pelvic MRI was performed, showing a perineal vascular malformation. This was originated in the urethral bulb and continues through 7 cm of spongy tissue, with up to 14 mm in diameter (Figure 4).

Currently, after almost two years of follow-up, our patient is asymptomatic, with no further episodes of urethral bleeding. In addition, regarding the urethral stricture, our patient is voiding properly presenting adequate uroflowmetry values, with no need for further procedures or dilatations and with a good quality of life.

3. Discussion

Urethral haemangiomas are uncommon benign vascular tumours [1]. They were initially described in 1895 [4]. Histologically, they are characterised by vascular spaces covered by endothelium. The aetiology is controversial, being unclear

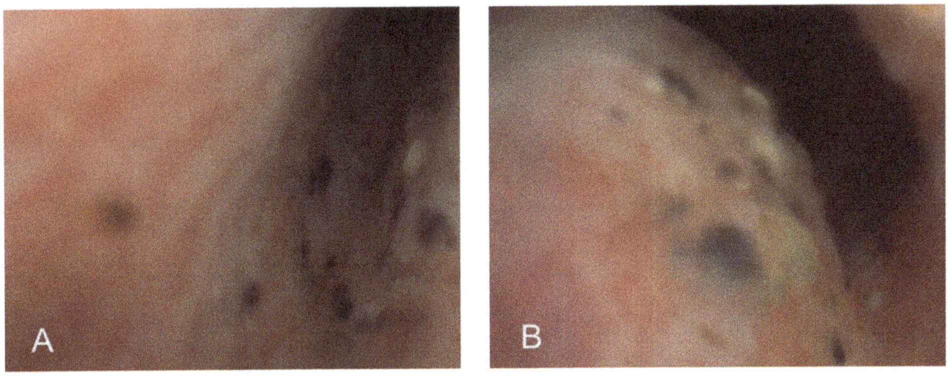

(a) (b)

Figure 3: Endoscopic aspect of the prostatic urethra.

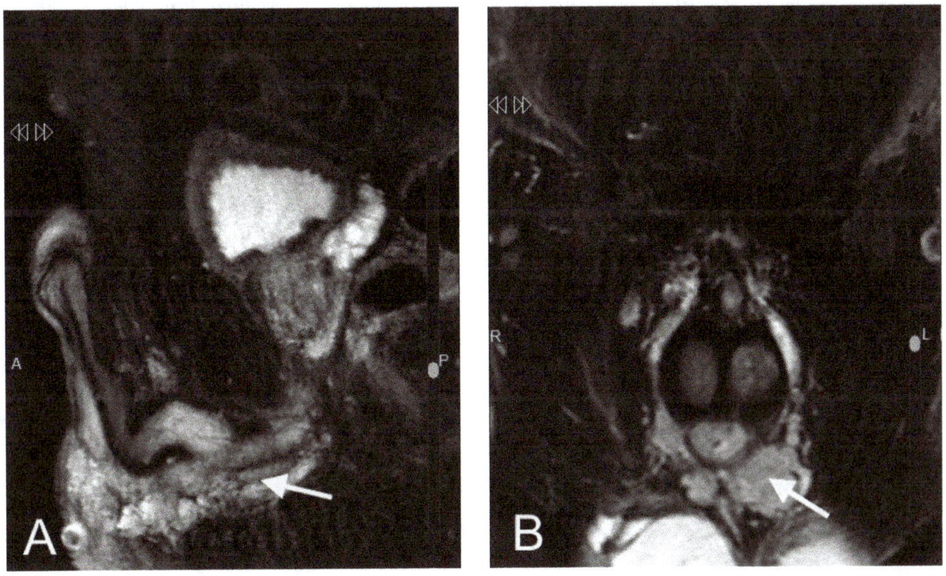

(a) (b)

Figure 4: MRI images in T2 sequence, showing periurethral hemangioma. (a) Sagittal section. (b) Coronal section.

if they are a congenital disease or are caused by vascular neoplasms. Their origin could be related to unusual differentiation of an unipotent angioblastic cell, but other hypotheses were suggested such as herniation of the cavernous bodies' constituent tissue, anomalous revascularization after a traumatism or chronic irritation, and local varicosities [1, 4].

Haemangiomas have been described in other locations, usually skin and liver [5]. Their presentation in the genitourinary system is uncommon, representing around 2% of overall haemangiomas [6]. They can appear in kidney, ureter, bladder, prostate, and urethra, which is the most infrequent location [1, 5].

It is possible to differentiate between different forms of haemangiomas. Those showing a low-flow are venous and cavernous capillary forms, opposed to arteriovenous malformations, which are high flow lesions [6, 7]. The most common haemangioma is the cavernous one [1, 2, 6, 8]. Despite their benign condition, urethral haemangiomas tend to recur despite applied treatments. In contrast, spontaneous regressions have also been reported [9].

Although cases affecting all ages have been described, they are diagnosed more often in males in the third decade of life [4, 5, 7].

Anterior urethral haemangiomas main symptom is urethral bleeding. Nevertheless, when the lesions are located in proximal urethral, they might usually cause haematuria, acute urinary retention, or haemospermia [1, 3, 5, 8]. When these lesions become bigger, they can produce obstructive urinary symptoms and even bulge out throughout external urethral meatus [1]. It is postulated that meatal urethral haemangiomas should bring up their differential diagnosis with condylomata, polyps, malign tumours, abscesses, and caruncles [2].

In our opinion, in spite of the association of both urethral stricture and haemangiomas in the case presented, we consider that there is not any relation between them, since they were not those that caused obstruction to the urinary flow. Due to the self-limited haematuria, we only applied active treatment on urethral stricture, deciding conservative management of urethral haemangiomas.

Urethral haemangiomas could be associated with cutaneous haemangiomas, as in our case, which have scrotal haemangiomas. On the other hand, urethral haemangiomas could be part of Klippel-Trenaunay syndrome, whose three typical features are varicose veins, cutaneous capillary malformations with Port wine colour, and bone and soft tissue hemihypertrophy [10–12]. Urethral haemangiomas affect 3-6% of patients diagnosed with this syndrome [10–12].

The diagnostic procedure of choice is urethrocystoscopy. It should allow identifying and defining the external appearance of lesions, ruling out other urethral bleeding aetiologies. Urethrocystoscopy would as well guide the best therapeutic choice in each case [1, 3]. MRI and doppler ultrasound can also help with diagnosis and characterisation of these lesions in cases with uncertain nature or extension [7].

A high variety of therapeutic options have been proposed for urethral haemangiomas. Treatments based on corticoids, radiotherapy, sclerotherapy, arterial embolization, or photoablation with different laser energies (Nd: YAG, argon, KTP, holmium) showed successful results, although urethrectomy could be required in certain cases. Conversely, lesions remaining asymptomatic would not require any treatment [1, 4, 5], as in our case. Location, size, and extension of haemangiomas should be considered, as well as available treatment options in each context. Above all, it is important to consider that urethral haemangiomas may be responsible for urinary obstruction according to their characteristics, although it did not happen in our patient. Therefore, a thorough preoperative planning together with suitable information to the patient is required.

4. Conclusion

The urethral haemangioma is an uncommon cause of urethral bleeding, haematospermia, and LUTS. It must be considered during differential diagnosis for these symptoms. The lesions are usually recognisable by urethrocystoscopy, but other imaging studies could be required to get an accurate diagnosis and delimitate their extension. Despite its benign nature, symptomatic cases would require treatment, with a great variety of successful therapeutic options.

Disclosure

All authors have approved the manuscript and gave their consent for the submission of this paper.

References

[1] I. Efthimiou, D. Kavouras, P. Vasilakis, and S. Katsanis, "Hemangioma of penile urethra-treatment with simple transurethral excision: a case report," *Cases Journal*, vol. 14, no. 2, p. 6199, 2009.

[2] H. Han, X.-G. Zhou, D.-D. Fan, L. Tian, and X.-D. Zhang, "An Unusual Etiology for Hematospermia and Treatments That Were Successful," *Urology*, vol. 86, no. 4, pp. 740–743, 2015.

[3] M. Abbinante, S. Crivellaro, P. Guaitoli, G. Mastrocinque, E. Ammirati, and B. Frea, "Cavernous hemangioma of the spongious body of the urethra: a case report," *Urologia*, vol. 79, no. 3, pp. 211–213, 2012.

[4] J. Ponce De León, J. Arce, L. Gausa, and H. Villavicencio, "Hemangioma of the prostatic urethra: Holmium laser treatment," *Urologia Internationalis*, vol. 80, no. 1, pp. 108–110, 2008.

[5] S. Parshad, S. P. Yadav, and B. Arora, "Urethral hemangioma: An unusual cause of hematuria," *Urologia Internationalis*, vol. 66, no. 1, pp. 43–45, 2001.

[6] V. I. Megías, F. S. Barranquero, L. E. R. Carmona, R. B. Parrilla, J. F. R. Escalante, and A. J. M. Moreno, "Hemangioma of the glans penis," *Archivos Españoles de Urología*, vol. 67, no. 4, pp. 357–359, 2014.

[7] J. T. White and R. J. Baverstock, "Eruption of blood: Arteriovenous malformation of the penile urethra," *Canadian Urological Association Journal*, vol. 11, no. 1-2, pp. E32–E34, 2017.

[8] S. Saito, "Posterior urethral hemangioma: one of the unknown causes of hematuria and/or hematospermia," *Urology*, vol. 71, no. 1, pp. 168.e11–168.e14, 2008.

[9] D. V. Singh and A. K. Mandal, "Unusual cause of urethral bleeding in an adolescent: A case in dilemma," *International Journal of Adolescent Medicine and Health*, vol. 26, no. 1, pp. 149–151, 2014.

[10] H. Lei, X. Guan, H. Han et al., "Painless urethral bleeding during penile erection in an adult man with klippel-trenaunay syndrome: a case report," *Sexual Medicine*, vol. 6, no. 2, pp. 180–183, 2018.

[11] N. Terada, R. Arakaki, Y. Okada, Y. Kaneko, and K. Nishimura, "Management of urethral hemangiomas associated with Klippel-Trenaunay-Weber syndrome by endoscopic sclerotherapy," *International Journal of Urology*, vol. 14, no. 7, pp. 658–660, 2007.

[12] A. Tepeler, Y. Yeilolva, A. Kln, T. Aktoz, and A. Nen, "A mild and rare form of Klippel-Trenaunay syndrome presenting with urethral bleeding due to penile hemangioma," *Urology*, vol. 77, no. 2, pp. 463–465, 2011.

32

Spontaneous Urethral Laceration in a Patient Experiencing Acute Ulcerative Colitis Flare

Ryan Morris,[1] John Barnard,[2] and Chad Morley[2]

[1]*Texas A&M Health Science Center, USA*
[2]*West Virginia University Health Science Center, USA*

Correspondence should be addressed to John Barnard; jbarnar4@hsc.wvu.edu

Academic Editor: Apul Goel

Spontaneous urethral laceration in the female without associated external trauma is an exceedingly rare phenomenon. Most cases are related to childbirth or the presence of a concomitant pelvic fracture or penetrating injury. Herein, we present a novel case of spontaneous urethral laceration in a female which happened to occur during an acute flare of her previously diagnosed ulcerative colitis. The diagnosis of spontaneous urethral laceration is rare, and underlying etiology is often uncertain.

1. Introduction

Urethral injuries are commonly secondary to well-defined traumatic events such as blunt trauma, penetrating injuries, or iatrogenic injuries including traumatic instrumentation [1]. The overall incidence of trauma-related pelvic injury is thought to be 5-10% when associated with a pelvic fracture making this type of injury not uncommon [2].

Ulcerative colitis is a chronic inflammatory condition affecting mainly the large colon from the rectum ascending proximally. The common symptoms and side effects of UC are well known and described in the medical literature including pain, diarrhea, hematochezia, and increased risk of colon cancer [3]. Of the known genitourinary manifestations of gastrointestinal disease, spontaneous urethral laceration has not been previously reported in conjunction with an acute UC flare [4].

2. Case Report

MA is a 49-year-old Caucasian female with a past medical history pertinent for ulcerative colitis who presented to the emergency department of our tertiary care, rural Level I trauma center for evaluation of periurethral pain and dysuria. She reported that her pain started 2 weeks prior to presentation while she was seated on the toilet straining to void. Due to symptoms of her UC, she had been experiencing frequent diarrhea. While attempting to void, she experienced a sudden onset of excruciating lower pelvic pain. Her pain persisted, and she was subsequently evaluated at an outside ED later that evening. She was diagnosed with a suspected ulcerative colitis flare given her history. Her dysuria was diagnosed as a urinary tract infection, and she was treated with empiric antibiotics. Over the next 3 days, despite adherence to antibiotic therapy, her symptoms persisted. She then presented to her primary care physician who agreed with the outside ED findings. She was additionally treated for hemorrhoids and advised to continue her antibiotic course. The following day, she had a new onset of gross hematuria for which she was again evaluated at an outside ED. Ultimately, she was admitted to the outside facility for 11 days before being discharged with a urology follow-up. After another 5 days elapsed, she was seen by her gynecologist who expressed concern for hematoma vs. abscess vs. malignancy due to an ulcerated, ecchymotic mass near the urethra. The patient was then advised to be evaluated at a tertiary care facility.

On presentation to our facility, she was found to be tachycardic with HR of 116, normotensive, normothermic, and nontachypneic with oxygen saturations of 98%. She denied any fever, chills, nausea, vomiting, or other abdominal signs

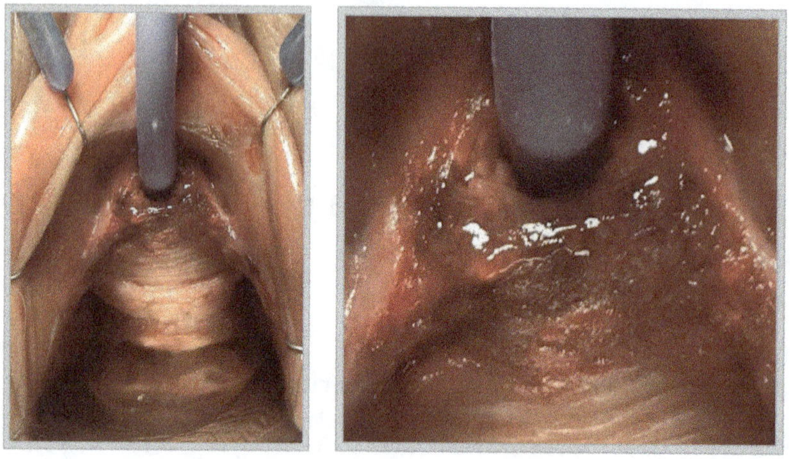

(a) (b)

Figure 1: (a) Vaginal physical exam at time of initial cystoscopy. A Foley catheter can be seen entering the urethra and lone star retractor hooks. (b) A blown-up image showing the periurethral hematoma in greater detail.

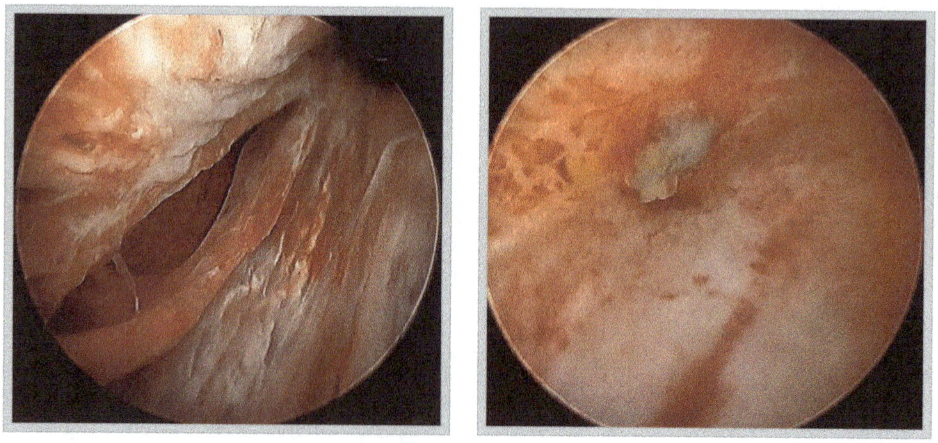

(a) (b)

Figure 2: (a) Image of urethral laceration taken at time of initial cystoscopy. Full thickness tear through the urethra is visualized with periurethral soft tissue visualized through the defect. (b) Image of the right anterior lateral bladder wall, area of concern for potential colovesical fistula formation.

or symptoms. A review of her medical history revealed depression and ulcerative colitis but no previous urological history. Her previous surgical history included cholecystectomy and an OB GYN history of cesarean delivery. She was a lifetime nonsmoker and denies heavy alcohol use or any other drug use. She is allergic to Macrobid. On genitourinary exam, an ecchymotic lesion was present circumferentially around the distal urethra with ulceration inferiorly transitioning into the anterior vaginal vault (see Figure 1).

She reported that she had initially noticed this lesion shortly after her pain started 2 weeks prior to presenting at our facility. The rest of her physical examination was without abnormality. The initial impression was that this may be due to urethral prolapse, and the urology service was consulted. After attempted examination by urology in the ED, the decision was made to perform genitourinary exam under anesthesia and cystourethroscopy due to the patient's inability to tolerate physical examination at the bedside.

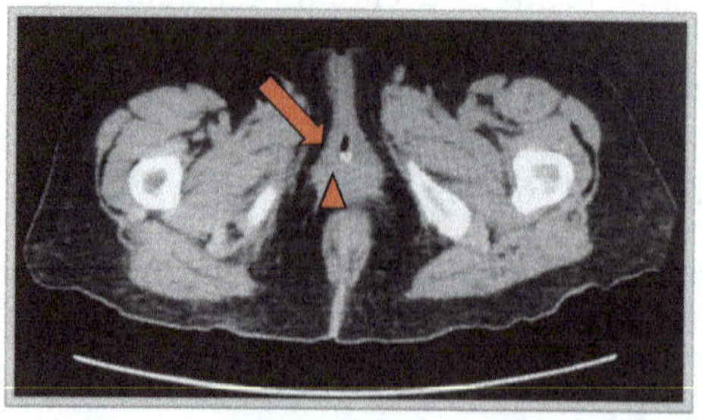

Figure 3: Axial cut CT image showing the urethral defect (*red arrow*) just anterior and slightly lateral to the Foley catheter (*arrowhead*) in place.

The examination under anesthesia revealed a firm indurated ecchymotic circumferential area around the urethra suspicious for hematoma with thrombosed urethral prolapse on the differential. Rigid cystourethroscopy was performed and showed a 1.0-1.5 cm longitudinal laceration of the urethra at the 7 o'clock position which would be the likely

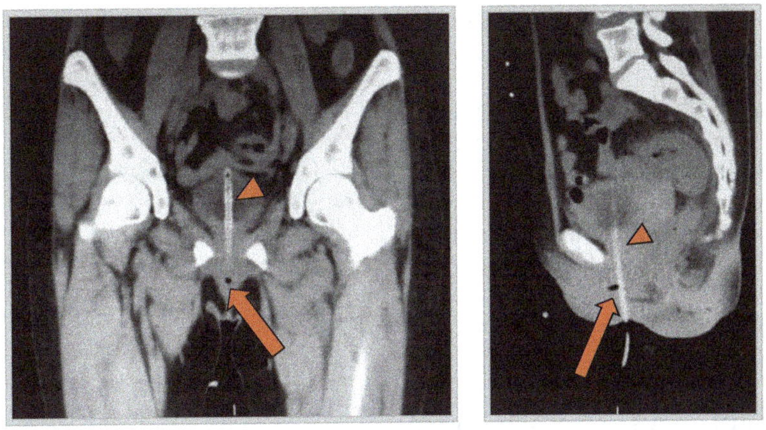

(a) (b)

FIGURE 4: (a, b) Coronal and sagittal CT sections demonstrating the urethral defect (*red arrow*) near the in place Foley catheter (*red arrowhead*).

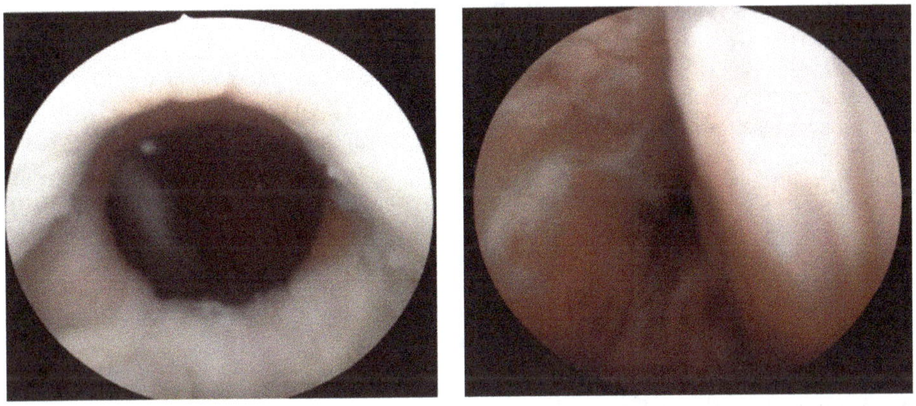

(a) (b)

FIGURE 5: Urethra visualized on follow-up cystoscopy 4 weeks after initial cystoscopy. (a) Bladder neck visualized and without abnormality. (b) Distal urethra with healed laceration and resolution of hematoma.

etiology of the hematoma (see Figure 2). Additionally, inspection of the bladder revealed numerous inflammatory lesions involving the trigone and bilateral lateral and anterior walls. Cold-cup biopsies were taken and sent to pathology, and the biopsy sites were fulgurated. Pathology later showed these lesions to be predominantly granulation tissue, blood clot, and inflammatory debris. There was also suspicion for colovesical fistula (see Figure 2) due do what appeared to be fecal material spilling into the bladder from some of the lesions. Hemostasis was achieved with spot coagulation, and an 18 Fr Foley catheter was placed at the end of the procedure which was maintained on discharge.

Her urine cultures from the operative intervention revealed Pseudomonas, and she was treated with culture-directed antibiotic therapy. A CT scan with and without contrast was ordered, and the patient was discharged with plans to follow up in the urology clinic in 2 weeks (see Figures 3 and 4).

She maintained her follow-up appointment and reported that she was doing well overall. She could not feel the hematoma like she could before, her pain was improving, and she denied any gross hematuria. She reported some drainage from around the catheter as well as some bladder spasms along with some mild fatigue. The physical exam confirmed significant improvement of her urethral and anterior vaginal wall hematoma. A repeat cystoscopy was scheduled for 2 weeks.

No other acute events occurred before the 2-week follow-up. On repeat cystoscopic examination, her urethra was found to have healed well (see Figure 5), and there was no residual hematoma appreciated on cystoscopy or on physical exam; the bladder was unremarkable. The Foley catheter was removed, and the patient was discharged from urology care. She has continued to follow with the GI service for 6 months postpresentation and has experienced one relapse of her genitourinary symptoms found to be attributable to a drug-resistant Pseudomonas UTI.

3. Discussion

This patient's atraumatic urethral laceration without a clear inciting event other than prolonged straining to void is consistent with a spontaneous urethral laceration. Among the evidence supporting this conclusion are the urethral hematoma formation as blood is seen at the vaginal introitus in 80% of female urethral injuries [5], physical exam evidence collected by several different physicians in various specialties, and ultimately direct visualization of urethral laceration on cystoscopic evaluation. The role of her ulcerative colitis flare is more unclear. A definitive cause-effect relationship is difficult to ascertain. It is possible that increased tissue friability from robust inflammatory response predisposed the patient to urothelial injury. However, it was only after a prolonged episode of straining to void that her laceration occurred. The pathological evidence consistent with fibrosis and granulomatous tissue seen within the bladder walls indicates an ongoing, prolonged inflammatory response involving the urothelium.

The diagnosis of interstitial cystitis (IC) was considered given the known association with GU ulceration (Hunner's Ulcers). IC is typically associated with pelvic pain and pressure with the frequent urge to urinate in the absence of positive culture results; it is a diagnosis of exclusion. The patient had positive urine results during the initial hospitalization (Pseudomonas aeruginosa) and developed drug-resistant Pseudomonas UTI 3 months postpresentation. She has been followed for 6 months since presentation and has experienced control of her GU symptoms with treatment of her GI disease, with relapse during her recurrent Pseudomonal UTI. Also, she underwent flexible sigmoidoscopy which revealed erythematous and friable colonic mucosa, and the biopsy revealed granulation tissue and inflammatory debris.

Overall, the presence of a urethral laceration or complete disruption in a female without concomitant pelvic fracture is exceedingly rare. Literature review showed only 3 cases which were all associated with trauma despite the absence of a pelvic fracture with fall from standing causing a straddle injury and MVC being the underlying causes [6–8]. Our case is particularly unique due to the absence not only of a pelvic fracture but also of an underlying traumatic etiology. Review of the literature did not reveal any such case described previously. The concomitant UC flare has an unknown significance with respect to any predisposition to urothelial injury but should also be noted.

4. Conclusion

Spontaneous urethral lacerations in females, defined as a urethral laceration in the absence of a clear, traumatic inciting event, are exceedingly rare as they are typically the result of significant blunt trauma causing a pelvic fracture. Above, we present a unique case of female urethral laceration not only in the absence of pelvic fracture but also without any traumatic mechanism. Based on a review of the literature, such cases are extremely rare and we could not find previous reports. The patient was also experiencing an acute flare of ulcerative colitis, and any predisposition to urothelial injury from the resultant inflammatory state remains to be elucidated. The case highlights the need for awareness that urethral laceration is possible in the female population even in the absence of pelvic trauma.

References

[1] A. A. Ter-Grigorian, G. R. Kasyan, and D. Y. Pushkar, "Urogenital disorders after pelvic ring injuries," *Central European journal of urology*, vol. 66, no. 3, pp. 352–356, 2013.

[2] C. M. Dixon, "Diagnosis and acute management of posterior urethral disruptions," in *Traumatic and Reconstructive Urology*, M. A. JW, Ed., pp. 347–355, Pa: WB Saunders, Philadelphia, 1996.

[3] C. Ford Alexander, M. Paul, and B. Haunauer Steven, "Ulcerative colitis," *BMJ*, vol. 346, no. feb05 2, p. f432, 2013.

[4] T. C. Demos and R. Moncada, "Inflammatory gastrointestinal disease presenting as genitourinary disease," *Urology Gold Journal*, vol. 13, no. 2, pp. 115–121, 1979.

[5] J. P. Kong, M. F. Bultitude, P. Royce, R. L. Gruen, A. Cato, and N. M. Corcoran, "Lower urinary tract injuries following blunt trauma: a review of contemporary management," *Revista de Urología*, vol. 13, no. 3, pp. 119–130, 2011.

[6] N. Bockolt, K. Nepple, C. Powell, and K. Kreder, "Traumatic urethral injury without pelvic fracture in an adult female," *The Scientific World Journal*, vol. 10, 310 pages, 2010.

[7] W. Al-Ashbahi, "Traumatic female urethral avulsion," *Saudi Medical Journal*, vol. 36, no. 4, pp. 366-367, 2015.

[8] A. McCool and D. Joseph, "Complete urethral disruption without pelvic fracture," *The Journal of Urology*, vol. 166, no. 4, p. 1425, 2001.

33

Stauffer's Syndrome in Patient with Metastatic Prostate Cancer

Andris Romašovs,[1] **Aldis Puķītis**,[1,2] **Viktorija Mokricka**,[1,2] **and Elina Frolova**[3]

[1] *University of Latvia, Riga, Latvia*
[2] *Center of Gastroenterology, Pauls Stradins Clinical University Hospital, Pilsoņu iela 13, Riga LV-1002, Latvia*
[3] *Medical Faculty, Riga Stradins University, Riga, Latvia*

Correspondence should be addressed to Andris Romašovs; andrisromashov@gmail.com

Academic Editor: Giorgio Carmignani

Cholestasis is a symptom that can be present in many conditions, such as bile duct obstruction by malignant mases, obstruction by gallstone, acute and chronic viral hepatitis, and autoimmune disorders, such as primary biliary and sclerosing cholangitis. Stauffer syndrome is a rare type of paraneoplastic syndrome that presents as cholestasis with absence of underlying disease. Classically Stauffer syndrome has been described in renal cell cancer patients. In literature cholestasis as manifestation of paraneoplastic syndrome has also been described in patients with prostate adenocarcinoma and pancreatic and bronchogenic carcinoma. *Conclusions.* Stauffer syndrome should be kept in mind in patients who present with cholestasis with no underlying cause. We advise to exclude any possible causes of cholestasis, for example, obstruction of bile duct.

1. Introduction

Stauffer syndrome is clinical diagnosis with unknown pathophysiology and incidence rate. Unfortunately there are no known diagnostic criteria. This syndrome was first described by the American gastroenterologist Maurice H. Stauffer, who worked at the Mayo Clinic in Rochester, MN, USA [1]. It was described as paraneoplastic syndrome in a patient with renal cell carcinoma, presenting with cholestatic disease in the absence of underlying liver disease. In a classical case, a patient with Stauffer syndrome would have elevated alkaline phosphatase, GGT (gamma-glutamyl transferase), erythrocyte sedimentation rate, α–2 globulin, thrombocytosis, and prolonged prothrombin time [2].

This case study was conducted in accordance with the Declaration of Helsinki. The protocol was approved by the Ethics committee of Pauls Stradins Clinical University Hospital on 8th November, 2018 (No. 081118-15L).

2. Case Presentation

An 80-year-old, white Caucasian man was presented to our hospital emergency department with one-month history of jaundice, pruritus, acholic feces, dark urine, unintentional weight loss, and worsening pain in the lumbar region. On the date of admission the urine was light yellow and the patient reported that feces were of normal color and consistence. He denied alcohol or illegal drug use and had no travel history within the last 10 years. He reported jaundice and pruritus progressing for one month prior to admission. He denied having pain, nausea, vomiting, or elevated temperature during the whole month. Pain in the lumbar region was progressing during the last 2 years, due to PCa metastasis. Patient had metastatic PCa and underwent palliative hormonal therapy in ambulatory settings; he also had moderate aortic stenosis found by echocardiography and angina pectoris of class II according to the classification system by Canadian Cardiovascular Society. In year 2016, metastatic process involving the lumbar spinal and thoracic region was diagnosed using skeletal scintigraphy. Starting from year 2016 he received androgen deprivation therapy in outpatient settings and testosterone level was controlled in conjugation with PSA. Testosterone remained at castrate level.

During physical examination, yellow skin, scratch marks on the back and thorax due to pruritus, and aortic murmur were revealed.

Table 1: Laboratory findings during hospitalization.

Analysis	Day 1	Day 7	Day 14	Reference range	5 months prior to admission date
ALT*,U/L	235	59	33	10-49	19
AST*, U/L	161	51	88	0-33	32
Bilirubin, umol/L	165	162	299	5-21	13
Direct-bilirubin, umol/L	132	133	237	0-5	4
Indirect-bilirubin, umol/L	33	29	63	0-16	9
Testosterone, ng/dL			12.76	86.49-788.22	
Alkaline phosphatase U/L	2513	1416	934	46-116	1356
Alkaline phosphatase bone fraction (ALP2), U/L			366	5.5-22.9	
LDH*, U/L		350	592	120-246	
GGT*, U/L	1174	515	361	0-72	
CRP*, mg/L	24.67	36.2	267.76	0-5	3.6
IL-6*, pg/mL			57	<3.4	
PSA*, ng/mL		66.01	91.78	0-3.99	
APTT*, sec.	36.3	41.8	46.1	26-36	39.5
Prothrombin index,%	87.6	18.4	20.7	70-120	74.5
INR*	1.06	3.16	2.88	0.8-1.2	1.14
Fibrinogen, g/L	5.73	8.58	8.68	0-0.5	1.68

*ALT- alanine aminotransferase; AST- aspartate transaminase; GGT- gamma-glutamyl transferase; CRP- C reactive protein; IL-6- interleukin 6; LDH- lactate dehydrogenase; PSA – prostate specific antigen; APTT – activated partial thromboplastin time; INR – international normalized ratio of prothrombin time of blood coagulation.

Blood tests indicated that the patient had cholestasis, elevated alanine aminotransferase, elevated aspartate transaminase, elevated gamma-glutamyl transferase, and elevated bilirubin (Table 1). Infectious disease such as hepatitis C and hepatitis B was excluded using testing for antibodies. Autoimmune causes were also excluded; anti-mitochondrial antibody, anti-glycoprotein antibody-210, and anti-sp100 antibodies, IgA and IgM, were all negative. Alpha-fetoprotein was also negative. Alkaline phosphatase (ALP) was significantly elevated; thus isoenzyme of bone origin ALP2 was determined to differentiate the source of elevated ALP (Table 1). Ultrasound examination of abdomen was performed, with no evidence of extrahepatic bile duct dilatation or cirrhosis. Magnetic resonance cholangiopancreatography showed no cholestasis, but 1.5 cm diameter cyst was found in hepatic parenchyma. The patient received supportive and symptomatic therapy.

Rapid deterioration of general health status occurred during hospitalization, with exitus letalis while in the hospital.

3. Discussion

Our data showed that the patient had the rare and underreported Stauffer syndrome. We have performed extensive investigation to determine a possible reversible cause of cholestasis in this case.

Most commonly Stauffer syndrome has been described relating to RCC (renal cell carcinoma), but its variants can be found in many different oncological conditions as paraneoplastic manifestation of the disease, for example, pancreatic cancer and prostate cancer (PCa) [3, 4]. It is considered that interleukin 6 has a role in the pathogenesis of paraneoplastic syndrome leading to cholestasis and liver damage with no other known causes [5]. Stauffer syndrome in patients with PCa has been reported in about 100 clinical cases since 1961 [3]. PCa remains one of the most common cancers in men, as one in five men with cancer will have PCa [6].

Recently Munveer et al. have reported a patient with newly diagnosed metastatic prostate cancer who developed paraneoplastic syndrome with cholestasis, and it resolved when androgen deprivation therapy was started. In this case PSA level was also significantly elevated and reached 4,130 ng/ml [7]. Min Kyu Kang et al. report a metastatic prostate cancer patient with paraneoplastic syndrome with cholestatic jaundice and effectiveness of androgen deprivation therapy [8]. In our case, watchful waiting with androgen deprivation therapy was started in outpatient setting and level of testosterone was maintained on castration level. Unfortunately we were unable to perform liver biopsy because of coagulopathy that developed during hospitalization.

The range of differential diagnoses for a patient presenting with cholestasis is very broad, and paraneoplastic syndrome should be kept in mind when the patient has a solid tumor with no metastases in liver or other possible causes of mechanical obstruction. By definition, paraneoplastic syndrome is triggered by the altered immune system response due to the primary tumor [9]. First of all, primary causes of liver damage should be excluded. We believe that patient had rare and underreported Stauffer syndrome, as possible mechanical, autoimmune, and infectious causes of cholestasis have been excluded. Unfortunately in this case we were unable to prolong patient life expectancy due to many comorbidities and acute progression.

References

[1] D. Kato, C. Okwara, C. Moreland, and A. Parker, "Hepatic dysfunction as a paraneoplastic manifestation of metastatic prostate adenocarcinoma," *Journal of Investigative Medicine High Impact Case Reports*, vol. 2, no. 2, 2014.

[2] G. S. Palapattu, B. Kristo, and J. Rajfer, "Paraneoplastic syndromes in urologic malignancy: the many faces of renal cell carcinoma," *Reviews in Urology*, vol. 4, no. 4, pp. 163–170, 2002.

[3] M. Fontes-Sousa, H. Magalhães, F. C. da Silva, and M. J. Maurício, "Stauffer's syndrome: A comprehensive review and proposed updated diagnostic criteria," *Urologic Oncology: Seminars and Original Investigations*, vol. 36, no. 7, pp. 321–326, 2018.

[4] G. P. Kranidiotis, P. T. Voidonikola, M. K. Dimopoulos, and M. I. Anastasiou-Nana, "Stauffer's syndrome as a prominent manifestation of renal cancer: A case report," *Cases Journal*, vol. 2, no. 1, p. 49, 2009.

[5] J.-Y. Blay, J.-F. Rossi, J. Wijdenes et al., "Role of interleukin-6 in the paraneoplastic inflammatory syndrome associated with renal-cell carcinoma," *International Journal of Cancer*, vol. 72, no. 3, pp. 424–430, 1997.

[6] J. Ferlay, I. Soerjomataram, R. Dikshit et al., "Cancer incidence and mortality worldwide: sources, methods and major patterns in GLOBOCAN 2012," *International Journal of Cancer*, vol. 136, no. 5, pp. 359–386, 2015.

[7] M. Bhangoo, B. Cheng, G. Botta, P. Thorson, and M. Kosty, "Reversible intrahepatic cholestasis in metastatic prostate cancer: An uncommon paraneoplastic syndrome," *Molecular and Clinical Oncology*, vol. 8, no. 4, pp. 613–616, 2018.

[8] M. K. Kang, J. G. Park, and H. J. Lee, "Cholestatic jaundice as a paraneoplastic manifestation of prostate cancer aggravated by steroid therapy," *Medical Principles and Practice*, vol. 27, no. 2, pp. 197–200, 2018.

[9] L. C. Pelosof and D. E. Gerber, "Paraneoplastic syndromes: an approach to diagnosis and treatment," *Mayo Clinic Proceedings*, vol. 85, no. 9, pp. 838–854, 2010.

34

A Rare Case of a Bladder Neck Abscess Masquerading as a Benign Mass

Victor A. Abdullatif, Jacob Novack, Philip J. Shalhoub, Todd G. Campbell, and Joel E. Abbott

Urology, Ascension Macomb-Oakland Hospital, Warren, 48093 MI, USA

Correspondence should be addressed to Victor A. Abdullatif; victor.abdullatif@westernu.edu

Academic Editor: Fumitaka Koga

Introduction. Bladder neck abscesses are rare urologic pathologies with very few cases published in modern literature. This report explores a case of a bladder neck mass incidentally found on computed tomography (CT) imaging in a patient with an iliopsoas abscess. *Case Presentation.* We present a case of a 60-year-old woman who was recently treated for sepsis secondary to an iliopsoas abscess in July of 2022. A CT scan revealed an indeterminate structure in the posterior inferior left paramedian bladder wall. During a cystoscopy with transurethral resection of the mass, an abscess was uncovered and evacuated. A postoperative Foley catheter was left in place, and the patient recovered without any complications. *Conclusion.* At the time of publication, the patient feels well and denies pain or lower urinary tract symptoms. Although bladder abscesses are exceptionally rare, incidental findings during cystoscopy may warrant further investigation in patients with comorbid abscesses.

1. Introduction

As a diagnostic entity, bladder neck abscesses are exceptionally rare anomalies. To date, there is only one report of a bladder wall abscess in the literature [1]. The etiology, epidemiology, clinical features, and management of these entities are not well defined as there are virtually no modern publications on the topic.

A thorough literature review revealed that intramural abscesses of the bladder wall and urachus are only slightly more common than bladder neck abscesses, with urachal abscesses representing a larger majority of these pathologies [2–4]. Due to the paucity of literature reporting their incidence, we describe a case of bladder neck abscess in a female patient. To the best of our knowledge, this is the first case report of bladder neck abscess uncovered incidentally during transurethral resection of a bladder mass. This case report serves to highlight a rare clinical phenomenon in urologic surgery.

2. Case Presentation

A 60-year-old Caucasian woman initially presented to the hospital emergency department complaining of a two-day history of right-sided inguinal pain and a fever of 103°F. The patient underwent workup in the emergency department. Laboratory workup was performed which showed a normal white blood cell count. Urinalysis was negative for pyuria or bacteriuria. Of note, the patient's C-reactive protein (CRP) was greater than 90 mg/L and erythrocyte sedimentation rate (ESR) was elevated at 47 mm/hr. A computed tomography (CT) scan of the abdomen and pelvis revealed inflammation of the iliopsoas muscle. Additionally, CT revealed an approximately 2 cm soft tissue density that appeared to lay dependently within or adjacent to a distended urinary bladder (Figure 1). An MRI of the pelvis was performed which revealed an undefined structure in the posterior inferior left paramedian bladder (Figure 2).

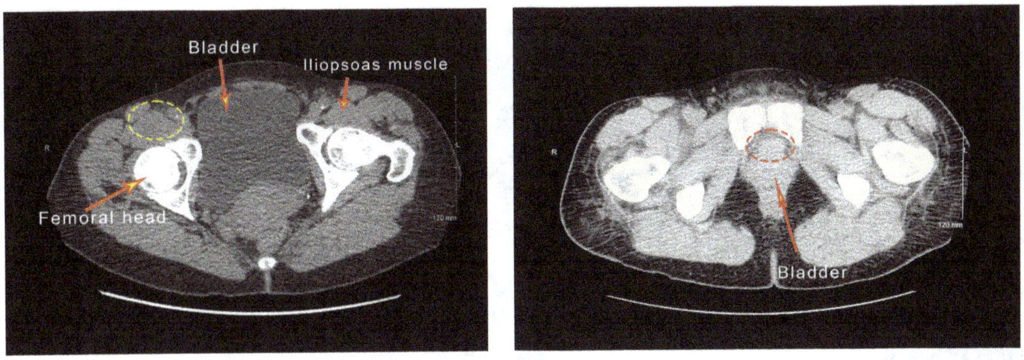

(a) (b)

Figure 1: CT scan of the abdomen and pelvis demonstrating a psoas abscess ((a) yellow circle) and a 20 × 15 × 14 mm soft tissue density in the inferior posterior left paramedian bladder wall ((b) red circle).

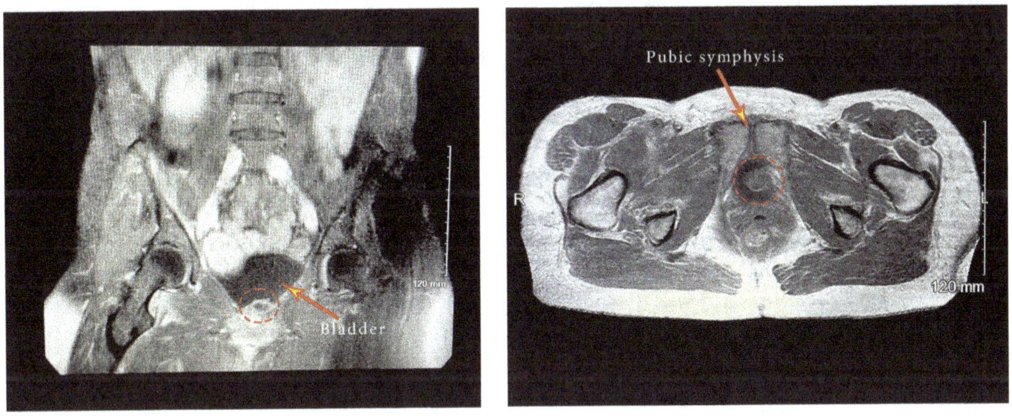

(a) (b)

Figure 2: MRI of the pelvis demonstrating an undefined structure in the posterior inferior left paramedian bladder wall protruding into the bladder (red circle). Image demonstrates decreased T1 with minimal increased T2 with questionable minimal enhancement of a thin rim with no internal enhancement.

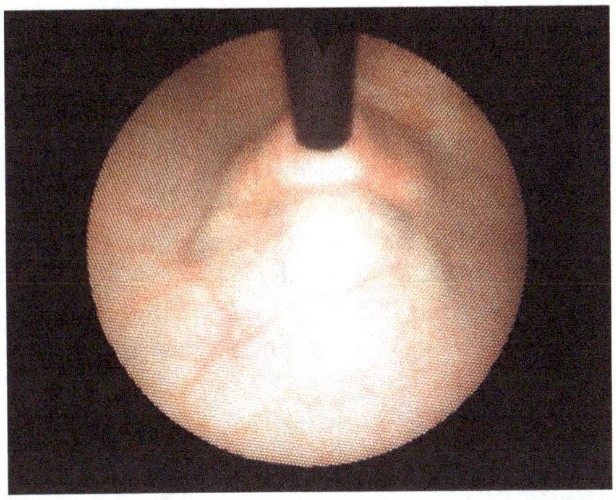

Figure 3: Cystoscopic photo of undefined, raised lesion in the bladder wall anterolateral to the urethra.

Following a diagnosis of sepsis secondary to a psoas abscess, the patient was admitted and treated with an intravenous course of vancomycin and piperacillin/tazobactam for four days. After completing her treatment course, the patients CRP and ESR had returned to baseline. The patient felt well, was hemodynamically stable, and was discharged 7 days after admission. She was instructed to follow-up with urology for further evaluation of the incidental bladder mass found on imaging.

The patient presented to the urology clinic feeling well. Her past medical history included hypothyroidism and myocarditis secondary to COVID-19. The patient was nondiabetic and was not taking any immunosuppressive medications. She is a nonsmoker, and her family history was noncontributory. Her physical exam was unremarkable. As the initial part of the urologic workup, a cystoscopy was performed which demonstrated an undefined, raised lesion in the bladder wall anterolateral to the urethra at the bladder base (Figure 3). The mass did not exhibit the physical characteristics of a traditional neoplastic growth of the bladder. To exclude malignancy, the patient was then scheduled for a transurethral resection of the mass to obtain a specimen for pathologic evaluation.

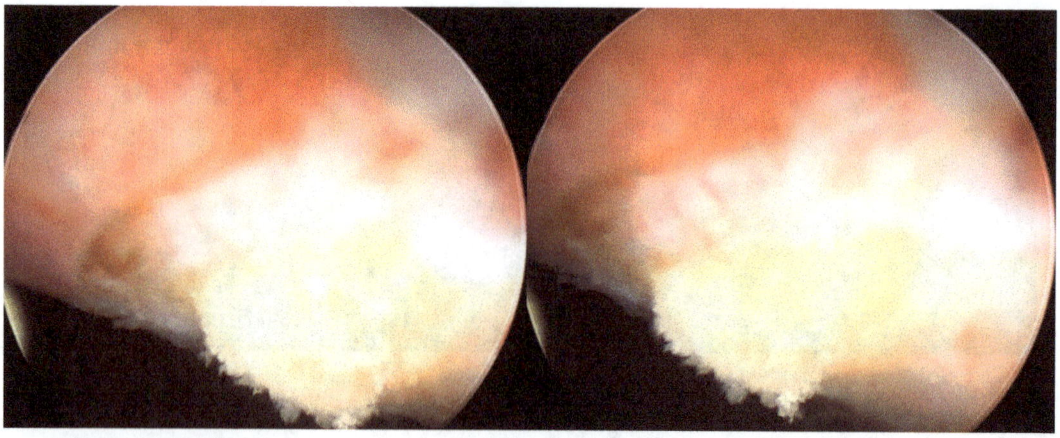

FIGURE 4: Photos taken during transurethral resection the bladder mass showing yellow, purulent fluid indicative of an abscess.

During transurethral resection of the mass, a yellow, purulent fluid was evacuated (Figure 4). The remainder of the bladder neck mass was shaved away in order to deroof the contents completely. The resectoscope was used to expel all residual pus until the bladder-wall cavity was cleared. A total of approximately 80 mL of purulent fluid was removed and sent for culture and cytology. Bladder tissue was sent for pathologic evaluation.

Following abscess deroofing and evacuation, a 16-French 2-way Foley catheter was placed. The patient was hemodynamically stable following the procedure and was discharged home where she completed a three-week course of trimethoprim/sulfamethoxazole. The patient was instructed to remove the Foley catheter at home, which she removed the day after the procedure.

Both wound and urine cultures demonstrated no growth. Cytology revealed mixed chronic and acute inflammatory cells in the background, mostly small lymphocytes with benign squamous and urothelial cells. Histologically, there was no significant smooth muscle tissue present. The surface urothelium showed focal small nests with bland cellular features, suggestive of mild proliferative chronic cystitis. Underlying connective tissues showed reactive fibrosis with some stromal hemorrhage. There was no evidence of papillary, in situ, or invasive malignancy.

Three weeks following deroofing of the bladder the abscess, the patient was reevaluated. She denied any lower urinary tract symptoms or suprapubic abdominal pain. Her physical exam was unremarkable.

3. Discussion

Bladder neck abscesses are an exceptionally rare finding. At the time of publication, the only case in the literature was reported in the Boston Medical and Surgical Journal in 1850 [1]. The patient described in this editorial was a young male who presented with significant dysuria, as well as a heavy, deep-seated pain in the perineum. Since then, there have only been reports of infected urachal cysts and intramural bladder-wall abscesses. Interestingly, bladder abscesses have a variable set of clinical features and presentations in healthcare settings as far as they have been reported.

In contrast to the aforementioned patient, our patient had no urologic history and was asymptomatic prior to being seen in the office. This difference could be explained by the anatomic differences between the female and male urinary tract. Obstructive lower urinary tract symptoms are much more common in men, and lesions that impact the area near the bladder neck are much more likely to cause symptoms [5]. In our patient, it is unclear how long she had the bladder lesion as she had no history of hospitalization or prior imaging. Her inguinal pain was most likely due to the iliopsoas abscess.

One possible explanation for the formation of multiple or recurrent abscesses is immunosuppression. It is well known that diabetic patients or those who are chronically immunocompromised from other conditions or medications are at a significantly increased risk for local and systemic infections [6]. However, our patient was nondiabetic and not on any immunosuppressive medications. Additionally, she had no history of organ transplantation or any condition that would have suppressed her immune system. Moreover, our patient had no history of urinary tract infections. This suggests that abscess formation in the urinary system may occur spontaneously in immunocompetent patients.

Due to the paucity of literature on bladder neck abscesses, it remains unclear what the disposition of our patient would have been without intervention. It is possible that following recovery from the psoas abscess, our patient could have remained asymptomatic for many years with the bladder abscess. Because her urine cultures were negative, it is unlikely that the bladder neck abscess would have led to hematogenous spread or sepsis without an obstruction. Our patient did well after the abscess evacuation indicating that surgical intervention may be a safe option in female with bladder neck abscesses.

4. Conclusion

Based on current evidence, the pathophysiological mechanism behind the formation of bladder abscesses is unclear. Drawing from the evidence of other abscesses, it may be appropriate to treat bladder abscesses with incision, drainage, and antibiotics. It remains unknown as to what the optimal treatment regimen is for bladder neck abscesses.

Patients with iliopsoas abscesses with undefined lesions on imaging may warrant further investigation and workup. Incidental findings during cystoscopy may warrant further investigation in patients with comorbid abscesses.

Consent

No written consent has been obtained from the patients as there is no patient identifiable data included in this case report.

References

[1] S. Mitchell, "Abscess in the Neck of the Bladder," *The Boston Medical and Surgical Journal*, vol. 43, no. 19, pp. 374-375, 1850.

[2] C. Walker, "A case report of urachal abscess: a rare differential in adult abdominal pain," *Hawaii Medical Journal*, vol. 69, no. 2, pp. 35-36, 2010, (In eng).

[3] H. Loertzer, S. O. Höhne, R. Finke, and P. Fornara, "Intramural bladder-wall abscess: a late complication arising after a urethro-cystoscopy?," *Pediatric Surgery International*, vol. 21, no. 4, pp. 323–325, 2005, (In eng).

[4] A. Elkbuli, K. Kinslow, J. D. Ehrhardt Jr., S. Hai, M. McKenney, and D. Boneva, "Surgical management for an infected urachal cyst in an adult: case report and literature review," *International Journal of Surgery Case Reports*, vol. 57, pp. 130–133, 2019, (In eng).

[5] L. Beland, C. Martin, and J. S. Han, "Lower urinary tract symptoms in young men-causes and management," *Current Urology Reports*, vol. 23, no. 2, pp. 29–37, 2022.

[6] L. K. Dropulic and H. M. Lederman, "Overview of infections in the immunocompromised host," *Diagnostic microbiology of the immunocompromised host*, vol. 4, no. 4, 2016(In eng).

Diffuse Leukoplakia of the Bladder Ostium-Sparing in Patient Treated with Leuprorelin for Breast Cancer

Antonio Nacchia,[1] Ferdinando di Giacomo,[1] Arcangelo Di Cerbo,[2] Massimo Dante Di Somma,[2] Giuseppe Patitucci,[2] Giuseppe Disabato,[1] and Giulia Vita[2]

[1]*Urology Department, IRCCS CROB, Rionero in Vulture (PZ), Italy*
[2]*Anatomical Pathology Department, IRCCS CROB, Rionero in Vulture (PZ), Italy*

Correspondence should be addressed to Antonio Nacchia; antonionacchia7@gmail.com

Academic Editor: Tun-Chieh Chen

Case. A 55-year-old woman came to our attention in April 2020 referring haematuria, frequency and urgency. The patient referred previous treatment with leuprorelin 3.75 mg/2 ml for breast cancer three years ago. Urine culture was performed and resulted always negative for pathogens. Cystoscopy revealed a whitish plaque lesion on the fundus, dome, trigone, and left lateral wall of the bladder. Histology of the biopsy confirmed the diagnosis of leukoplakia of the bladder. The plan is to follow her up repeating a cystoscopy every three months and biopsy in 6 months. Literature search revealed very little information on pathogenesis and prognosis of this condition due to its rare occurrence. The main objective of our case study was to describe individual situation of a woman affected by diffuse leukoplakia of the bladder ostium-sparing with a previous treatment with leuprorelin 3.75 mg/2 ml for breast cancer and to show safety of follow-up by cystoscopy and biopsy. *Conclusions.* We showed a case of a woman treated with leuprorelin and with diffuse leukoplakia of the bladder. We support the recommended long-term follow-up and surveillance based on the literature review by cystoscopy with or without biopsy.

1. Introduction

Leukoplakia vesicae (LV), also known as keratinizing squamous metaplasia, is a rare histological change of the bladder predisposing the individual to a possible high risk of bladder carcinoma in the background of prolonged exposure to a chronic irritant [1, 2]. It is rarely encountered in urological practice with an incidence of 1 : 10000. In areas where schistosomiasis is uncommon, it usually occurs due to chronic irritation of the inflamed bladder mucosa by bacteria. Risk factors include chronic catheterization, neurogenic bladder, vitamin A deficiency, urinary fistulas, and bladder outlet obstruction [3, 4]. Literature search revealed few reported cases of LV. We are reporting one case of this histological change in the bladder not secondary to chronic irritation due to infection. The main objective of our case study was to describe individual situation of a woman affected by diffuse leukoplakia of the bladder ostium-sparing with previous treatment with leuprorelin 3.75 mg/2 ml for breast cancer and to show safety of follow-up by cystoscopy and biopsy.

2. Case Report

A 55-year-old woman presented gross haematuria for several days. She had history of storage lower urinary tract symptoms (LUTS) since undergoing quadrantectomy surgery for breast cancer 3 years previously. She referred previous treatment with leuprorelin 3.75 mg/2 ml. She was an ex-smoker with a cigarette consumption of maximum ten a day. She interrupted smoking when she was diagnosed breast cancer. She referred past episodes of haematuria and storage LUTS that she always treated with antibiotics even if urine culture was negative. In April 2020, she came to our ambulatory of urology. She showed us a recent urine culture negative for infections and urinary cytology negative for malignant cells. Cystoscopy was performed, and it demonstrated an extensive

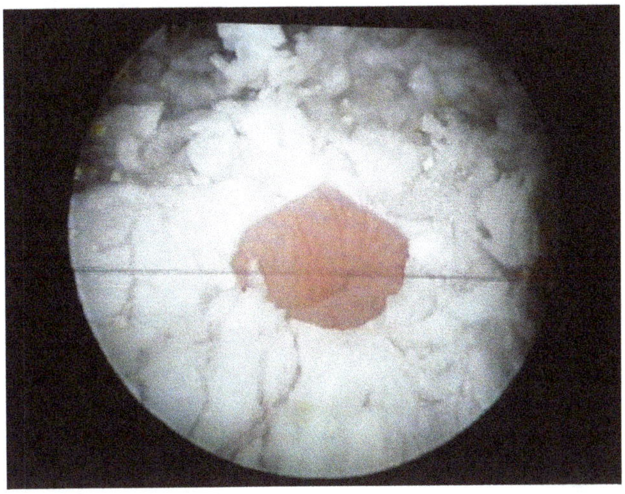

FIGURE 1: Whitish plaque extended near the left ureteric orifice without interesting it.

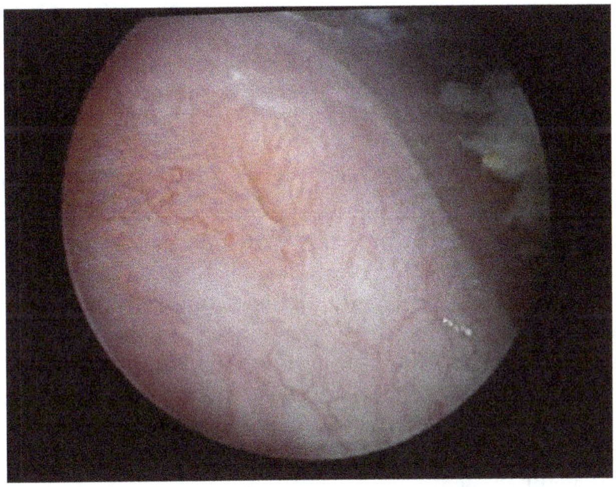

FIGURE 2: Right orifice was completely spared by plaques.

whitish plaque area on the fundus, the dome, left emi-trigone, and left bladder wall. It extended near the left ureteric orifice without interesting it (Figure 1). Right orifice was completely spared (Figure 2). The efflux from both the ureteric orifices was normal. The mucosa underneath the plaques was inflamed *(*Figure 3*)*. Multiple biopsies were performed. A net margin separated sane mucosa from pathological plagues. The histology of the affected area revealed keratinizing squamous metaplasia and focal low grade epithelial dysplasia (Figure 4). With these collected data, the main objective of our case study was to describe individual situation of a woman affected by diffuse leukoplakia of the bladder ostium-sparing with previous treatment with leuprorelin 3.75 mg/2 ml for breast cancer and to show safety of follow-up by cystoscopy and biopsy.

3. Discussion

A women of 55 years old came to our attention for LUTS, especially urgency and frequency, associated with haematuria

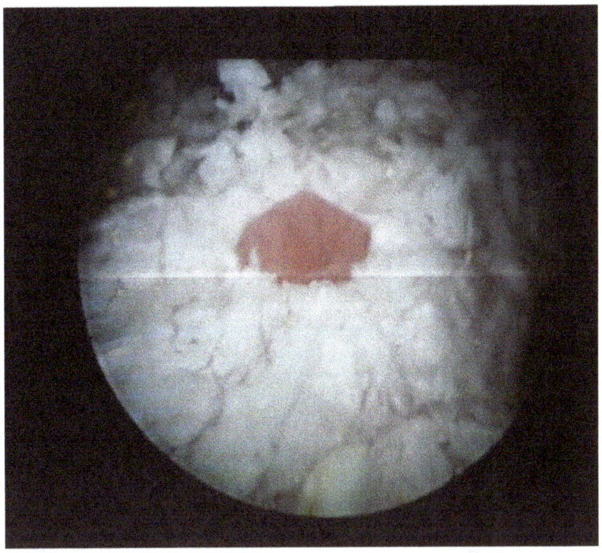

FIGURE 3: The mucosa underneath the plaques was inflamed.

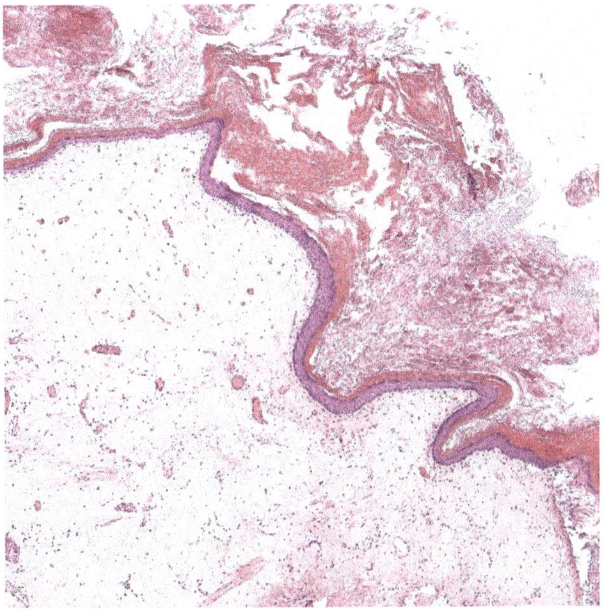

FIGURE 4: Replacement of the urothelium with stratified keratinized squamous epithelium.

in April 2020. Urine culture was negative. Urinary cytology was negative for malignant cells. Cystoscopy was performed showing a diffuse white plague ostium-sparing. Left orifice was circumferentially spared by LV (Figure 1). Dedicated informed consent for surgery and for this article was given by subject, and her anonymity is totally preserved. Multiple biopsies were performed with a LV diagnosis. According to some evidences in literature [1–3], the patient was managed with medical treatment. Antibiotics, pain killers, and antimuscarinics were given to manage her storage LUTS. She repeated a cystoscopy at six months from first cystoscopy in October 2020, and mapping of the bladder was performed in December 2020 confirming keratinizing squamous metaplasia (Figures 4 and 5).

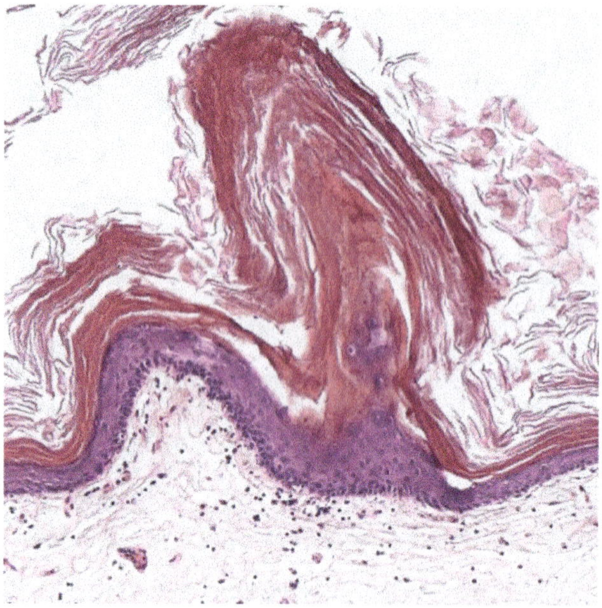

FIGURE 5: Hyperkeratotic, acanthotic squamous epithelium lining the lumen of the bladder with papillomatosis.

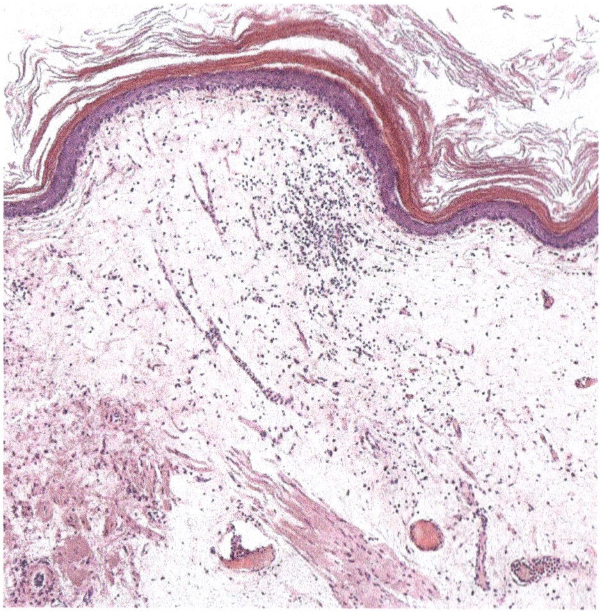

FIGURE 6: Loose subepithelial connective tissue rich in small vessels with chronic inflammation infiltrate.

Leukoplakia signifies "white plaque": the pathogenesis being cornification of normally noncornifying membrane due to a chronic inflammation (Figure 6) triggered by various risk factors [5]. It is encountered in urological practice with an incidence of 1 : 10000 and with the highest incidence in women between 50 and 70 years old [1, 5]. Trigone is the commonest site of occurrence sparing the ureteric orifice as in our case, but the condition can also be seen in the other walls of the bladder. Risk factors include chronic catheterization, neurogenic bladder, vitamin A deficiency, urinary fistulas, and bladder outlet obstruction [3].

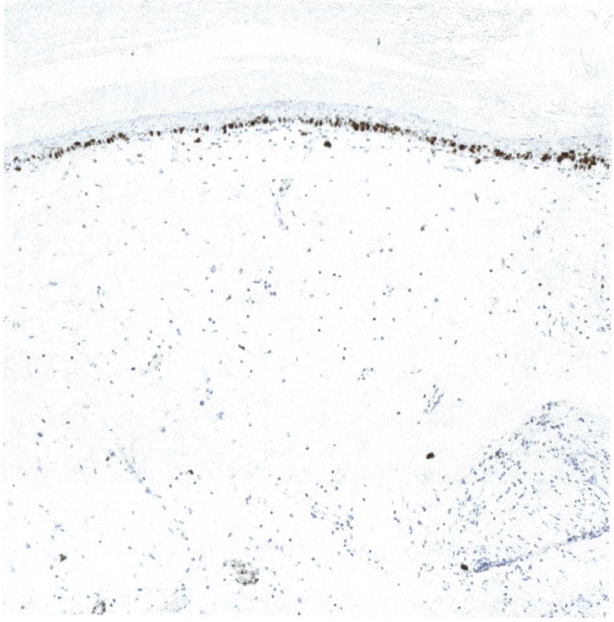

FIGURE 7: Staining for Ki67 (cell proliferation index) limited to the basal layer of the epithelium supports the benign nature of leukoplakia.

The etiology is not known exactly, but according to Eyup et al. [2], possible hypotheses are embryological dispersal of ectoderm or spontaneous transformation or secondary epithelial response to appropriate stimuli.

Diagnosis is histological. Microscopically, the normal urothelium is replaced by squamous epithelium with an overlying layer of keratin (Figures 5 and 7). It is considered as a risk factor for squamous cell carcinoma. Based on available literature, the current recommendation is for close cystoscopic monitoring annually to look for any subsequent malignant changes [4].

No consensus on management and treatment is actually available. Antibiotics are the most common therapy used in clinical practice, and they may help symptomatic remission, but efficacy is not durable. Transurethral resection of the bladder therapy significantly relieves urinary symptoms in women with LV. Improvement of quality of life has a success rate of 57.6%. Considering the very low complication rate, our study supports transurethral resection as an alternative treatment for patients who are resistant to medical therapy [6]. Recently, Benelli et al. [7] manage a man affected by LV with hyaluronic acid instillations with resolution of clinical symptoms. It could be considered the starting point and the gold standard in the follow-up of our patient. However, at present, further studies are required to formulate an adequate policy for therapeutic management of this unusual lesion of the bladder mucosa [7].

The woman of this case report was previously treated with leuprorelin 3.75 mg/2 ml for breast cancer. Leuprorelin is in the gonadotropin-releasing hormone (GnRH) analogue family of medications. There are two works evaluating the efficacy of the GnRH-analogue, leuprolide acetate, on NK cell activity. The first one suggests an increased NK cell activity in peripheral blood samples determined by 51Cr release assay

[8], and the second one reported that NK cell cytotoxicity from control and patients was significantly decreased with leuprolide acetate [9]. These findings suggest a direct immunomodulatory role of GnRH on NK cell activity.

There is a report where the immunomodulation exerted by GnRH on freshly isolated primary peritoneal macrophages is clearly observed. In this work, the authors found that the production of nitric oxide, costimulated with lipopolysaccharide (LPS) and interferon-γ (IFNy), and the activity of NF-κB were suppressed by GnRH exposure. These results demonstrate that GnRH participates in macrophage function and indicate that the NF-κB signaling pathway may be responsible for GnRH-mediated immune modulation [9].

In some studies, leuprorelin was associated with interstitial lung diseases, granulomas, or other kinds of cutaneous eruptions (erythematous macules, infiltrated plaques, subcutaneous nodules, and sterile abscesses) [10–14], but no case reports of LV associated with leuprorelin are reported, so our manuscript should be considered innovative as first article on this topic. Possible association between leuprorelin treatment and LV could be related to alterations on immune system as proposed for interstitial lung disease by Shioi et al. [10]. This possible explanation about immune reactivity was supported for granulomas leuprorelin-related by Yasukawa et al. too [12]. However, etiology and pathogenesis about this association are actually not clear and should be clarified in the future.

Additional Points

Learning Points. LV is a rare condition which aetiology is not known exactly. Leuprorelin was associated with interstitial lung diseases, granulomas, or other kinds of cutaneous eruptions (erythematous macules, infiltrated plaques, subcutaneous nodules, and sterile abscesses). Leuprorelin use could be associated with LV too through immune system pathways. Recommended long-term follow-up and surveillance by cystoscopy with or without biopsy are safety and should be performed in LV.

References

[1] C. G. Roehrborn, C. M. Teigland, and H. M. Spence, "Progression of leukoplakia of the bladder to squamous cell carcinoma 19 years after complete urinary diversion," *The Journal of Urology*, vol. 140, no. 3, pp. 603-604, 1988.

[2] G. Eyup, Y. Banu, and M. Cengiz, "Extensive bilateral renal pelvis, ureter and bladder leukoplakia-case report," *International Journal of Urology*, vol. 9, no. 11, pp. 653–655, 2002.

[3] M. B. Amin, J. K. McKenney, G. P. Paner et al., "ICUD-EAU International consultation on bladder cancer 2012: pathology," *European Urology*, vol. 63, pp. 16–35, 2013.

[4] T. Pandey, S. Pandey, A. Goel, and A. Aggarwal, "Leukoplakia of the urinary bladder: keratinising squamous metaplasia," *BMJ Case Reports*, vol. 2018, article 227019, 2018.

[5] A. Kasianandan and K. Kannan, "Leukoplakia of the bladder: a case report and literature review," *International Urogynecology Journal*, vol. 23, no. 1, pp. 131–133, 2012.

[6] H. Wang, T. Chong, X. Y. Tang, and W.-B. Zhang, "Transurethral resection in women with symptomatic keratinizing squamous metaplasia of urinary bladder: a retrospective study of 92 cases," *May*, vol. 12, no. 2, pp. 137–142, 2020, Epub 2019 Nov 24.

[7] A. Benelli, V. Varca, and C. Vaccaro, "Keratinizing squamous metaplasia of the bladder: our experience and current approaches," *Urologia*, vol. 87, no. 2, pp. 97–100, 2020, Epub 2018 Dec 3.

[8] T. Tanaka and N. Umesaki, "Novel intermittent GnRHa therapy for patients with endometriosis Nihon Rinsho," vol. 59, Supplement 1, pp. 124–128, 2001.

[9] M.-G. Kang, D.-W. Gwak, H.-J. Cho, Y.-S. Min, and J.-S. Park, "Effect of leuprorelin in bulbar function of spinal and bulbar muscular atrophy patients: observational study for 1 year," *Journal of Neurology*, 2021.

[10] K. Shioi, M. Yoshida, and N. Sakai, "Interstitial pneumonitis induced by bicalutamide and leuprorelin acetate for prostate cancer," *International Journal of Urology*, vol. 10, no. 11, pp. 625-626, 2003.

[11] K. Maeda, T. Osafune, Y. Masuda et al., "Drug-induced interstitial lung disease during combined androgen blockade with bicalutamide and leuprorelin acetate for prostate cancer Nihon Hinyokika Gakkai Zasshi," vol. 110, no. 1, pp. 36–40, 2019.

[12] K. Yasukawa, D. Sawamura, and H. Sugawara, "Leuprorelin acetate granulomas: case reports and review of the literature," *The British Journal of Dermatology*, vol. 152, no. 5, pp. 1045–1047, 2005.

[13] N. Kluger, S. Hahtola, and T. Lempinen, "Granulomes cutanes apres injections sous-cutanees d'acetate de leuproreline," *Presse Médicale*, vol. 46, no. 10, pp. 966–968, 2017, Epub 2017 Sep 14.

[14] C. A. de Salins, I. Kupfer-Bessaguet, and C. Fleuret, "Fixed drug eruption induced by leuprorelin," *Annales de Dermatologie et de Vénéréologie*, vol. 142, no. 12, pp. 780-781, 2015, Epub 2015 Aug 4.

36

Long-Term Undesirable Consequences of Penile Skin Island Flap to Correct Penoescrotal Transposition: A Case Report and Review of Literature

Raquel Varea-Malo,[1] **Daniel Martínez Revuelta**,[2] **Felix Campos-Juanatey**,[1,3] **Paola Calleja Hermosa**,[1] **and Miguel Angel Correas Gómez**[1,4]

[1]*Urology Department, Marqués de Valdecilla University Hospital, Santander, Cantabria, Spain*
[2]*GP Department, Marqués de Valdecilla University Hospital, Santander, Cantabria, Spain*
[3]*Valdecilla Research Institute (IDIVAL), Santander, Cantabria, Spain*
[4]*School of Medicine, University of Cantabria, Santander, Cantabria, Spain*

Correspondence should be addressed to Raquel Varea-Malo; raquelvareamalo@gmail.com

Academic Editor: Mohamed A. Ghoneim

Hypospadias is a congenital malformation of the male lower urinary tract, consisting of a ventral urethral opening proximal to the glans penis. This condition is corrected surgically in the paediatric age, with a great variety of techniques available. Traditionally, a tubularized genital skin was used for one- or two-stage repairs. Nowadays, the tendency is to use preputial or oral mucosa grafts, dorsally located, to avoid diverticula formation and prevent hair growth in the neourethra. We present a case of a patient born with proximal hypospadias with penoscrotal transposition, surgically corrected in his childhood, using dorsal penile skin island flap. The patient is referred to urology consultation in his adulthood for a weak urinary stream, recurrent infections, and a large amount of hair exiting through the urethral meatus.

1. Introduction

Hypospadias is the most common congenital malformation of the male lower urinary tract [1]. In this condition, the urethral opening is ventrally located, proximal to the tip of the penis. Its position ranges from a glandular position—located in the ventral aspect of the glans—to more proximal locations—proximal penile, penoscrotal, or even perineal. In severe cases, it is associated with penoscrotal transposition, where the scrotal insertion is above the penile base.

The hypospadias is corrected surgically during the early years of life, with different techniques depending on meatal location. There are more than 300 procedures described for the surgical treatment of hypospadias. Traditionally, preputial or genital skin was used as a tube for performing repairs in one surgical time. Nowadays, the tendency shifted towards using preputial or oral mucosa grafts, dorsally located, in single or staged repairs [2]. In most cases, there is a lack of adequate long-term follow-up of patients. All this variety reflects the absence of consensus among paediatric surgeons and urologists about which techniques are the most suitable ones.

Our objective is to describe the long-term undesirable consequences of the surgical repair by dorsal penile island flap [3] for proximal hypospadias with penoscrotal transposition. Additionally, we will review the literature and discuss the main complications potentially developed by hypospadias patients in adolescence and adulthood and the variety of current treatments. We followed the CARE guidelines for case report communication [4].

2. Clinical Case

A 38-year-old male was referred to our clinic for lower urinary tract symptoms (LUTS) and hair growth protruding through the external urethral meatus. The patient was diagnosed as a newborn of proximal penile hypospadias with penoscrotal transposition. His condition was corrected by when he was 3 years old by ventral transposition of dorsal penile skin flap in a single surgical time, according to the technique described by Perovic and Vukadinovic [3].

He complained of recurrent episodes of urinary tract infections (UTI) for several months, weak urinary stream, and difficulty in sexual intercourse.

Physical examination confirmed the growth of large amounts of hair through the urethral opening (Figure 1). Urine culture was performed, yielding a negative result. Uroflowmetry showed a maximum flow rate (Qmax) of 11.1 ml/s, and an average flow rate of 7.9 ml/s for a voiding volume of 309 ml. The voiding curve evidenced a plateau shape, corresponding with urethral stricture. A retrograde urethrography (RUG) was performed, confirming the existence of a very short segment of urethral stricture, located at the junction of the penile and bulbar urethra (Figure 2). Flexible urethroscopy using a 16F cystoscopy was conducted, allowing for good passage through the penile neourethra to the penoscrotal angle, where the visualization of the stricture was not possible due to a large amount of hair.

After completing the diagnostic workout and offering a surgical approach for reconstruction, the patient rejected further interventions. He is being monitored, with voiding parameters maintained (Qmax above 10 ml/s) and no UTIs. His main complaints are related to sexual intercourse, due to penile curvature 45° downwards, and cosmetic alteration caused by severe scarring associated with the presence of hair through the urethra.

3. Discussion

Hypospadias is a congenital malformation of the male lower urinary tract, consisting of a urethral meatus opening proximally to the normal location at the distal end of the glans. Its incidence is approximately 1 in 300 men (0.3-0.45%) [1], with a family-specific genetic predisposition. It presents a great variability in terms of its severity, and the meatus can be located at various levels from the distal part of the penile shaft to the perineal area. It is frequently associated with ventral penile curvature, both at rest and in erection. There are several classifications for hypospadias. Classically, they are divided into proximal and distal. The proximal hypospadias (PH) are the most complex and can be perineal, interscrotal, penoscrotal, or midshaft. The distal hypospadias (DH), which are more frequent, can be subcoronal, coronal, or glandular. Additionally, the GMS classification (Glans, Meatus and Shaft) lists from 1 to 4 each item: G (glans size and urethral plate quality), M (meatal location), and S (penile curvature). Applying this classification before surgery is recommended since it has been correlated with the appearance of surgical complications [5].

The treatment of hypospadias is surgical, performing surgery preferably before the age of 5 [6]. The purpose of the interventions is threefold: bring the neomeatus to the tip of the glans to achieve correct urination and ejaculation, achieve cosmetic appearance suitable and satisfactory for the patient, and correct penile curvature in erection [7]. There is no ideal surgical technique, with more than 300 options described, making it very difficult to establish a standardized guide for treatment and follow-up.

Repair of hypospadias in childhood can lead to certain postoperative complications involving urinary urethra, bulbar or penile stricture, fistula, diverticulum, growth of hair, cavernous bodies, ventral chordee, axial torsion, glans, dehiscence or partial necrosis, and morphology of the penis and scrotal skin [8]. In most patients, short-term complications of primary repair are caused by surgical errors of design, technique, or postoperative care such as infection, suture dehiscence, urine extravasation, hematoma, ischemia, or postoperative necrosis in transplanted tissue [9]. However, they can also provide complications many years later, with successful functional and cosmetic results in primary repair and urethral stricture development decades after initial surgery [9]. There are not many studies on the long-term outcomes of hypospadias surgery, with patients lost to follow-up usually being higher than 50% [10]. In addition, only a few cases maintained an established protocol of prolonged routine checks over time. This is important since pubertal growth can change the cosmetic and functional aspects of the penis, with the appearance of new curvatures, affecting psychosexual development [11]. This is especially relevant in repairs using hair-bearing skin, like scrotal tubes or dorsal penile skin as in our case [3]. We have not found any specific study in the literature about the growth of large amounts of hair through the urethra, following a surgical repair of hypospadias with penoscrotal transposition by island skin flap of the dorsum of the penis.

Classical evaluation of the outcomes after hypospadias surgery is performed by comparing the early development of fistulas, diverticula, and strictures. However, there is usually no long-term follow-up for these patients [6, 12]. If the urinary function is resolved, there is usually no follow-up in terms of cosmetic result or sexual function. Often during the transition to adulthood, these patients are not referred to a urologist, and on the other hand, not all urologists are prepared to attend to the failed hypospadias, which aggravates the problem. It is estimated that 1 in 15 patients followed over 3 years will need reintervention [12].

With only one surgical intervention, about 75% of good results are obtained [12]. In the case of PH, these results are even worse, with complications reaching 58% (including 55.7% fistulas) in a series of 115 patients [10]. In other series, complications are less common, reporting 3.5-10% restrictures and 11-20% fistulas in patients with DH. In HP, an average of 3.7 surgeries (from 1 to 15) are required until a full resolution is achieved. Reinterventions occur during the first year in nearly 50% of the cases, but up to 37.7% are needed more than 2 years after the initial surgery [12].

In the follow-up of patients after hypospadias surgery, voiding pattern should be assessed to rule out obstructive symptoms. It is recommended to complete an evaluation with uroflowmetry, an objective, reliable, noninvasive, and inexpensive test. Flow rates could be altered in up to 1 in 3 patients, being a suitable test for screening of recurrences or other anatomic alterations, such as diverticula or hairballs [10].

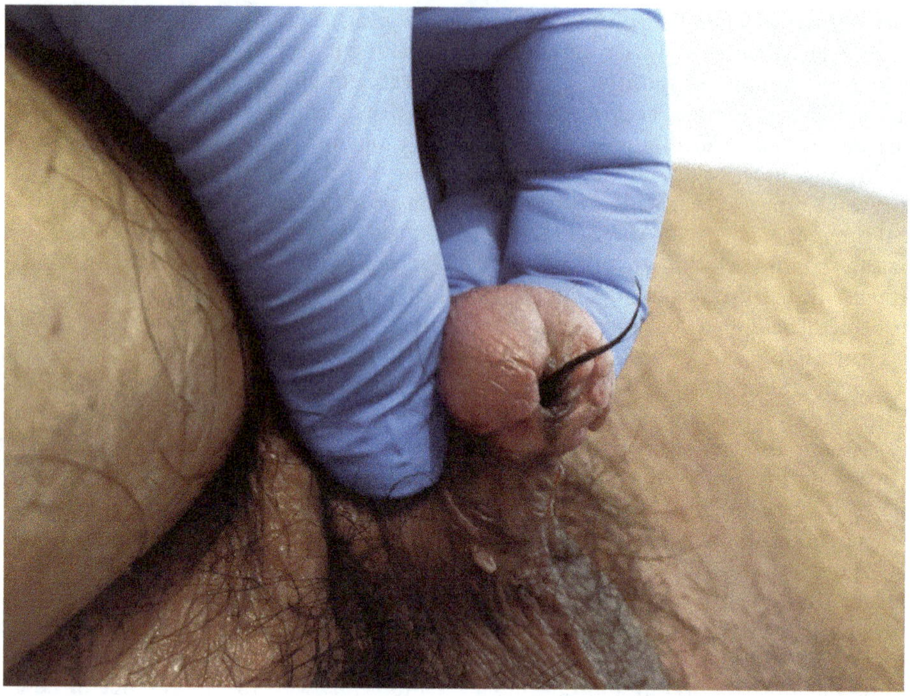

Figure 1: External appearance after dorsal penile island flap presenting a large amount of hair exiting the external meatus.

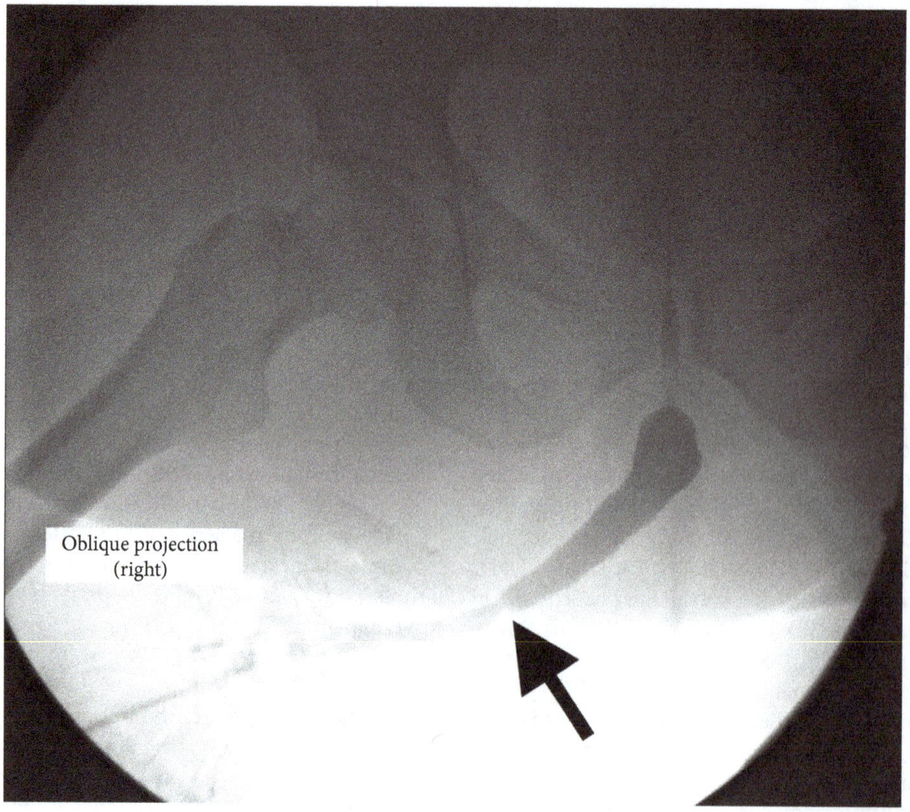

Figure 2: Retrograde urethrogram showing a stricture in the junction between the neourethra and the native bulbar urethra (arrow).

Up to 60% of patients present long-term problems, being more prevalent in PH and in those operated using multistage techniques [7]. "Spraying," or dispersion of the urine stream when leaving the urethral neomeatus, is usually the most reported symptom [6]. Another common symptom, reported by up to 50% of severe hypospadias, is postmicturition dribbling, due to the characteristics of the neourethra, which lacks adequate musculature for its complete emptying after voiding [7]. RUG usually associated with voiding cystourethrography or flexible urethroscopy is used to diagnose urethral complications, as we evidenced in our case. Targeted questionnaires are also used to specifically assess voiding quality. Ideally, they should be performed pre- and postsurgery to compare the results. From the voiding point of view, we can use the IPSS (International Prostate Symptoms Score) and urethral stricture PROM (Patient Reported Outcome Measure) questionnaires [10].

The cosmetic outcome should also be evaluated after hypospadias correction [13]. Several strategies and tools have been proposed. The HOSE (Hypospadias Objective Scoring Evaluation) [14] questionnaire, GPS-J (Junior Genital Perception Scale) [15], and PPS (Penile Perception Score) [16] are the most widespread questionnaires. PPS was first described for the paediatric population, being the first validated instrument for evaluation of the aesthetic result after hypospadias surgery [17]. A good correlation was found between evaluations by patients, parents, and urologists [16]. Another useful tool for comparing and evaluating the results is standardized photography, which has also been applied for developing rating scales [18].

Sexual problems in these patients are often present. They can be functional due to genital scarring or residual or relapsed penile curvature causing painful intercourse. Also, the body image disorder related to previous genital surgeries could lead to erectile dysfunction or ejaculation problems [7]. In addition, if the neomeatus has remained proximal to the balanopreputial sulcus, alterations in fertility may occur by not reaching the ejaculation in the cervix. This could be associated with weak ejaculation due to a lack of contractility of the neourethra.

The most common aspects to correct in adulthood are strictures, fistulas, diverticula, and persistent hypospadic location of the neomeatus [8]. Several aspects made the reconstruction complex [11]: poorly vascularized tissues after previous surgeries, congenital absence of corpus spongiosum, lack of skin and coverage tissues, and psychological issues of patients, avoiding further interventions, as we presented in our case.

Strictures are usually located at the junction of the native hypospadic urethra with the reconstructed area or in the distal neourethra. We should discuss whether urethral dilations are suitable for maintaining long-term patency or a new surgical intervention is required. In some cases, increasing urethral calibre by dorsal or ventral augmentation using grafts or flaps is feasible [11]. However, it is usually required to perform a complete urethral reconstruction after removing previous repairs. This complete substitution could be done in selected cases with oral mucosa grafts in a single procedure [19], but in most situations would require a staged approach using oral mucosa, preputial, or extragenital skin [11]. As a general rule, it is safer to remove all the fibrotic tissues, put wide grafts of oral mucosa—or other tissue—to cover the defect, and bring the new urethral plaque to the tip of the glans in a first procedure. After a period of 3 to 6 months, this graft can be tubularized to shape the neourethra, but the placement of more grafts prior to tubularization is required in approximately 20% of cases. For this reason, the term "multistage surgery" is preferred over the classic term of two-stage surgery. As the most common sexual problem is penile curvature, this aspect should be evaluated during reconstructive procedures, especially in PH. If necessary, dorsal albuginea application techniques could be used in paediatric population to correct curvatures [10]. In adulthood, releasing of the scarred tissues and ventral corpora cavernosum incisions at the time of reconstruction are preferred, to preserve penile length.

4. Conclusion

Long-term complications of hypospadias repair are common, but a large amount of hair growing in the neourethra is a rare consequence of penoscrotal transposition repairs. During a diagnostic workout, other alterations, as strictures, fistulas, or diverticula, should be considered. Long-term follow-up after hypospadias surgery should be offered, ideally until puberty or adulthood.

Authors' Contributions

All authors have approved the manuscript and gave their consent for the submission to the Case Reports in Urology.

Acknowledgments

The authors would like to express their gratitude to Dr. José Antonio Portillo Martín, for his kind assistance during the article production.

References

[1] J. E. H. Bergman, M. Loane, M. Vrijheid et al., "Epidemiology of hypospadias in Europe: a registry-based study," *World journal of urology*, vol. 33, no. 12, pp. 2159–2167, 2015.

[2] E. M. Gong and E. Y. Cheng, "Current challenges with proximal hypospadias: we have a long way to go," *Journal of pediatric urology*, vol. 13, no. 5, pp. 457–467, 2017.

[3] S. Perovic and V. Vukadinovic, "Penoscrotal transposition with hypospadias: 1-stage repair," *The Journal of urology.*, vol. 148, 5 Part 1, pp. 1510–1513, 1992.

[4] D. S. Riley, M. S. Barber, G. S. Kienle et al., "CARE guidelines for case reports: explanation and elaboration document," *Journal of clinical epidemiology*, vol. 89, pp. 218–235, 2017.

[5] L. S. Merriman, A. M. Arlen, B. H. Broecker, E. A. Smith, A. J. Kirsch, and J. M. Elmore, "The GMS hypospadias score: assessment of inter-observer reliability and correlation with post-operative complications," *Journal of pediatric urology*, vol. 9, no. 6, pp. 707–712, 2013.

[6] C. C. Hoag, G. T. Gotto, K. B. Morrison, G. U. Coleman, and A. E. Macneily, "Long-term functional outcome and satisfaction of patients with hypospadias repaired in childhood," *Canadian Urological Association journal = Journal de l'Association des urologues du Canada*, vol. 2, no. 1, pp. 23–31, 2008.

[7] C. Jiao, R. Wu, X. Xu, and Q. Yu, "Long-term outcome of penile appearance and sexual function after hypospadias repairs: situation and relation," *International urology and nephrology*, vol. 43, no. 1, pp. 47–54, 2011.

[8] G. Barbagli, S. Perovic, R. Djinovic, S. Sansalone, and M. Lazzeri, "Retrospective descriptive analysis of 1,176 patients with failed hypospadias repair," *The Journal of urology*, vol. 183, no. 1, pp. 207–211, 2010.

[9] G. Barbagli, M. De Angelis, E. Palminteri, and M. Lazzeri, "Failed hypospadias repair presenting in adults," *European urology*, vol. 49, no. 5, pp. 887–895, 2006.

[10] A. Springer, "Assessment of outcome in hypospadias surgery - a review," *Frontiers in pediatrics*, vol. 2, 2014.

[11] F. B. S. Campos-Juanatey, S. L. Ivaz, A. Frost, D. E. Andrich, and A. R. Mundy, "Management of penile urethral strictures: challenges and future directions," *World Journal of Clinical Urology*, vol. 5, no. 1, p. 1, 2016.

[12] A. F. Spinoit, F. Poelaert, L. A. Groen, E. Van Laecke, and P. Hoebeke, "Hypospadias repair at a tertiary care center: long-term followup is mandatory to determine the real complication rate," *The Journal of urology*, vol. 189, no. 6, pp. 2276–2281, 2013.

[13] M. A. Mureau, F. M. Slijper, A. K. Slob, F. C. Verhulst, and R. J. Nijman, "Satisfaction with penile appearance after hypospadias surgery: the patient and surgeon view," *The Journal of urology*, vol. 155, no. 2, pp. 703–706, 1996.

[14] A. J. Holland, G. H. Smith, F. I. Ross, and D. T. Cass, "HOSE: an objective scoring system for evaluating the results of hypospadias surgery," *BJU international*, vol. 88, no. 3, pp. 255–258, 2001.

[15] M. A. M. Mureau, F. M. E. Slijper, A. K. Slob, and F. C. Verhulst, "Genital perception of children, adolescents, and adults operated on for hypospadias: a comparative study," *The Journal of Sex Research*, vol. 32, no. 4, pp. 289–298, 1995.

[16] D. M. Weber, M. A. Landolt, R. Gobet, M. Kalisch, and N. K. Greeff, "The Penile Perception Score: an instrument enabling evaluation by surgeons and patient self-assessment after hypospadias repair," *The Journal of urology*, vol. 189, no. 1, pp. 189–193, 2013.

[17] D. M. Weber, V. B. Schonbucher, M. A. Landolt, and R. Gobet, "The Pediatric Penile Perception Score: an instrument for patient self-assessment and surgeon evaluation after hypospadias repair," *The Journal of urology*, vol. 180, no. 3, pp. 1080–1084, 2008.

[18] M. Ververidis, A. P. Dickson, and D. C. Gough, "An objective assessment of the results of hypospadias surgery," *BJU international*, vol. 96, no. 1, pp. 135–139, 2005.

[19] A. R. Mundy, F. Campos-Juanatey, S. Bugeja et al., "Single-stage tubular urethral reconstruction using oral grafts is an alternative to classical staged approach for selected penile urethral strictures," *Asian journal of andrology*, vol. 22, no. 2, pp. 134–139, 2020.

37

Prune Belly Syndrome Associated with Interstitial 17q12 Microdeletion

Surasak Puvabanditsin, Miry Shim, Jeffrey Suell, Jeffrey Manzano, Kristin Blackledge, Avram Bursky-Tammam, and Rajeev Mehta

Department of Pediatrics, Rutgers Robert Wood Johnson Medical School, New Brunswick, New Jersey, USA

Correspondence should be addressed to Surasak Puvabanditsin; surasak1@aol.com

Academic Editor: Tun-Chieh Chen

We report a term male neonate presenting with a "prune belly," bilateral hydronephrosis, hydroureter, posterior urethral obstruction, and bilateral undescended testes. Analysis with the whole genome SNP microarray revealed an interstitial deletion of about 1.49 megabase (MB) at chromosome 17q12. We present a rare association of prune belly syndrome with a chromosomal deletion in this same region.

1. Introduction

Interstitial deletions involving terminal 17q12 (17q12-qterm) are rare chromosomal abnormalities associated with variable phenotypes. Previous case reports of 17q12 microdeletion characterized the patients with structural and/or functional disorders of the kidney and urinary tract, maturity-onset diabetes of the young type 5 (MODY5), and neurodevelopmental or neuropsychiatric disorders (e.g., developmental delay, intellectual disability, autism spectrum disorder, schizophrenia, anxiety, and bipolar disorder) [1–3]. To date, there are few reported cases of prune belly syndrome (PBS) and associated chromosomal abnormalities. We report a new case of PBS associated with 17q12 microdeletion, and we review the literature.

2. Case Report

A term Hispanic male neonate was born at 40-week gestation to an 18-year-old primigravida by cesarean section. Apgar scores were 9 and 9 at 1 and 5 minutes, respectively. Pregnancy was complicated by an abnormal prenatal ultrasound at 20-week gestation which revealed bilateral renal pelvis dilation, dilated ureters, thickened bladder with keyhole sign, and dilated urethra. Subsequent sonography revealed progression of the hydronephrosis and hydroureters. Genetic studies that were performed during the pregnancy had shown 17q12 microdeletion, a de novo mutation. The family history was negative for congenital anomalies, and there were no history of in utero exposure to any known teratogens and no history of consanguinity.

Physical examination revealed a weight of 3470 grams (45th centile), length of 50 cm (40th centile), and head circumference of 35 cm (45th centile). Anomalies noted at birth included marked abdominal distension with a thin, wrinkled, and flaccid abdominal wall and bilateral undescended testes (shown in Figures 1 and 2). A Foley catheter was placed on day of life (DOL) 0, and the infant was started on amoxicillin for urinary tract infection (UTI) prophylaxis. Ultrasound of the kidneys and bladder on DOL 0 showed severe right hydroureteronephrosis, moderate left hydroureteronephrosis, thick-walled urinary bladder, and dilatation of the posterior urethra. There was a cystic structure noted in the prostate (shown in Figure 3). An abdominal ultrasound found bilateral testes in the midabdomen. Voiding cystourethrogram (VCUG) performed on DOL 2 revealed grade 5 left vesicoureteral reflux and grade 1 right vesicoureteral reflux. The cystic structure in the prostate represented the prostatic utricle cyst on VCUG. The posterior urethral

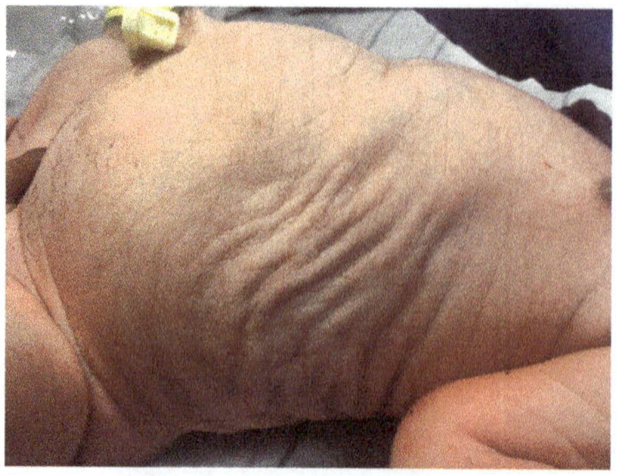

Figure 1: Note the wrinkled, flaccid, and thin abdominal wall.

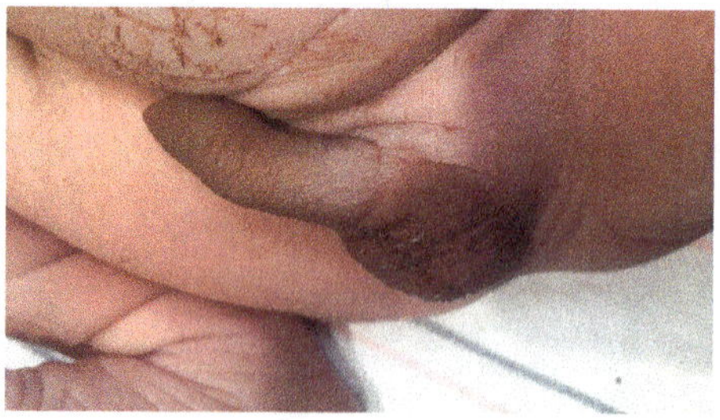

Figure 2: Note few rugae and undescended testes.

dilatation was noted which was probably the result of prostatic hypoplasia. The anterior urethral dilatation was also noted secondary to anterior urethral valve (shown in Figure 4). A MAG-3 renogram with Lasix on DOL 6 revealed split function of 43% in the left kidney and 57% in the right kidney without significant clearance after Lasix administration, which was consistent with bilateral obstruction. Echocardiogram showed a small patent ductus arteriosus and patent foramen ovale, and a neurosonogram was normal. The serum creatinine was monitored daily for the first few days of life and then twice weekly, peaking at 1.1 mg/dL on DOL 2 and 8.

Right and left nephrostomy tubes were placed on DOL 8 and 15, respectively. After the procedures, he developed *Enterobacter cloacae* pyelonephritis despite UTI prophylaxis. Upon discharge on DOL 21, serum creatinine was 0.8 mg/dL. The infant's feeds consisted of breastmilk or Similac PM 60/40. Bilateral nephrostomy tubes remained in places upon discharge; he was prescribed daily oral amoxicillin for the prevention of urinary tract infection. He was discharged to a subacute hospital for continued management of nephrostomy tubes until planned bilateral pyelostomy and orchiopexy at 1 month.

3. Cytogenetic and Molecular Studies

Whole genome SNP (single-nucleotide polymorphism) microarray analysis was performed using the SNP oligonucleotide microarray analysis (SOMA) CytoScan HD platform which uses over 743,000SCN probes and 1,953,000 NPCN probes with median spacing of 0.88 kilobase (kb). Total genomic DNA was extracted from the patient's blood sample and digested with NspI and ligated to NspI adaptors. Polymerase chain reaction (PCR) products were purified and quantified. Purified DNA was fragmented and biotin labeled and hybridized to the CytoScan HD GeneChip. There was a 1.49 megabase (MB) interstitial deletion of the long arm of chromosome 17: arr [hg19] 17q22 (34,822, 465-36, 307,773) x1 and 826 kilobase (kb) interstitial duplication in the long arm of chromosome 7: 7q12.1 (98,230,688-99, 056,822) x3.

The SNP microarray analysis identified an interstitial deletion of 17q22.1, and this deleted interval includes numerous Online Mendelian Inheritance in Man (OMIM) genes starting from *ZNHIT3* to *TBC1D3H*. Deletion of this region has been reported to be associated with the following phenotypes: cystic renal disorders, pancreatic atrophy, liver abnormalities, cognitive impairment and structural brain abnormalities, maturity-onset diabetes of the young (MODY), Müllerian aplasia/Mayer-Rokitansky-Küster-Hauser syndrome in females, and epilepsy (OMIM 189907).

Whole genome SNP microarray (Reveal) analysis identified an interstitial duplication of 7q12.1; this interval includes 10 OMIM genes (NPTX2, TRRAP, SMURF1, KPNA7, ARPC1A, ARCP1B, PDAP1, BUD31, PTCD1, and CPSF4). There has been no report of clinically established disorders with duplication of this region.

4. Discussion

Aplasia of the abdominal wall muscle was described by Froehlich in 1939, which is considered the first description of PBS [1]. The incidence of PBS is estimated about 1/30,000 to 1/50,000 live births [2–4], with the incidence decreasing likely due to improvement of prenatal detection and elective termination of affected pregnancies. Most of the cases of PBS are male (3-5% being female), prevalence is higher in the black population, and incidence is higher in infants born to younger mothers [5, 6]. The triad of PBS manifestation included (1) dysgenesis and partial or complete aplasia of muscle of the abdominal wall, (2) undescended testes, and (3) complex malformations of the urinary tract [7].

There are other findings apart from the triad, which are present in 75% of the PBS cases. Pulmonary abnormalities, e.g., pulmonary hypoplasia (not parenchymal lung disease), are present and related to prenatal oligohydramnios. Gastrointestinal complications included malrotation, intestinal atresia/stenosis, volvulus, and obstruction occurring in about 30% of PBS patients [8]. 10% of PBS cases have associated cardiac anomalies: septal defects, tetralogy of Fallot, and patent ductus arteriosus [3]. Musculoskeletal abnormalities, usually lower extremities: club feet, congenital hip dislocation, and hypoplasia of the leg or foot, were seen in 5% of the PBS cases [2, 9].

The pathogenesis of PBS has been debated and currently proposed with two prominent thoughts: mesenchymal developmental failure or urinary tract obstruction [10]. Higher incidence in males and cases of familial PBS lead to the speculation of a possible sex-influenced inheritance pattern. Murray et al. and Haeri et al. reported 2 cases of PBS

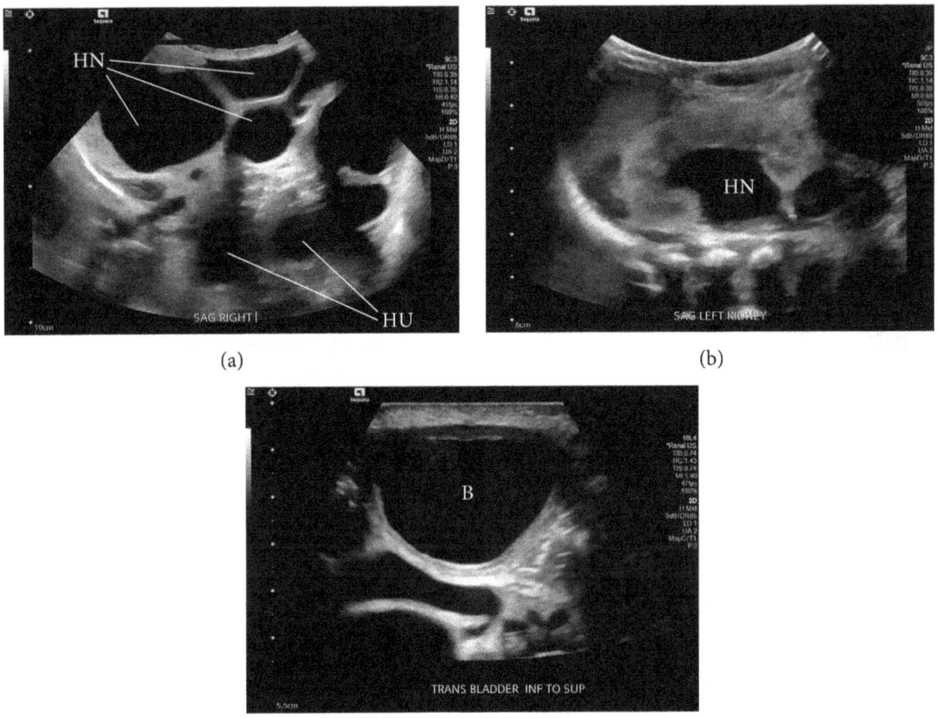

FIGURE 3: Renal and bladder sonography showed a severe (a) right hydroureteronephrosis, (b) moderate left hydroureteronephrosis, and (c) thick wall urinary bladder. HN: hydronephrosis; HU: hydroureter; B: urinary bladder.

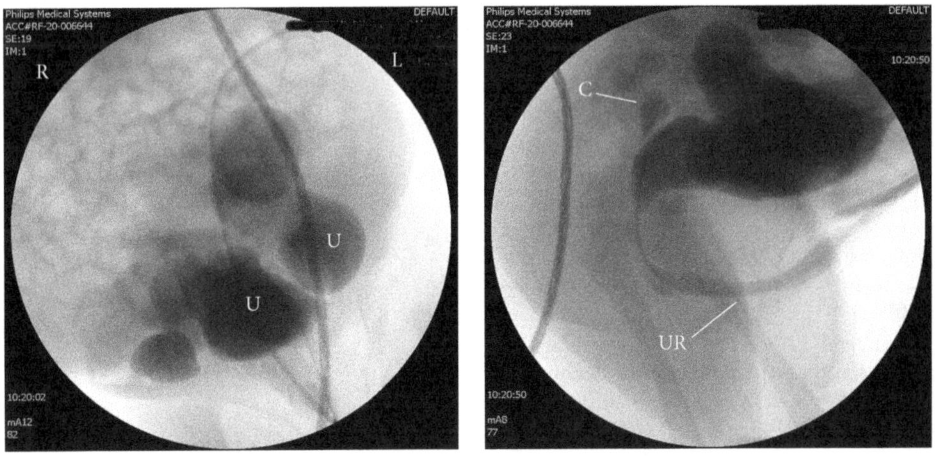

FIGURE 4: (a) Voiding cystourethrogram showed grade 5 left vesicoureteral reflux (ureter (U)). (b) Dilatation of the posterior and anterior urethra and cystic structure posterior to the urinary bladder (utricle cyst) (cyst (C), urethra (UR)).

with interstitial deletions of chromosome 17q12, suggesting the role of *HNF1B* (*TCF2*), a gene that is responsible for mesodermal and endodermal development in different tissues, in PBS [11–13]. However, 17q12 deletion has also been reported in association with other congenital abnormalities of the kidney and urinary tract (CAKUT) without the PBS phenotype: agenesis, hypoplasia, dysplasia, multicystic dysplastic kidney (MCDK), and horseshoe kidney, collecting system abnormalities (duplicated collecting systems, ureteropelvic junction obstruction, isolated hydronephrosis, or hydroureter) and tubulointerstitial disease of the kidney [14–18].

5. Conclusion

We report a case of a neonate with 17q12 microdeletion that is associated with PBS. Our report supports the genetic basis in PBS, and the screening for HNF1B gene mutations/deletions on chromosome 17q12 could help identify the patient of PBS and lead to preventing and improving the treatment of this rare disease.

Consent

Written informed consent was obtained from the parents of the patient for publication of this case report and any accompanying images. A copy of the written consent is available for review by the editor-in-chief of this journal.

Authors' Contributions

All authors are equally involved in drafting, literature search, and writing the paper.

References

[1] F. Froehlich, "Der Mangel der Muskeln, insbesondere der Seitenbauchmuskeln.," Zürn, Wuerzburg, 1839.

[2] F. J. Greskovich and L. M. Nyberg, "The prune belly syndrome: a review of its etiology, defects, treatment and prognosis," *Journal of Urology*, vol. 140, no. 4, pp. 707–712, 1988.

[3] R. S. Sutherland, R. A. Mevorach, and B. A. Kogan, "The prune-belly syndrome: current insights," *Pediatric Nephrology*, vol. 9, no. 6, pp. 770–778, 1995.

[4] T. Hoshino, Y. Ihara, H. Shirane, and T. Ota, "Prenatal diagnosis of prune belly syndrome at 12 weeks of pregnancy: case report and review of the literature," *Ultrasound in Obstetrics & Gynecology*, vol. 12, no. 5, pp. 362–366, 1998.

[5] S. Hassett, G. H. Smith, and A. J. Holland, "Prune belly syndrome," *Pediatric Surgery International*, vol. 28, no. 3, pp. 219–228, 2012.

[6] G. Tonni, V. Ida, V. Alessandro, and M. P. Bonasoni, "Prune-belly syndrome: case series and review of the literature regarding early prenatal diagnosis, epidemiology, genetic factors, treatment, and prognosis," *Fetal and Pediatric Pathology*, vol. 31, no. 1, pp. 13–24, 2013.

[7] R. E. Stevenson, J. G. Hall, and R. M. Goodman, *Human Malformations and Related Anomalies*, Oxford University Press, New York, 1st edition, 1993.

[8] V. Zugor, G. E. Schott, and A. P. Labanaris, "The prune belly syndrome: urological aspects and long-term outcomes of a rare disease," *Pediatric Reports*, vol. 4, no. 2, article e20, 2012.

[9] R. T. Loder, J. P. Guiboux, D. A. Bloom, and R. N. Hensinger, "Musculoskeletal aspects of prune-belly syndrome. Description and pathogenesis," *American Journal Disease of Childhood*, vol. 146, no. 10, pp. 1224–1229, 1992.

[10] A. M. Arlen, C. Nawaf, and A. J. Kirsch, "Prune belly syndrome: current perspectives," *Pediatric Health Medicine and Therapeutics*, vol. Volume 10, pp. 75–81, 2019.

[11] P. J. Murray, K. Thomas, C. J. Mulgrew, S. Ellard, E. L. Edghill, and C. Bingham, "Whole gene deletion of the hepatocyte nuclear factor-1 gene in a patient with the prune-belly syndrome," *Nephrology, Dialysis, Transplantation*, vol. 23, no. 7, pp. 2412–2415, 2008.

[12] S. Haeri, P. L. Devers, K. A. Kaiser-Rogers et al., "Deletion of hepatocyte nuclear factor-1-beta in an infant with prune belly syndrome," *American Journal of Perinatology*, vol. 27, no. 7, pp. 559–563, 2010.

[13] C. F. Granberg, S. M. Harrison, D. Dajusta et al., ""Genetic basis of prune belly syndrome," screening for HNF1β gene," *Journal of Urology*, vol. 187, no. 1, pp. 272–278, 2012.

[14] M. W. Mitchel, D. Moreno-De-Luca, S. M. Myers et al., ""17q12 recurrent deletion syndrome", Dec 8, 2016 [Updated 2020 Oct 15]," in *Gene Reviews®*, M. P. Adam, H. H. Ardinger, R. A. Pagon, S. E. Wallace, L. J. H. Bean, K. W. Gripp, G. M. Mirzaa, and A. Amemiya, Eds., University of Washington, Seattle, Seattle (WA), 1993-2021, https://www.ncbi.nlm.nih.gov/books/NBK401562/.

[15] C. P. Chen, S. D. Chang, T. H. Wang et al., "Detection of recurrent transmission of 17q12 microdeletion by array comparative genomic hybridization in a fetus with prenatally diagnosed hydronephrosis, hydroureter, and multicystic kidney, and variable clinical spectrum in the family," *Taiwan Journal of Obstetetrics & Gynecology*, vol. 52, no. 4, pp. 551–557, 2013.

[16] R. Li, F. Fu, Y. L. Zhang, D. Z. Li, and C. Liao, "Prenatal diagnosis of 17q12 duplication and deletion syndrome in two fetuses with congenital anomalies," *Taiwan Journal of Obstetetrics & Gynecology*, vol. 53, no. 4, pp. 579–582, 2014.

[17] Y. L. Jiang, Q. W. Qi, X. Y. Zhou et al., "Prenatal diagnosis of 17q12 microdeletion syndrome in fetal renal abnormalities," *Zhonghua Fu Chan Ke Za Zhi*, vol. 52, no. 10, pp. 662–668, 2017.

[18] X. Y. Jing, L. Y. Huang, L. Zhen, J. Han, and D. Z. Li, "Prenatal diagnosis of 17q12 deletion syndrome: a retrospective case series," *Journal of Obstetetrics & Gynaecology*, vol. 39, no. 3, pp. 323–327, 2019.

38

Primary Adenosquamous Carcinoma of the Prostate with Rectal Invasion

Pierre Azzi,[1] Dominique Bossé,[2] Ilias Cagiannos,[3] Paul Borowy-Borowski,[4] and David Tiberi[5]

[1]*Faculty of Medicine, University of Ottawa, Ottawa, Ontario, Canada*
[2]*Division of Medical Oncology, The Ottawa Hospital Cancer Center, Ottawa, Ontario, Canada*
[3]*Division of Urology, The Ottawa Hospital, Ottawa, Ontario, Canada*
[4]*Department of Pathology and Laboratory Medicine, The Ottawa Hospital, Ottawa, Ontario, Canada*
[5]*Division of Radiation Oncology, The Ottawa Hospital Cancer Center, Ottawa, Ontario, Canada*

Correspondence should be addressed to David Tiberi; davidatiberi@gmail.com

Academic Editor: Fumitaka Koga

Prostate adenosquamous carcinoma (pASC) is a rare form of prostate cancer accounting for <1% of all cases. It is generally considered an aggressive variant often presenting with significant symptom burden and/or metastatic disease. Given its rarity, optimal management of this cancer is unknown. We present a case of a patient with pASC treated with radiotherapy and chemotherapy with excellent symptomatic improvement and local control.

1. Introduction

Prostate cancer is the most common malignancy (excluding skin cancers) in men accounting for 20% of all new cancer cases in men [1]. The vast majority of prostate cancers (roughly 95%) are of the adenocarcinoma subtype [2].

Prostate adenosquamous carcinoma (pASC) is a rare subtype accounting for <1% of all prostate cancers. It is a very aggressive malignancy that frequently metastasizes to the bone, liver, and lung [3].

Data regarding the optimal management of pASC is lacking given its rarity.

2. Case Presentation

We present the case of a 62-year-old man who presented to his family physician with lower urinary tract symptoms (LUTS), rectal bleeding, and pain. A digital rectal exam (DRE) was performed which revealed a bulky and indurated prostate, and the patient was referred to urology for investigation and placement of a urinary catheter.

Total prostate-specific antigen (PSA) was 3.11 ng/ml and urinalysis was negative. A staging workup consisting of computed tomography (CT), bone scan, and pelvic magnetic resonance imaging (MRI) was ordered.

Bone scan revealed no evidence of skeletal metastases. Pelvic MRI showed extensive partially necrotic right-sided prostatic carcinoma with definite extracapsular spread, seminal vesicle invasion, and involvement of the neurovascular bundles. There was also invasion into the mesorectal fat with suspected involvement of the caudal aspect of the rectal serosa/upper aspect of anal canal (Figure 1). CT of the chest, abdomen, and pelvis demonstrated a 2.8 cm mass centered in the right peripheral prostate, inseparable from the right seminal vesicle and abutting the anterior rectal wall. There was no evidence of distant metastatic disease.

The patient underwent transrectal ultrasound-guided prostate biopsy (TRUS) which revealed a poorly differentiated squamous cell carcinoma moderately that was positive

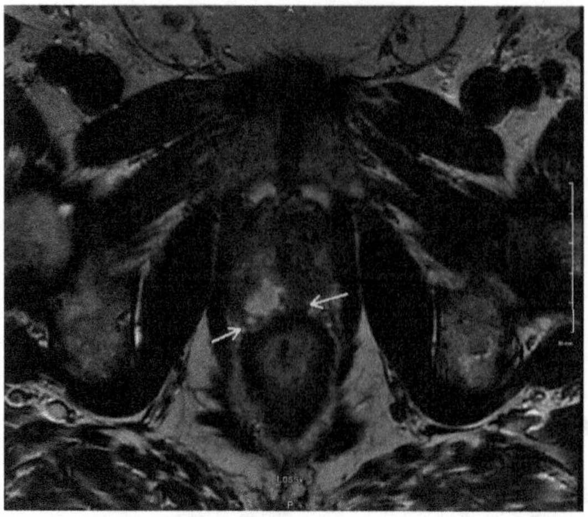

Figure 1: Axial T2-weighted MRI image showing the caudal aspect of the tumor abutting the caudal aspect of the rectum/upper aspect of the anal canal with possible serosal invasion.

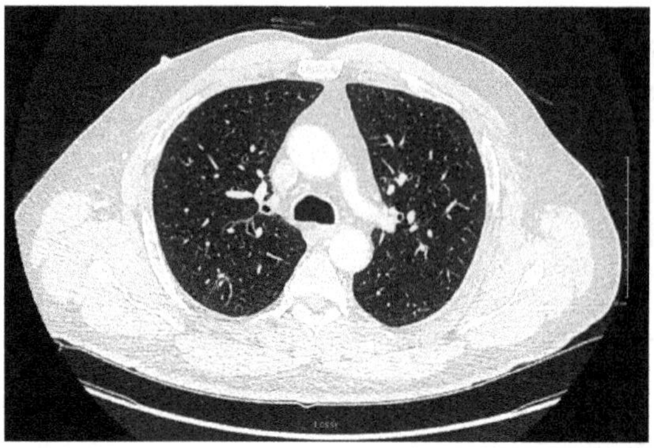

Figure 2: Representative histopathologic slides from transrectal prostate biopsy showing squamous cell carcinoma intimately mixed with glandular structures encircling a nerve (×400 magnification). IHC: immunohistochemistry; DPIN4 cocktail consisting of racemase, Ker903 (high-molecular weight cytokeratin), and p63.

for p63 and Ker903 (Figure 2). This was present in all 16 of the sampled cores and periprostatic fat invasion was present. There was a very small component of synchronous Gleason 6 acinar adenocarcinoma in 2 out of the 16 cores, representing at most 1% over the overall sampled tissue. The patient also had a cystoscopy to investigate for possible urethral mass or bladder mass which did not reveal any suspicious lesions.

This case was presented at our institutional tumor board for discussion. Pathology review by our dedicated genitourinary pathology team concluded that this was likely an adenosquamous carcinoma due to the small acinar adenocarcinoma component.

Due to the locally invasive primary tumor invading the rectum, the patient was deemed inoperable. The proposed management plan consisted of local radiotherapy followed by chemotherapy.

External beam radiotherapy using volumetric modulated arc therapy (VMAT) to a dose of 40.05 Gy in 15 fractions was administered to the pelvic disease. Within 10 days of starting radiotherapy, the rectal bleeding had stopped, and the patient began having a significant reduction in his rectal/pelvic pain.

Restaging CT scans 2 months later demonstrated response at the level of the primary lesion treated with radiotherapy. Unfortunately, there was evidence of a new lung nodule suspicious for metastasis (Figure 3). The patient was started on docetaxel chemotherapy at a dose of 75 mg/m^2 intravenously every 3 weeks. Follow-up CT scans 3 months after starting chemotherapy demonstrated disease progression with new, bilateral lung nodules and a new liver lesion consistent with metastatic disease. There was no evidence of bony disease on bone scan and PSA levels remained <4 ng/ml.

Currently, the patient is jointly followed by our institution's outpatient palliative care clinic in order to optimize management. Now, nearly 9 months from initial presentation his symptoms are much improved. His rectal pain has diminished significantly since radiotherapy and his narcotic medication has been tapered down and he no longer requires breakthrough doses. He was able to have his urinary catheter removed.

3. Discussion

Prostate adenosquamous cell carcinoma is a rare form of cancer that makes up 0.5%-1% of all prostate carcinomas. Only 25 cases were reported in the Surveillance, Epidemiology, and End Results (SEER) database [4]. Useful histopathological tests can include stains such as Ker903, whose presence rules out typical prostate adenocarcinoma and usually stains tumors with squamous differentiation [5]. These tumors can also have negative staining for PSA and PAP (prostatic acid phosphatase).

pASC patients often present with symptoms including dysuria, rectal/pelvic pain, acute urinary retention, urinary tract infection, hematuria, and bony pain due to metastases. These tumors can also have normal serum PSA and PAP. Risk factors for the development of prostatic adenosquamous carcinoma can include prior radiation and/or hormonal therapy [6], none of which our patient had received. There have been several documented cases of pASC in the absence of hormonal or radiotherapy, and some authors have suggested that this may reflect pluripotent cells capable of multidirectional differentiation [7].

Unfortunately, these forms of prostate cancer carry a poor prognosis with a median survival estimated at 12-14 months [6]. The disease is also frequently metastatic at diagnosis most commonly spreading to bones and lymph nodes.

Due to the small number of cases present in the literature, optimal treatment for this malignancy is controversial. Hennessey et al. recently reported a case of de novo pASC treated with a multimodal approach including surgery, androgen-deprivation therapy (ADT), docetaxel chemotherapy, and radiation with a good radiologic and clinical improvement 20 months post treatment [7].

Due to the lack of data regarding systemic therapy regimens, it is unclear what the expected response rate to chemotherapy or what the role of immunotherapy may be.

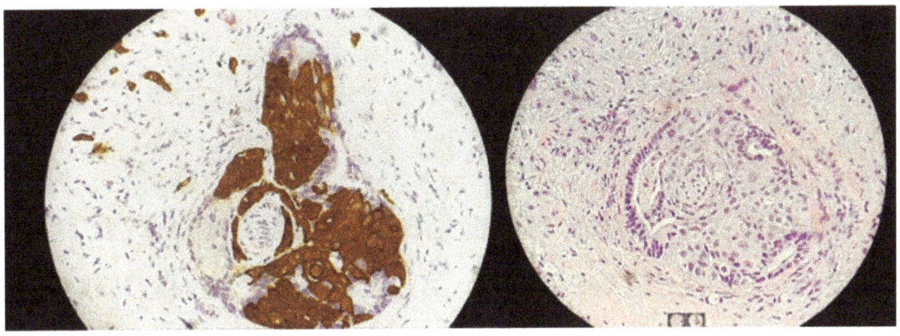

FIGURE 3: Axial chest CT scan showing a 5 mm solid pulmonary nodule suspicious for metastatic disease.

Some have hypothesized that response to ADT is poor when there is a predominant squamous carcinoma component in the tumor. As a result, we elected not to prescribe ADT in our case due to the very minimal adenocarcinoma component.

Little et al. used an aggressive surgical approach, radical cystoprostatectomy, to treat 2 patients. One of the patients remained cancer free 40 months after initial diagnosis, and the other died 25 months after diagnosis from lung metastases [8].

Our patient was deemed inoperable due to the rectal involvement after tumor board review, so a decision to use sequential radiotherapy followed by chemotherapy was made. Due to the very significant bulk of local disease, the tumor board felt that radical chemoradiation would be unlikely to cure the patient and recommended a more moderate approach to balance local control and toxicity. Therefore, we selected a 3-week course of radiotherapy with a total dose (40.05 Gy) which is higher than what would typically be used for pure palliation but slightly lower than for radical-intent therapy. This treatment provided excellent symptomatic relief with an improvement in quality of life.

Based on the cases presented in the literature, radiation therapy and chemotherapy may be a useful multimodal approach for locally advanced and metastatic squamous cell carcinoma. Continued follow-up of our patient is needed to determine overall symptomatic benefit more long-term.

4. Conclusion

Prostate adenosquamous carcinoma is a rare and aggressive malignancy with a paucity of data to guide management. Published case reports suggest that surgery is reasonable for early-stage disease, while chemotherapy +/- radiotherapy may be used for more advanced stages. We present a case of pASC treated with sequential radiotherapy and multiagent chemotherapy with excellent symptomatic relief and local control.

Hopefully, continued follow-up of our current case and future case series will help refine the optimal management of pASC.

References

[1] C. C. S. A. Committee, *Canadian Cancer Statistics: A 2020 Special Report on Lung Cancer*, Canadian Cancer Society, Toronto, 2020.

[2] T. L. Randolph, M. B. Amin, J. Y. Ro, and A. G. Ayala, "Histologic variants of adenocarcinoma and other carcinomas of prostate: pathologic criteria and clinical significance," *Modern Pathology*, vol. 10, no. 6, pp. 612–629, 1997.

[3] F. Munoz, P. Franco, P. Ciammella et al., "Squamous cell carcinoma of the prostate: long-term survival after combined chemo-radiation," *Radiation Oncology*, vol. 2, no. 1, pp. 1–7, 2007.

[4] J. Wang, F. W. Wang, C. A. LaGrange, and G. P. Hemstreet, "Clinical features and outcomes of 25 patients with primary adenosquamous cell carcinoma of the prostate," *Rare Tumors*, vol. 2, no. 3, pp. 130–134, 2010.

[5] A. V. Parwani, J. D. Kronz, E. M. Genega, P. Gaudin, S. Chang, and J. I. Epstein, "Prostate carcinoma with squamous differentiation: an analysis of 33 cases," *The American Journal of Surgical Pathology*, vol. 28, no. 5, pp. 651–657, 2004.

[6] J. O. Long and J. T. Moncur, "Adenosquamous carcinoma of the prostate: a unique presentation of a rare entity and review of the literature," *AJSP: Reviews & Reports*, vol. 25, no. 3, pp. 123–126, 2020.

[7] A. Hennessey, D. Buller, S. Sama, E. Girard, J. Clement, and B. T. Ristau, "Case report: adenosquamous carcinoma of the prostate with greater than 20 month response to multimodal therapy," *Urology Case Reports*, vol. 29, p. 101084, 2020.

[8] N. A. Little, J. S. Wiener, P. J. Walther, D. F. Paulson, and E. E. Anderson, "Squamous cell carcinoma of the prostate: 2 cases of a rare malignancy and review of the literature," *The Journal of Urology*, vol. 149, no. 1, pp. 137–139, 1993.

Actual Management of Anterior Calyceal Diverticular Calculi: A Challenging Flexible Retrograde Endoscopic Approach

Ali Barki and Anouar El Moudane

Department of Urology, Mohammed IV University Medical Center Oujda, Morocco

Correspondence should be addressed to Anouar El Moudane; anouar.elmoudane@gmail.com

Academic Editor: Yankai Xia

Calyceal diverticula is a cavity that communicates with the collecting system through a narrow isthmus of the kidney. The incidence of the formation of stones in calyceal diverticula is 10-50%. This paper reports three cases of two females and one male who presented with calyceal diverticular calculi; the patients have been, arbitrarily, selected between August and February 2019 at the urology department of our university hospital. A minimally invasive treatment includes extracorporeal lithotripsy (ESWL), and F-URS (flexible ureteroscopy) was performed. We report this case series.

1. Introduction

Calyceal diverticula constitute a cavity, which communicates with the collecting system through a narrow isthmus of the kidney. 0.21-0.45% of routine intravenous studies showed calyceal diverticula, which makes them uncommon [1]. Calyceal diverticula are usually asymptomatic but can eventually cause infection and become painful [2]. The incidence of stone formation in calyceal diverticula is 10-50% [3].

Asymptomatic calyceal diverticular calculi with no signs of infection can be managed just with surveillance. In other cases, the choice of the treatment will depend on the location of the calyceal diverticular calculi.

We report three different cases of two females and one male, who presented calyceal diverticular calculus treated with (F-URS) after the failure of ESWL; we performed a review of literature about the management of this kind of stones.

2. Case 1

A 61-year-old woman, with an unremarkable medical history, presented with bilateral lumbar pain evolving for two years. Physical examination was unremarkable, with no fever; the blood pressure was 120/70 mmHg. The laboratory test results were within the normal range with a serum creatinine level at 8.5 mg/l and a white blood cell count at 7.000 per microliter.

CT scan with contrast demonstrated three stone-bearing diverticula, in the middle calyces of the left kidney measuring respectfully 5, 6, and 8 mm, whereas the right kidney was damaged on long-standing obstruction.

ESWL was performed first; radiographic control did not show any progress. A double pigtail stent (CH6) was placed to dilate the ureter 3 weeks preoperatively (Figure 1). The retrograde pyelogram showed the stone contained in the calyceal diverticula with its neck opacified (Figure 2). The infundibulum of the caliceal diverticulum was incised with a calculase II holmium laser (230 microoptical fiber, 1.0 J-10 Hz), and the calculi were pulverized with low energy and high frequency (0.8 J-25 Hz) (Figure 3). The evolution was marked by the disappearance of symptoms, with no residual at a three-month follow-up.

3. Case 2

A 68-year-old woman, with no medical history, presented with right lumbar pain since one year ago with intermittent hematuria. Physical examination was unremarkable with no fever; the blood pressure was 130/70 mmHg. The laboratory test results were within the normal range with a serum

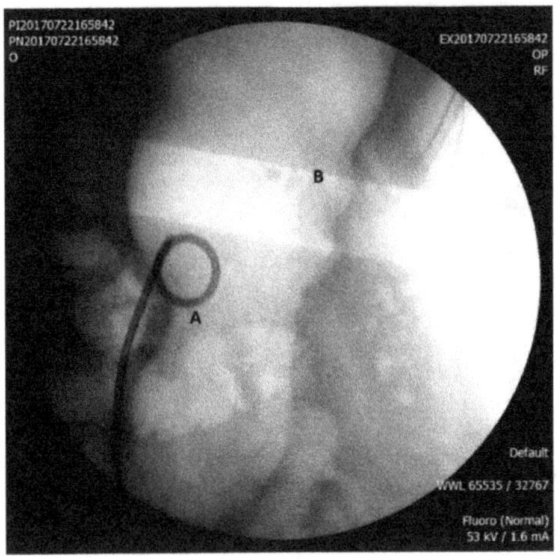

FIGURE 1: A: double pigtail stent (CH6) placed to dilate the ureter. B: 3 stone-bearing diverticula in middle calyces.

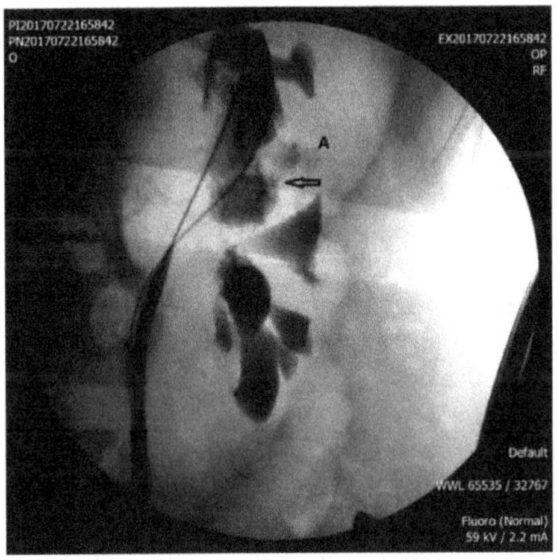

FIGURE 2: A: stone-containing calyceal diverticula. Arrow: opacified neck of a calyceal diverticulum.

creatinine level at 7 mg/l and a white blood cell count at 8.000 per microliter.

CT scan with contrast demonstrated a 10 mm stone-bearing diverticulum with 750 UH of density situated in the upper pole (Figure 4).

A double pigtail stent (CH6) was placed to dilate the ureter 3 weeks preoperatively. The retrograde pyelogram showed the stones contained in the calyceal diverticula, with its neck opacified. The infundibulum of the caliceal diverticulum was incised with a calculase II holmium laser (230 μm optical fiber) (Figure 5), and the calculi were fragmented, with high energy and low frequency (1.2 J-6 Hz) into gravel less than 2 mm, and the rest of fragments were removed with a small caliber basket (Figure 6). In order to ensure that the kidney drains urine well after F-URS, a ureteral stent was left in place and then removed the following morning. The evolution was marked by the disappearance of symptoms, with no residual calculi at a three-month follow-up.

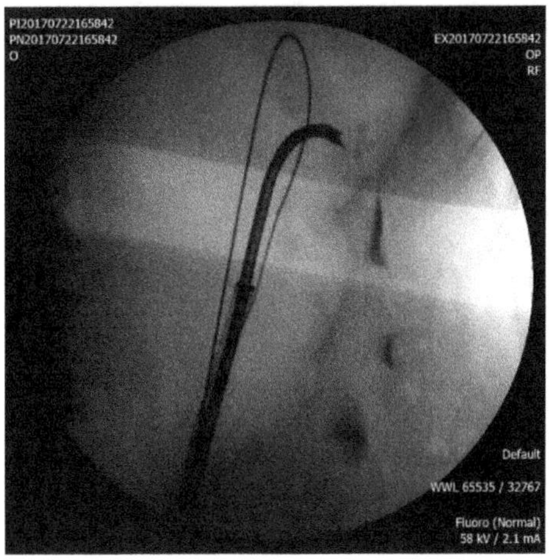

FIGURE 3: Pulverized calculi with the holmium laser.

4. Case 3

A 57-year-old man, with an unremarkable medical history, presented with recurrent bilateral lumbar pain evolving for three years. Physical examination was unremarkable, with no fever; the blood pressure was 120/70 mmHg. The laboratory test results were within the normal range, with a serum creatinine level at 9.84 mg/l and a white blood cell count at 5020 per microliter.

CT scan with contrast and with 3D reconstruction demonstrated a 9.8 mm stone-bearing diverticulum with 1200 UH of density, located in both the anterior and middle calyces.

A double pigtail stent (CH6) was placed to dilate the ureter for 4 weeks. The retrograde pyelogram showed stone-containing calyceal diverticula with an opacified neck of the calyceal diverticulum (Figures 7 and 8). The infundibulum of the caliceal diverticulum was incised with a calculase II holmium laser (230 μm optical fiber), and the calculi were fragmented, with high energy and low frequency (1.2 J-6 Hz) into gravel less than 2 mm, and the rest of the fragments were removed with a small caliber basket. In order to ensure that the kidney drains urine well after F-URS, a ureteral stent was left in place and then removed the following morning. The evolution was marked by the disappearance of symptoms with no residual calculi at a three-month follow-up.

The follow-up of all patients at six months was uneventful.

5. Discussion

The congenital abnormality caused by the failure of regression of the ureteric buds leads rarely to calyceal diverticula, and it occurs equally with the same frequency in both sexes [4].

Calyceal diverticula are in general asymptomatic before stone formation [4, 5]. Asymptomatic calyceal diverticular calculi with no signs of infection can be managed just with surveillance: once the patient becomes symptomatic with the occurrence of hematuria and flank pain due to stone formation or development of recurrent urinary tract infection [6], several options of treatment can be used to manage

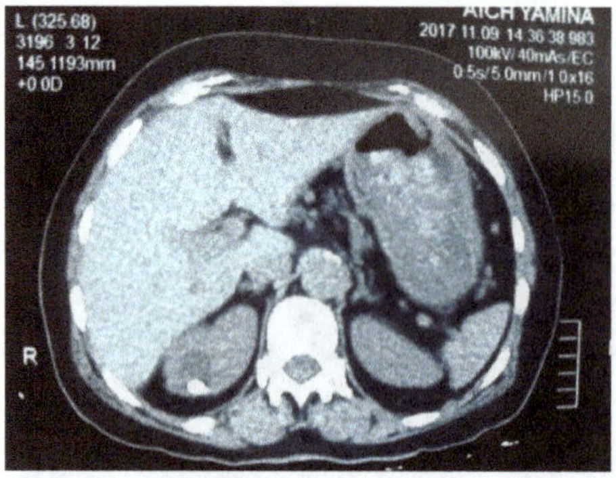

FIGURE 4: CT demonstrates a 10 mm stone-bearing diverticulum with 750 UH of density situated in the pole with the holmium laser.

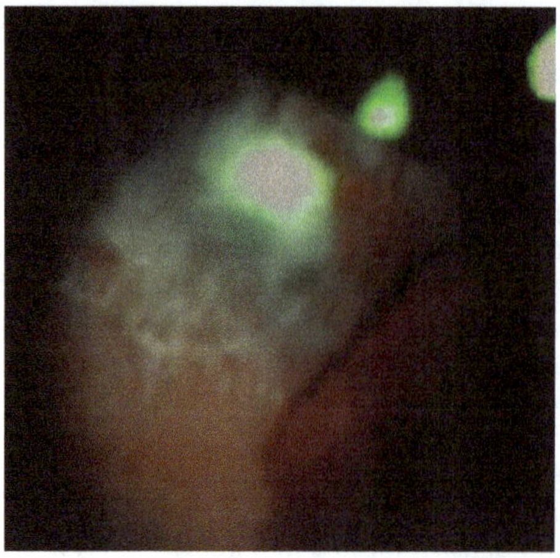

FIGURE 5: (F-URS) the infundibulum of diverticulum the calyceal diverticulum incised upper.

symptomatic calyceal diverticular calculi. However, the choice of the treatment is established based on the diverticular location and size, the presence or absence of evident infundibulum, and the quality of overlying parenchyma.

The principal minimally invasive modalities, for managing calyceal diverticular calculi, are ESWL, PCNL (percutaneous nephrolithotomy), F-URS, and laparoscopy [2].

5.1. Extracorporeal Lithotripsy (ESWL). The first choice of treatment can be the extracorporeal lithotripsy (ESWL) for all diverticular calculi whatever their location in the kidney, but a narrow diverticular neck blocks the free passage of stone fragments. It is difficult to demonstrate how adequate the fragmentation of stone is in calyceal diverticulum or dilated calyx for patients treated with ESWL [4]. ESWL can reach stone-free rates of only 4-20% and gives symptomatic amelioration in 36-70% of patients [7, 8]. Patients with small-sized superior calyceal diverticular calculi treated with ESWL present a high stone-free rate.

Streem and Yost suggested that the stone-free rate can be higher if ESWL was limited to the patients with small calculi (<1.5 cm) and evident infundibulum [9, 10]. Treating stone-bearing calyceal diverticula with ESWL should be practiced with attention even with these reports of admissible stone-

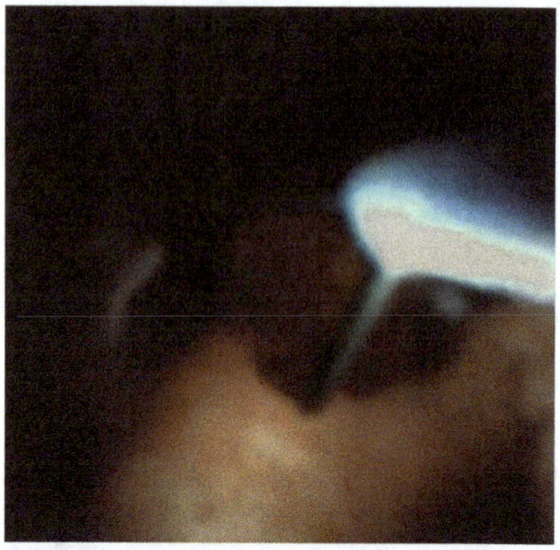

FIGURE 6: A fragment of calculi removed with a small caliber basket.

free rates and amelioration of symptoms [9]. Jones et al. proved that even if initially patients are symptom-free, afterward they will need a retreatment [7].

5.2. Percutaneous Nephrolithotomy (PCNL). The percutaneous approach has been used in diverse small series. The management of the calyceal diverticulum by the percutaneous route is challenging because the cavity is usually small and the identification of the diverticular neck is often difficult [9]. It is recommended to puncture the calyceal diverticulum directly [11]. The percutaneous approach is considered to be the most minimally invasive approach used in treating calyceal diverticula [4].

In the literature, the rate of stone-free in PCNL treatment for stone-bearing calyceal diverticula is about 70-100% [12]. Despite the good results of the PCNL approach, the risk postoperative of recurrence case of calyceal diverticula and residual calculi is not insignificant [1, 2, 4–11, 13], using PCNL which increases the risk of complications as severe hemorrhage, damage to the surrounding organs or the kidney parenchyma, sepsis, or even death [2]. The anterior location of the diverticulum can cause a difficult puncture, so the anatomical position of the diverticulum is major [14].

This approach allows fulguration and destruction of the walls of the diverticulum; the other techniques do not allow it [15]. If the diverticulum is in a superior and anterior calyx, the flexible ureterorenoscopy is recommended.

5.3. Flexible Ureteroscopy (F-URS). Ureterorenoscopic (URS) management of diverticular stones is more effective than SWL monotherapy and can allow avoiding the complications and discomfort of the more invasive therapies like percutaneous or laparoscopic techniques.

With the advancement of the flexible ureterorenoscopy, and the appliance of the holmium laser energy, this technique can be suitable for the treatment of calyceal diverticulum. The rates of success and long-term symptom-free are higher with the F-URS approach. Thus, the F-URS approach has more advantages with a short duration of hospitalization and low risk of complications [16, 17].

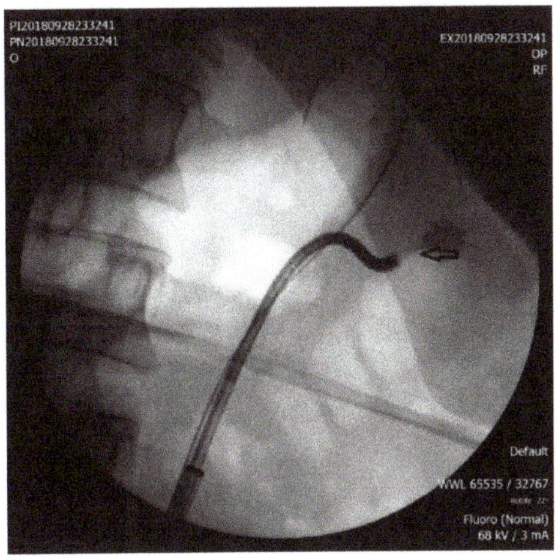

FIGURE 7: Arrow: opacified neck of a calyceal diverticulum.

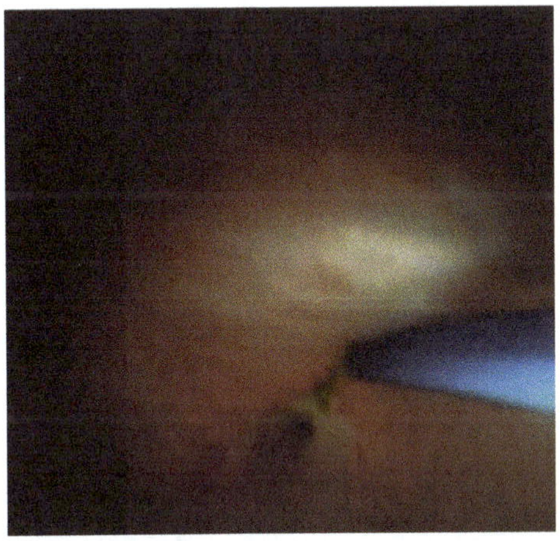

FIGURE 8: With F-URS, the infundibulum of the calyceal diverticulum is incised with the holmium laser.

Flexible ureteroscopy can be used for every location of the diverticulum but with a small burden with a short accessible diverticular neck. The significant problems that the urologist can face when using F-URS are maintaining adequate deflection and identification of the diverticular neck.

5.4. Laparoscopy and Retroperitoneoscopy. In 1994, Ruckle and Segura described the laparoscopic management of a stone-filled calyceal diverticulum [18]. Laparoscopic surgery is reserved for cases with large stones in anteriorly located diverticula, with a narrow neck and complex branched calculi, with thin overlying parenchyma [11]. Compared to ESWL, percutaneous nephrolithotomy and ureteroscopic management of laparoscopic surgery are considered to be the most invasive approach. This should be the last choice, only when the other options are not feasible.

6. Conclusion

The F-URS with the holmium laser is an effective option to manage stone-bearing calyceal diverticula mainly for the upper and mid, anterior, or posterior diverticula. This technique proved that F-URS is effective with a high rate of success and symptom-free, but we need many series to compare it with the other techniques.

References

[1] J. C. Hulbert, P. K. Reddy, D. W. Hunter, W. Castaneda-Zuniga, K. Amplatz, and P. H. Lange, "Percutaneous techniques for the management of caliceal diverticula containing calculi," *The Journal of Urology*, vol. 135, no. 2, pp. 225–227, 1986.

[2] X. Ding, S.-T. Xu, Y.-H. Huang et al., "Management of symptomatic caliceal diverticular calculi: minimally invasive percutaneous nephrolithotomy versus flexible ureterorenoscopy," *Chronic Diseases and Translational Medicine*, vol. 2, no. 4, pp. 250–256, 2016.

[3] J. W. Timmons Jr., R. S. Malek, R. R. Hattery, and J. H. Deweerd, "Caliceal diverticulum," *The Journal of Urology*, vol. 114, no. 1, pp. 6–9, 1975.

[4] A. J. Gross and T. R. W. Herrmann, "Management of stones in calyceal diverticulum," *Current Opinion in Urology*, vol. 17, no. 2, pp. 136–140, 2007.

[5] A. J. Gross and M. Fisher, "Management of stones in patients with anomalously sited kidneys," *Current Opinion in Urology*, vol. 16, no. 2, pp. 100–105, 2006.

[6] J. M. Wogan, "Pyelocalyceal diverticulum: an unusual cause of acute renal colic," *The Journal of Emergency Medicine*, vol. 23, no. 1, pp. 19–21, 2002.

[7] J. A. Jones, J. E. Lingeman, and C. P. Steidle, "The roles of extracorporeal shock wave lithotripsy and percutaneous nephrostolithotomy in the management of pyelocaliceal diverticula," *The Journal of Urology*, vol. 146, no. 3, pp. 724–e727, 1991.

[8] K. E. Psihramis and S. P. Dretler, "Extracorporeal shock wave lithotripsy of caliceal diverticula calculi," *The Journal of Urology*, vol. 138, 4 Part 1, pp. 707–711, 1987.

[9] B. Turna, A. Raza, S. Moussa, G. Smith, and D. A. Tolley, *Management of calyceal diverticular stones with extracorporal shock wave lithotripsy and percutaneaous nephrolithotomy: long-term outcome*, Department of Urology and Scottish Lithotriptor Centre, Western General Hospital, Edinburgh, 2007.

[10] S. B. Streem and A. Yost, "Treatment of caliceal diverticular calculi with extracorporeal shock wave lithotripsy: patient selection and extended followup," *The Journal of Urology*, vol. 148, 3 Part 2, pp. 1043–1046, 1992.

[11] B. Canales and M. Monga, "Surgical management of the calyceal diverticulum," *Current Opinion in Urology*, vol. 13, no. 3, pp. 255–260, 2003.

[12] J. E. Lingeman, B. R. Matlaga, and A. P. Evan, "Surgical management of upper urinary tract calculi," in *Campbell-Walsh Urology*, A. J. Wein, L. R. Kavoussi, A. C. Novick, A. W. Partin, and C. A. Peters, Eds., Saunders-Elservier, Philadelphia, 9th edition, 2005.

[13] M. Monga, R. Smith, H. Ferral, and R. Thomas, "Percutaneous ablation of caliceal diverticulum: long-term followup," *The Journal of Urology*, vol. 163, no. 1, pp. 28–32, 2000.

[14] S. C. Kim, R. L. Kuo, W. W. Tinmouth, S. Watkins, and J. E. Lingeman, "Percutaneous nephrolithotomy for caliceal diverticular calculi: a novel single stage approach," *The Journal of Urology*, vol. 173, no. 4, pp. 1194–1198, 2005.

[15] H. Hedelin, K. Geterud, L. Grenabo, C. Henriksson, S. Pettersson, and B. F. Zachrisson, "Percutaneous surgery

for stones in pyelocaliceal diverticula," *British Journal of Urology*, vol. 62, no. 3, pp. 206–208, 1988.

[16] M. Sejiny, S. Al-Qahtani, A. Elhaous, B. Molimard, and O. Traxer, "Efficacy of flexible ureterorenoscopy with holmium laser in the management of stone-bearing caliceal diverticula," *Journal of Endourology*, vol. 24, no. 6, pp. 961–967, 2010.

[17] O. Bas, E. Ozyuvali, Y. Aydogmus et al., "Management of calyceal diverticular calculi: a comparison of percutaneous nephrolithotomy and flexible ureterorenoscopy," *Urolithiasis*, vol. 43, no. 2, pp. 155–161, 2015.

[18] H. C. Ruckle and J. W. Segura, "Laparoscopic treatment of a stone-filled, Caliceal diverticulum: a definitive, minimally invasive therapeutic option," *The Journal of Urology*, vol. 151, no. 1, pp. 122–124, 1994.

40

Thoracoabdominal Approach for Large Retroperitoneal Masses: Case Series and Review

Siv Venkat, Andre Matteliano, and Darrel Drachenberg

Section of Urology, University of Manitoba, Winnipeg, MB, Canada

Correspondence should be addressed to Siv Venkat; siva.venkat@medportal.ca

Academic Editor: David Duchene

The thoracoabdominal incision was first described in 1946 as an approach to concomitant abdominal, retroperitoneal, and thoracic injuries. In urology, this technique was popularized in 1949 for the resection of large renal tumours. Today, it is reserved for complex cases where optimal exposure of the renal hilum and adrenal and superior pole of the kidney is necessary. We present four consecutive cases in which this approach was taken by a single surgeon at our tertiary surgical centre. The outcomes, postoperative course, and pathology are described. We provide a comprehensive literature review and outline the indications, advantages, and disadvantages of this approach. *Objectives.* To present a case series outlining the efficacy and safety of the thoracoabdominal incision in complex oncologic procedures in urology. *Methods.* Four cases utilizing the thoracoabdominal incision, performed by a single surgeon at our tertiary care center, were reviewed. Case history, preoperative imaging, intraoperative experience, postoperative course, final pathology, and complications were examined. A thorough literature review was performed and comparison made with historical cohorts for estimated blood loss, length of stay, and complications encountered versus other common surgical approaches. The indications, advantages, and disadvantages of the thoracoabdominal approach were outlined. *Results.* All patients had large retroperitoneal masses of varying complexity, requiring maximal surgical exposure. Surgery was straightforward in all cases, without any significant perioperative or postoperative complications. Postoperative pain, length of hospital stay, estimated blood loss, and analgesia requirements were all similar to open and mini-flank approaches in review of historical case series cohorts. Laparoscopic approaches had lower estimated blood loss and length of stay. *Conclusions.* The thoracoabdominal approach is rarely utilized in urological surgery, due to the perceived morbidity in violating the thoracic cavity. These cases outline the benefit of the thoracoabdominal approach in select cases requiring maximal surgical exposure, and the generally benign postoperative course that appropriately selected patients may hope to endure. Postoperative pain, length of hospital stay, estimated blood loss, and analgesia requirements can be expected to be similar open and mini-flank approaches. As expected, laparoscopic approaches had lower estimated blood loss and length of stay.

1. Case 1

A 66-year-old Aboriginal male presented to his family physician with a 2-month history of early satiety, nausea, and abdominal distension. An abdominal CT scan revealed a 20 cm Bosniak IV left renal mass. This occupied much of the left hemiabdomen and displaced the great vessels laterally. No evidence of metastatic disease was found on further workup (Figure 1).

The patient underwent a radical left nephrectomy. A thoracoabdominal approach was selected due to size and superior polar location of the renal mass. No intraoperative complications were encountered, and the procedure was well tolerated. A 28 Fr chest tube was placed prior to the closure of the thoracic cavity and was connected to low suction. A nasogastric tube (NGT) was placed in anticipation of a postoperative ileus. Intraoperative estimated blood loss (EBL) was 400cc.

The patient's NGT was clamped on postoperative day 2 and removed on postoperative day 3. The epidural was discontinued on postoperative day 2, and the patient was weaned off intravenous analgesia on postoperative day 4. The following day, on postoperative day 5, the chest tube was removed. The patient was subsequently discharged on postoperative day 6 without incident for a total length of stay (LOS) of 6 days.

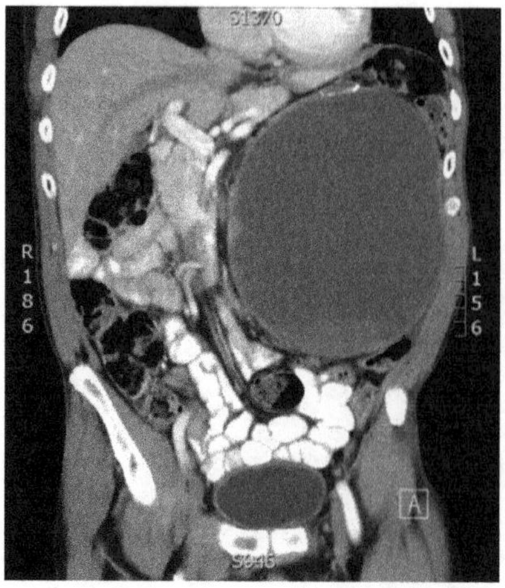

FIGURE 1: CT abdomen coronal view showing a large left cystic renal mass displacing great vessels laterally.

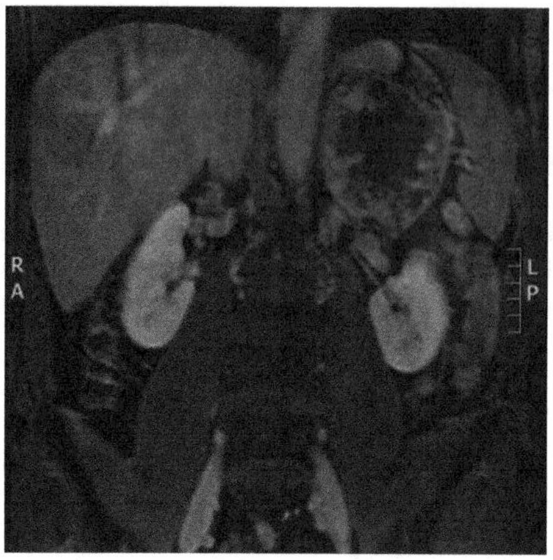

FIGURE 2: Gadolinium-enhanced T1 abdominal MRI, coronal view, showing a large heterogeneous left adrenal mass.

Final pathological analysis confirmed a type 1 papillary renal cell carcinoma. Surgical margins were negative with no evidence of lymphovascular invasion (LVI), corresponding to pathological stage T2bNxMx. Tumour grade was recorded as Fuhrman nuclear grade 2/4.

2. Case 2

A 50-year-old Caucasian male with a history of hypertension and benign prostatic hypertrophy was found to have microscopic hematuria on his annual urinalysis. An abdominal MRI found an incidental 12 cm left adrenal mass involving the superior pole of the left kidney, and possibly the splenic hilum and distal pancreas. Imaging findings were concerning for a locally invasive adrenocortical carcinoma (Figure 2).

There was no evidence of lymphadenopathy or distant metastases on further workup. The patient had serum DHEAS, 17-ketosteroid, and cortisol functionality tests drawn, which were negative. Urine metanephrines were also negative, confirming a nonfunctional adrenal mass.

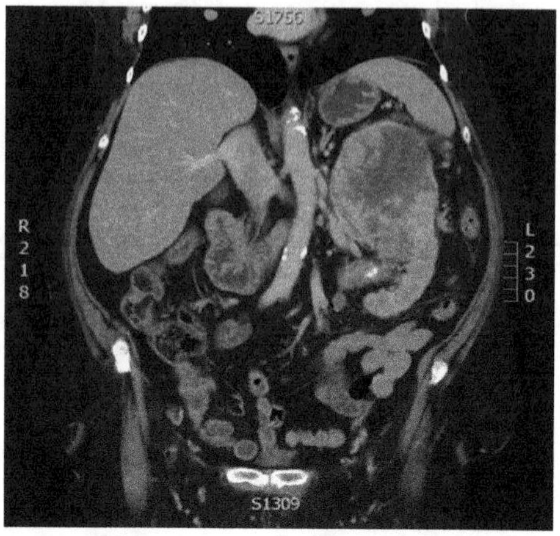

FIGURE 3: CT abdomen coronal view showing a large heterogeneous left renal mass with suspected splenic hilar invasion.

The patient subsequently underwent left nephroadrenalectomy. A thoracoabdominal approach was favoured due to the size, location, and locally invasive appearance of the mass. Intraoperatively, the spleen and pancreas were found to be uninvolved and did not require resection. No complications were encountered and EBL was 150cc. A 28 Fr chest tube was placed prior to the closure of the thoracic cavity and connected to low suction.

The chest tube was removed on postoperative day 3, and a follow-up radiograph confirmed the absence of a pneumothorax. The patient experienced modest difficulty weaning the epidural, which was discontinued on postoperative day 5. He was discharged on postoperative day 6 when pain was well managed with oral analgesia.

On pathological analysis, microscopic inspection revealed extensive fibrosis, hyalinization, focal dystrophic calcification, and ossification. Immunohistochemical studies (cytokeratin, S100, vimentin, and EMA) did not show evidence of neoplastic changes. Final pathological diagnosis confirmed an adrenal pseudocyst. No further follow-up was necessary.

3. Case 3

A 67-year-old Aboriginal female with a history of hypertension and diabetes presented to her family physician with a 3-month history of 20 pound weight loss, early satiety, and fatigue. A CT scan of her abdomen revealed a 14 cm mass in the superior pole of the left kidney with suspected splenic hilar invasion. There was evidence of an enhancing soft tissue mass in the tail of the pancreas, suspicious for metastasis. Further metastatic workup revealed a small burden of pulmonary disease (Figure 3).

After a thorough discussion with medical oncology and a full assessment of her functional status, the patient was enrolled in a tumour vaccine trial, which required cytoreductive nephrectomy. With the assistance of the general surgery team, she underwent a left radical nephrectomy, splenectomy, distal pancreatectomy, and retroperitoneal lymph node dissection (RPLND). A 28 Fr chest tube was placed prior to the

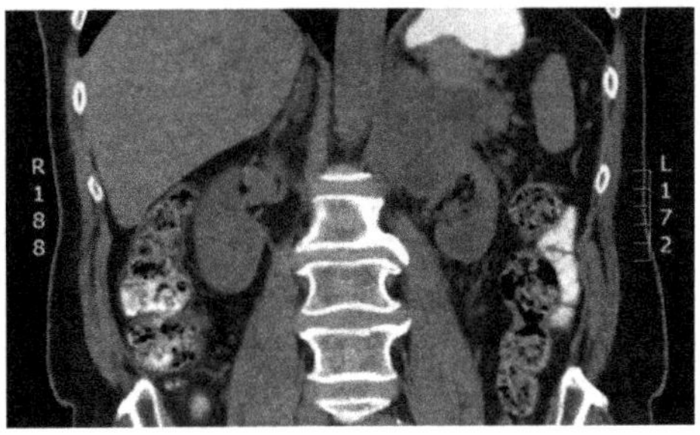

FIGURE 4: CT abdomen coronal view showing a large cystic left renal mass with suspected splenic hilar invasion.

closure of the thoracic cavity and connected to low suction. Due to the size and location of the tumour, and the suspected local invasion, a thoracoabdominal approach was pursued. No complications were encountered intraoperatively and EBL was 400cc.

The patient's postoperative course was uneventful. The epidural and chest tube were discontinued on postoperative day 4. She was weaned off intravenous analgesia by postoperative day 6 and was discharged on postoperative day 8 when fully mobile.

Final pathological analysis confirmed a clear cell renal cell carcinoma. Surgical margins were negative with no evidence of LVI. As suspected, a metastatic lesion in the distal pancreas was confirmed. Two lymph nodes were included in the analysis, both of which were negative for malignancy. Final pathological stage was defined as T3aN0M1. The tumour grade was recorded as Fuhrman nuclear grade 3/4.

4. Case 4

A 61-year-old Caucasian male had previously seen a urologist for recurrent low-grade bladder cancer, which required multiple resections. Unfortunately, he was lost to follow-up and presented to his family physician several years later with abdominal discomfort and weight loss. An abdominal CT scan was ordered, which found a 10 cm cystic mass in the superior pole of the left kidney, concerning for malignancy with suspected splenic hilar invasion. A full metastatic workup was undertaken. No evidence of metastatic disease was identified (Figure 4).

The patient underwent a radical left nephrectomy, splenectomy, distal pancreatectomy, completion nephroureterectomy, and RPLND. In anticipation of a difficult resection, the thoracoabdominal approach was selected to maximize surgical exposure. Intraoperatively, the tumour was found to involve the distal pancreas, which was resected with assistance from the general surgery team. During the kidney dissection, an incidental left upper ureteric mass was identified. Given the patient's history of recurrent bladder cancer, urothelial malignancy was suspected, and a completion nephroureterectomy was performed. A 28 Fr chest tube was placed prior to the closure of the thoracic cavity and connected to low suction. No complications were encountered during the procedure and EBL was 4000cc. Three units of packed red blood cells and 1 L of fresh frozen plasma were administered intraoperatively.

The patient's postoperative course was slow, but uneventful. The epidural and chest tube were discontinued on postoperative day 5, and he was discharged on postoperative day 9, once deemed physically fit for independent living by physiotherapy and occupational therapy.

Final pathological analysis confirmed high-grade transitional cell carcinoma (TCC) with extensive tumour necrosis. Tumour was found to be invading peripelvic fat, renal parenchyma, perinephric fat, and the tail of the pancreas. The resection margins, including the pancreatic margin and the bladder cuff resection margin, were involved by TCC. Two lymph nodes were included in the specimen, which were negative for malignancy. Final pathological stage was defined as T4N0M1. The patient was referred to medical oncology for consideration of systemic therapy.

5. Discussion

The thoracoabdominal approach involves incision of the eighth, ninth, or tenth rib, with transpleural, transdiaphragmatic, and transabdominal exposure of retroperitoneal structures and the pleural and peritoneal cavities [1]. This method is particularly useful in right-sided cases, where hepatic veins limit exposure and control of the renal vascular supply [2]. Mobilizing the colon medially and kocherizing the duodenum allow a straightforward approach to the right kidney and early vascular control of the great vessels. For left sided renal masses, the colon and the tail of the pancreas are mobilized, providing excellent exposure of the renal pedicle [3]. This approach is advantageous in cases involving large retroperitoneal masses. In cases where surrounding structures are involved, it provides optimal exposure to allow meticulous resection [3, 4]. Specific indications for this method have been proposed, which include complex renal malignancies with inferior vena cava involvement or with local spread, a large upper pole tumour greater than 7 cm, and surgeon preference [1]. It has also been described in cases of partial nephrectomy involving upper pole masses [4].

Due to the violation of the thoracic cavity, some surgeons perceive the added morbidity of this approach as a deterrent to its use. However, there are certain advantages that this approach offers over a standard flank or transabdominal or lumbar incision. The incomparable exposure of the kidney and adrenal and renal hilum allows for early primary ligation of the renal vasculature before tumour manipulation. It also allows for easier resection of Gerota's fascia, the ipsilateral adrenal gland, and surgical extirpation of the lymphatic field [1]. Violation of the thoracic cavity also permits biopsy and resection of pulmonary lesions [2].

A commonly described disadvantage of this approach is the incision of multiple muscle layers when accessing the abdominal and thoracic cavities [1]. Inherently, this carries the risk of injuring the phrenic nerve and compromising diaphragmatic function [2, 4]. Potential injury to adjacent structures is also described. Splenic injury is possible, occurring most often during division and resection of the diaphragm. Other potential injuries include ureteric injury

TABLE 1: Comparison of case series and surgical approaches.

Series	Approach used	Number of patients	EBL (range), cc	LOS (range), days	Clavien I-III complications, %
Venkat et al., 2018	Thoracoabdominal	4	1237 ± 1598 (150-4000)	7.3 ± 1.3 (6-9)	0
Yang et al., 2009	Thoracoabdominal	60	150 ± 10	9.5 ± 1.6	3
Kumar et al., 1999	Thoracoabdominal	42	-	4.2 ± 1.0 (3-7)	7
Yang et al., 2009	Open Flank	56	209 ± 13	9.4 ± 1.6	0
Kumar et al., 1999	Open Flank	52	-	4.0 ± 1.0 (3-7)	0
Wang et al., 2014	Open Flank	111	226 ± 265 (10-3000)	8.2 ± 3.9 (3-39)	13
Stifleman et al., 2001	Open Flank	23	364 ± 449	4.5 ± 1.2	13
Parra et al., 1995	Open Flank	13	295 (75-750)	8.0 (3-16)	15
Wang et al., 2014	Mini-flank, supra 12th rib	41	103 ± 88 (20-500)	6.8 ± 2.1 (5-17)	12
DiBlasio et al., 2005	Mini-flank, supra 11th rib	167	400 (50-2400)	5.0 (3-28)	4
Wang et al., 2014	Laparoscopic	42	119 ± 150 (20-800)	6.65 ± 2.5 (3-16)	21
Stifleman et al., 2001	Laparoscopic, hand assisted	40	83 ± 62	3.5 ± 0.7	8
Parra et al., 1995	Laparoscopic	12	141 (50-200)	3.5 (2-6)	16

during retroperitoneal dissection and left first lumbar vein injury during mobilization of the left kidney. Postoperative pain is a proposed drawback of this approach, due to the transection of the cartilaginous costal arch [5].

A recent study by Yang et al. [6] compared the morbidity of various surgical incisions. In this retrospective study, the thoracoabdominal approach was compared to the flank incision for radical nephrectomy and found no significant difference in operative time, removal of surgical drains, postoperative pain scores, amount of analgesia use, length of hospital stay, and time from surgery to return to work. The only significant difference was estimated blood loss, with volumes of 150.2 cc and 209.9 cc for flank and thoracoabdominal approaches, respectively. Of note, there was a significant difference in the size of the tumours, with maximum diameters of 21.8 cm and 13.8 cm for the thoracoabdominal and flank approaches, respectively.

Kumar et al. [4] directly also compared the thoracoabdominal approach to the flank incision for radical nephrectomy through retrospective review and questionnaires. Again, there was no significant difference found in LOS, pain severity, both immediate and delayed, discontinuation of pain medication, time for patients to return to work, or complication rates. Mean length of stay was 4.0 ± 1.0 days (range 3 to 7) for the flank approach, and 4.2 ± 1.0 days (range 3 to 7) in the thoracoabdominal approach ($p = 0.37$), which was not statistically significant. A mix of epidural and patient controlled analgesia was used across both groups. This study failed to show a difference in morbidity of the thoracoabdominal incision as compared to the flank incision, but did recommend further prospective studies to be performed. This study also demonstrated compelling results for *not* placing a chest tube in patients unless there was evidence of a parietal pleural injury. In this study, patients without chest tubes had a significantly shorter postoperative recovery course, despite an increased incidence of asymptomatic pneumothoraces and pleural effusions.

Our four cases presented had EBL values of 400, 150, 400, and 4000cc, respectively, for a mean of 1237 ± 1598cc (Table 1). The large variance in this small series is due to the 4000cc blood loss in the rather complex Case 4, described above. Other studies have also looked at estimated blood loss with various approaches. Wang et al. [7] retrospectively reviewed 194 patients who underwent partial nephrectomy, comparing a mini-flank supra-12th rib approach to traditional open and laparoscopic approaches. Average EBL was 103 ± 88cc for the mini-flank, 226 ± 264cc for open, and 119 ± 150cc for laparoscopic approaches. DiBlasio et al. [8] retrospectively reviewed a mini-flank supra-11th rib incision for open partial and radical nephrectomy. Average EBL was 400cc. Stifleman et al. [9] reviewed a series comparing hand-assisted laparoscopic donor nephrectomy to an open flank approach. Average EBL was 83 ± 62cc for the hand-assisted laparoscopic approach and 364 ± 449cc for the flank approach. Parra et al. [10] retrospectively compared open flank and laparoscopic approaches for radical nephrectomy. Average EBL was 140cc for the laparoscopic and 295cc for the flank approach. These compare favorably with our series of thoracoabdominal cases, excluding Case 4 as described previously. As expected, the laparoscopic series did have a lower EBL. Given the small size of our series, more robust statistical analysis did not reach significance.

Our four cases had LOS values of 6, 6, 8, and 9 days, for a mean of 7.2 ± 1.3 days (Table 1). In considering postoperative length of stay, Wang et al. [7] had a mean LOS of 6.8 ± 2.1 days for mini-open approaches, 8.2 ± 3.9 days for open approaches, and 6.7 ± 2.5 days for laparoscopic approaches. DiBlasio et al. [8] had a median LOS of 5 days for their mini-flank supra 11th rib incision. Stifleman et al. [9] had an average LOS of 3.5 ± 0.7 days for the hand-assisted laparoscopic approach and 4.5 ± 1.2 days for their open flank approach. Parra et al. [10] had an average LOS of 3.5 days for laparoscopic and 8 days for their open flank approach. These values are similar to our series of thoracoabdominal cases. Again, as expected, the laparoscopic series had a shorter LOS.

The four cases presented here had no complications, early or late (Table 1). Yang et al. [6] had a complication rate of 0% in the flank group and 3% in the thoracoabdominal group, with all being unrelated to the incision. Kumar et al. [4] had a complication rate of 0% in the flank group and 7% in the thoracoabdominal group, with all being unrelated to the incision. Wang et al. [7] found a complication rate of 12% for the mini-flank supra-12th approach, 13% for the open, and 21% for laparoscopic, with all complications being Clavien I-III. DiBlasio et al. [8] had no intraoperative complications, with a 4% rate of late complications, all related to surgical site hernias. Stifleman et al. [9] had a total complication rate of 13% for the open group, and a total complication rate of 8% for the laparoscopic group, all Clavien II or III, with one intraoperative complication in the open group and the rest all postoperative. Parra et al. [10] had a complication rate of 16% for the laparoscopic approach, with all of these being Clavien III, and a rate of 15% for the open flank approach, with all of these being Clavien II. These series again compare favorably to our small series of thoracoabdominal cases.

6. Conclusion

These case reports represent clinical scenarios where the thoracoabdominal surgical approach was indicated. All patients had large retroperitoneal masses of varying complexity, requiring maximal surgical exposure. The thoracoabdominal approach is rarely utilized in urological surgery, due to the perceived morbidity in violating the thoracic cavity. However, comparison with several retrospective series examining open and mini-flank approaches suggests no difference between thoracoabdominal and the open flank approaches in terms of postoperative pain, length of hospital stay, EBL, analgesia requirements, return to work, and complication rates. As expected, laparoscopic approaches had lower EBL and LOS. Although a small series, our cases outline the benefit of the thoracoabdominal approach in select cases, and the generally benign postoperative course that appropriately selected patients may hope to endure. In the era of robotic assisted and minimally invasive surgery, urologists should be reminded of this effective and safe approach to address challenging retroperitoneal masses.

Disclosure

This study was undertaken while all authors were under employment at the University of Manitoba, Winnipeg, Manitoba, Canada.

Authors' Contributions

Siv Venkat and Andre Matteliano conceived the idea, acquired, reviewed, and analyzed chart details, performed the literature review, and wrote the manuscript. Darrel Drachenberg supervised the project.

References

[1] C. J. Rosser, D. L. McCullough, and M. C. Hall, "Thoracoabdominal radical nephrectomy: Is a postoperative thoracostomy tube necessary?" *Urology*, vol. 55, no. 6, pp. 847–851, 2000.

[2] P. Kenney, C. Wotkowicz, and J. Libertino, "Contemporary open surgery of the kidney," in *Campbell-Walsh Urology*, A. J. Wein, L. R. Kavoussi, A. C. Novick, A. W. Partin, and C. A. Peters, Eds., vol. 2 of *chapter 54*, Elsevier, Philadelphia, Pa, USA, 10th edition, 2012.

[3] M. Cookson, "Radical Nephrectomy," in *Glenn's Urologic Surgery*, S. D. Graham and J. F. Glenn, Eds., chapter 7, pp. 116–129, JB Lippincott Company, Philadelphia, Pa, USA, 5th edition, 1998.

[4] S. Kumar, J. L. F. Duque, K. C. O. Guimaraes, J. Dicanzio, K. R. Loughlin, and J. P. Richie, "Short and long-term morbidity of thoracoabdominal incision for nephrectomy: A comparison with the flank approach," *The Journal of Urology*, vol. 162, no. 6, pp. 1927–1929, 1999.

[5] A. B. Lumsden, G. L. Colborn, S. Sreeram, and L. J. Skandalakis, "The surgical anatomy and technique of the thoracoabdominal incision," *Surgical Clinics of North America*, vol. 73, no. 4, pp. 633–644, 1993.

[6] M. Yang and X. Zhao, "Retrospective study of the efficacy and complication of thoracoabdominal incision for nephrectomy: A comparison with flank approach," *Frontiers of Medicine in China*, vol. 3, no. 2, pp. 191–196, 2009.

[7] H. Wang, L. Zhou, J. Guo et al., "Mini-flank supra-12th rib incision for open partial nephrectomy compared with laparoscopic partial nephrectomy and traditional open partial nephrectomy," *PLoS ONE*, vol. 9, no. 2, 2014.

[8] C. J. DiBlasio, M. E. Snyder, and P. Russo, "Mini-flank supra-11th rib incision for open partial or radical nephrectomy," *BJU International*, vol. 97, no. 1, pp. 149–156, 2006.

[9] M. D. Stifelman, D. Hull, R. E. Sosa et al., "Hand assisted laparoscopic donor nephrectomy: A comparison with the open approach," *The Journal of Urology*, vol. 166, no. 2, pp. 444–448, 2001.

[10] R. O. Parra, M. G. Perez, J. A. Boullier, and J. M. Cummings, "Comparison Between Standard Flank Versus Laparoscopic Nephrectomy for Benign Renal Disease," *The Journal of Urology*, vol. 153, no. 4, pp. 1171–1174, 1995.

41

A Case of Traumatic Catheterisation leading to Rectal Perforation and Periprostatic Abscess

Orla Cullivan, Silviu David, and Syed Jaffry

Department of Urology, Galway University Hospital, Galway, Ireland

Correspondence should be addressed to Orla Cullivan; orla.cullivan@gmail.com

Academic Editor: Tun-Chieh Chen

A 79-year-old gentleman presented to the Emergency Department (ED) with catheter-related issues on a background of a long-term catheter for previous urinary retention, Hartmann's procedure for colorectal cancer, and brachytherapy for prostate cancer. A 3-way silicone catheter was placed by ED staff and bladder irrigation commenced. The urine draining following catheterisation was found to be dark and thick, and irrigation fluid was noted to be draining per rectum. CT imaging was performed and demonstrated the catheter tip extending through the posterior wall of the urethra and into the rectum. The patient was admitted under the urology team, and urinary diversion was achieved with a suprapubic catheter. Subsequent imaging demonstrated a periprostatic abscess, which was initially managed with antimicrobial therapy, followed by attempted image-guided drainage. Repeat imaging following a 6-week course of antibiotics failed to show an improvement in the collection. During his inpatient stay, he contracted COVID-19 and passed away suddenly. This case demonstrates the potential catastrophic consequences associated with urethral catheterisation.

1. Introduction

Urinary catheterisation represents a relatively common healthcare procedure that can be associated with a variety of complications. This case explores a case of traumatic catheterisation and the resulting consequences for the patient and challenges for the treating healthcare team.

2. Case History

A 79-year-old gentleman presented to the Emergency Department (ED) reporting symptoms of bypassing from his urinary catheter, bleeding from his urethral meatus, and dark urine in his catheter bag. Four months prior to this attendance, he developed urinary retention requiring catheterisation. He subsequently failed two voiding trials. Past history included prostate cancer treated with brachytherapy 11 years ago, urethral stricture disease, and T4N1 colorectal cancer for which he underwent a Hartmann's procedure 4 years ago. Endoscopy of his rectal stump one month prior to his presentation demonstrated proctitis. The patient himself denied a history of passing urine per rectum. The patient had a normal flexible cystoscopy one year previously and a normal CTTAP 3 years previously.

The patient's indwelling catheter was changed to a 20 French 3-way catheter by ED staff, and bladder irrigation was commenced. Blood was noticed in the catheter bag immediately following catheterisation. Subsequently, the urine draining was described as thick and dark in appearance, and irrigation fluid was noted to be draining from the patient's rectum. Blood results demonstrated mildly raised inflammatory makers with white cells of 11.8×10^9/L(RR 4-10×10^9/L) and a C-Reactive Protein of 68 mg/L (RR 0-5 mg/L). Creatinine was at the patient's baseline of 130 μmol/L (RR 64-104 μmol/L). CT imaging demonstrated a malpositioned catheter with the catheter tip extending through the posterior wall of the prostatic urethra and into the rectum, creating a rectourethral fistula (Figures 1 and 2). The bladder was also noted to be thick-walled secondary to chronic outflow obstruction and radiotherapy.

The patient was admitted under the urology team, and urinary diversion was achieved with a suprapubic catheter.

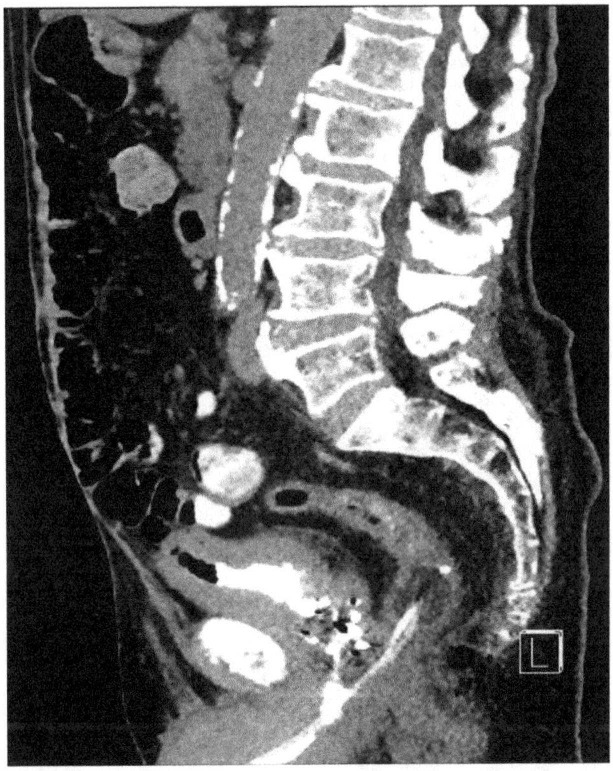

FIGURE 1: Sagittal CT demonstrating catheter placement in rectum.

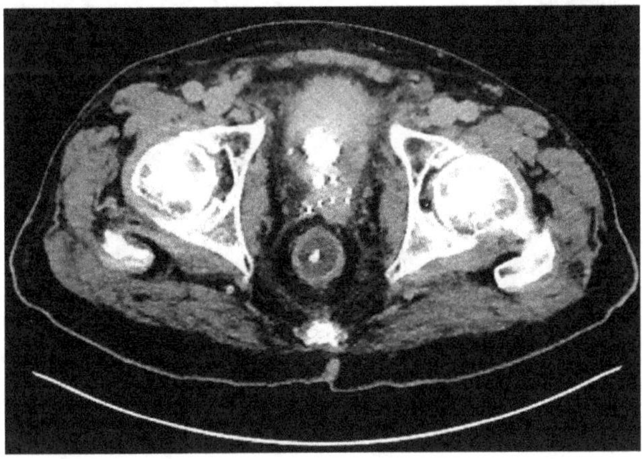

FIGURE 2: Axial CT demonstrating catheter placement in rectum.

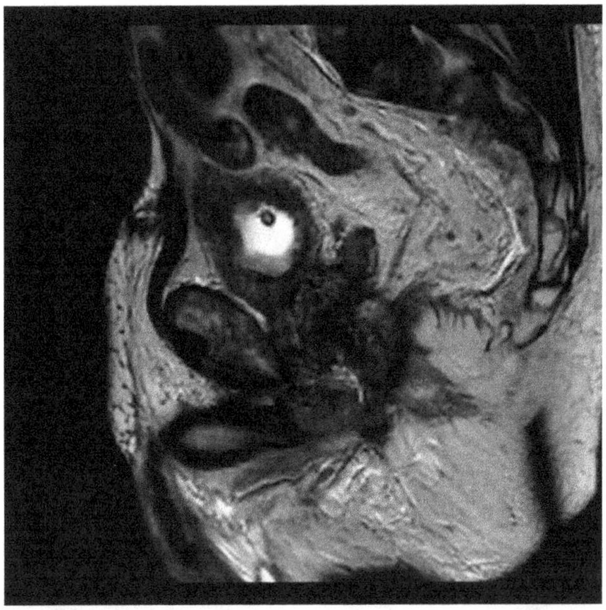

FIGURE 3: Sagittal MRI of periprostatic collection.

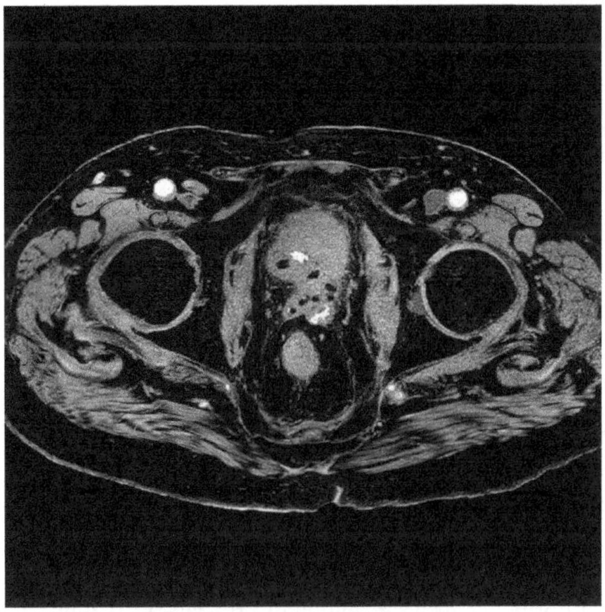

FIGURE 4: Axial CT of periprostatic collection.

He was reviewed by the colorectal team, who were happy that no surgical intervention was needed as an inpatient, and would arrange outpatient follow-up. The patient reported persistent rectal pain, so pelvic MRI imaging was arranged. This demonstrated an extensive pelvic abscess involving the prostate with concerns for early osteomyelitis of the inferior left pubic ramus (Figures 3 and 4). Urine cultures grew Klebsiella pneumonia. The patient was initially treated with Augmentin, then switched to Piperacillin-Tazobactam on the advice of microbiology colleagues due to rising inflammatory markers. Inflammatory markers failed to improve following 10 days of this, and treatment was changed to oral Ciprofloxacin and Metronidazole, with a 6-week total course advised.

The patient remained in the hospital to complete his antibiotic course and became acutely unwell approximately 5 weeks into his admission. He was reviewed by the medical, intensive care, and microbiology teams. The impression was that the patient had a septic event related to his abscess. CT pulmonary angiogram and COVID-19 tests were performed and were both negative. There was no growth on repeat urine and blood cultures. Antibiotics were changed to Meropenem, Vancomycin, and Daptomycin. CT TAP was performed which demonstrated thickening of the wall of the transverse colon. A repeat MRI pelvis was obtained which demonstrated an unchanged pelvic abscess (Figures 5 and 6). The patient was then arranged for transrectal image-guided

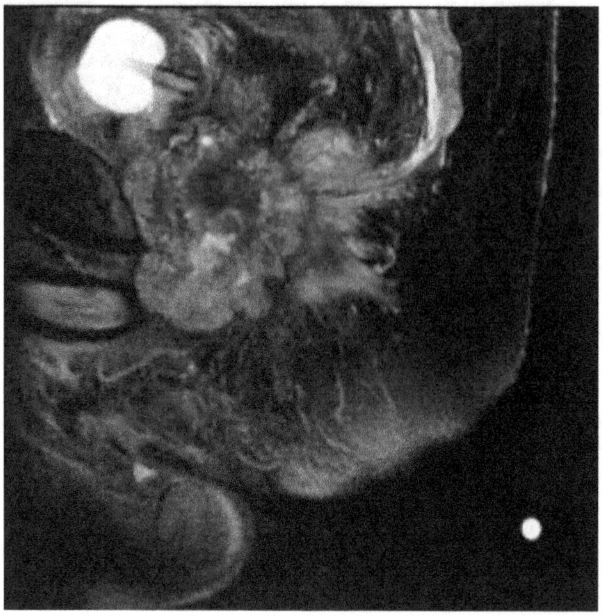

Figure 5: Saggital MRI imaging demonstrating persistence of collection post-antibiotic treatment.

drainage of the abscess with interventional radiology. A small amount of blood-stained material was aspirated, and a 10Fr drain was sited, but it was deemed that the collection was mostly solid and necrotic therefore not amenable to drainage. Enterococcus faecium sensitive to Vancomycin was isolated from the aspirate. The drain dislodged 2 days postinsertion and was not replaced as the preceding output had been minimal.

The patient contracted COVID-19 during his stay and was taken over by the Infectious Diseases team as per the hospital policy. He developed a hypoactive delirium secondary to his COVID-19 infection and subsequently passed away, likely due to COVID-19-related complications.

3. Discussion

Urinary catheterisation is a common intervention performed for a variety of reasons including urinary retention, monitoring of urinary output in critically ill patients and selected surgical cases, and in prolonged immobilisation [1]. Although there is variation in the figures reported in the literature, it is estimated that approximately 25% of patients admitted to hospital have a urinary catheter during their inpatient stay [2]. A UK study performed in 2017 found that 18.6% of hospital inpatients had a urinary catheter at any one time [3]. Despite the relative ubiquity of catheterisation as an intervention, there are several complications associated with this process, including infection, trauma, malignancy, hypersensitivity, blockage, and fistula formation [4, 5].

It has been recorded that genitourinary trauma due to catheterisation occurs in 1.5% of catheter days [5]. A review of iatrogenic urethral catheterisation injuries performed across two Irish tertiary centres calculated the total cost of managing 37 injuries over a 6 month period as

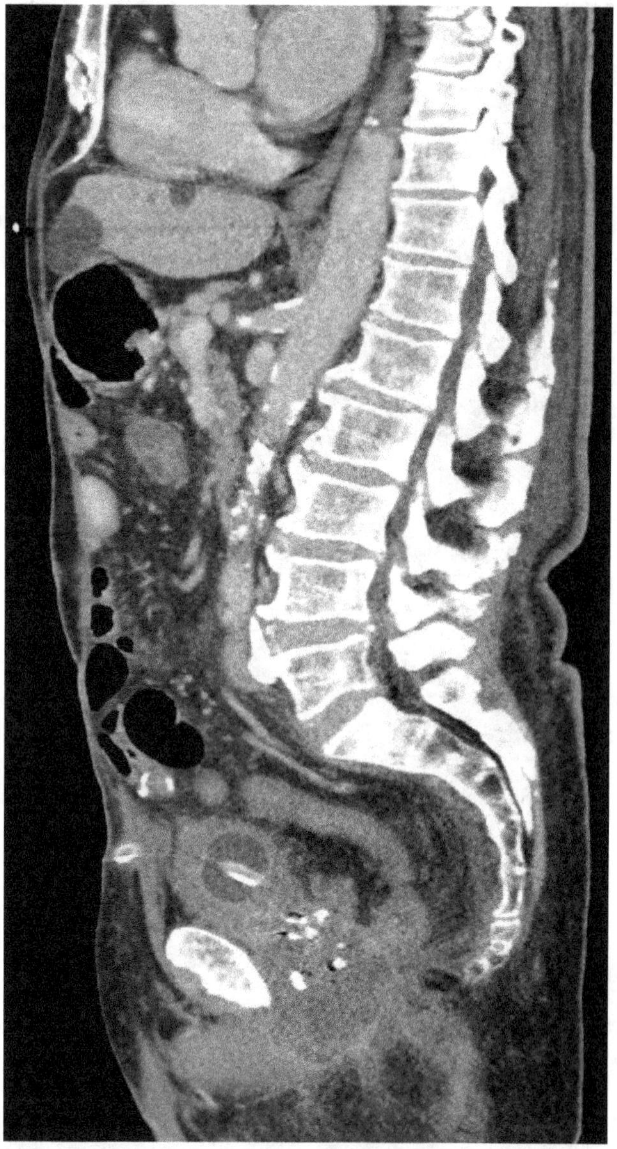

Figure 6: Saggital CT imaging demonstrating persistence of collection post antibiotic treatment.

€335,377 [6]. Clearly, urethral catheterisation represents a significant burden of cost and morbidity. Dellimore et al. [4] describe how severe urethral trauma, which includes perforation, is directly related to mechanical interaction between the catheter and urethra, with additional catheter characteristics such as shape and physical properties as possible contributing factors. As a potential strategy to combat this, they recommend alterations to catheter manufacturing to produce catheters that have a hydrophyllic, antibacterial, low-friction, and durable coating, with a less-rigid tip, stiff shaft, and a structure that allows minimal contact between the catheter and urethra [4].

Rectal perforation is indeed a rare complication of urethral catheter insertion, with few previous cases reported in the literature [7]. Therefore, little is known about such an occurrence. We attribute the cause of our patient's rectal perforation to his previous brachytherapy treatment and known proctitis. Brachytherapy is a common treatment choice for localised prostate cancer [8]. However, it is associated with several adverse effects including radiation proctitis, sexual dysfunction, incontinence, urethral stricture, and haematuria [9]. Rectourethral fistula is also a recognised complication of brachytherapy treatment [10]. However, given that this patient had a recent endoscopy which only demonstrated proctitis and denied a history of passing urine per rectum, it is unlikely that he had a preceding rectourethral fistula. Radiation proctitis can induce tissue changes of endarteritis, inflammation, and fibrosis [11, 12]. This can result in friable and ulcerated tissue, which can be more susceptible to injury, as happened to this patient. This case is a cautionary tale about the potential harms that can result from what is considered a common and relatively straightforward procedure.

Consent

Informed, written consent was obtained from the patient prior to the submission of this manuscript; however, no identifiable patient information is included in this document.

References

[1] J. Meddings, M. A. M. Rogers, S. L. Krein, M. G. Fakih, R. N. Olmsted, and S. Saint, "Reducing unnecessary urinary catheter use and other strategies to prevent catheter-associated urinary tract infection: an integrative review," *Safety*, vol. 23, no. 4, pp. 277–289, 2014.

[2] S. Saint, J. Wiese, J. K. Amory et al., "Are physicians aware of which of their patients have indwelling urinary catheters?," *The American Journal of Medicine*, vol. 109, no. 6, pp. 476–480, 2000.

[3] M. Giles, L. Graham, J. Ball et al., "Variations in indwelling urinary catheter use in four Australian acute care hospitals," *Journal of Clinical Nursing*, vol. 28, no. 23-24, pp. 4572–4581, 2019.

[4] K. H. Dellimore, A. R. Helyer, and S. E. Franklin, "A scoping review of important urinary catheter induced complications," *Journal of Materials Science: Materials in Medicine*, vol. 24, no. 8, pp. 1825–1835, 2013.

[5] A. M. Leuck, D. Wright, L. Ellingson, L. Kraemer, M. A. Kuskowski, and J. R. Johnson, "Complications of Foley catheters–is infection the greatest risk?," *The Journal of Urology*, vol. 187, no. 5, pp. 1662–1666, 2012.

[6] N. F. Davis, M. R. Quinlan, N. R. Bhatt et al., "Incidence, cost, complications and clinical outcomes of iatrogenic urethral catheterization injuries: a prospective multi-institutional study," *The Journal of Urology*, vol. 196, no. 5, pp. 1473–1477, 2016.

[7] A. Zachariou, A. Kolynou, and M. Filiponi, "Rectal perforation: a rare complication of indwelling urethral catheterization," *Hippokratia*, vol. 21, no. 1, p. 58, 2017.

[8] A. R. Mundy and D. E. Andrich, "Posterior urethral complications of the treatment of prostate cancer," *BJU International*, vol. 110, no. 3, pp. 304–325, 2012.

[9] T. J. Wilt, R. MacDonald, I. Rutks, T. A. Shamliyan, B. C. Taylor, and R. L. Kane, "Systematic review: comparative effectiveness and harms of treatments for clinically localized prostate cancer," *Annals of Internal Medicine*, vol. 148, no. 6, pp. 435–448, 2008.

[10] D. Shakespeare, D. M. Mitchell, B. M. Carey et al., "Recto-urethral fistula following brachytherapy for localized prostate cancer," *Colorectal Disease*, vol. 9, no. 4, pp. 328–331, 2007.

[11] M. Venerito, K. Mönkemüller, S. Rickes, and P. Malfertheiner, "Gastrointestinal: radiation proctitis," *Journal of Gastroenterology and Hepatology*, vol. 22, no. 5, p. 761-, 2007.

[12] F. Ali and K. Y. Hu, "Evaluation and management of chronic radiation proctitis," *Diseases of the Colon and Rectum*, vol. 63, no. 3, pp. 285–287, 2020.

Permissions

All chapters in this book were first published by Hindawi Publishing Corporation; hereby published with permission under the Creative Commons Attribution License or equivalent. Every chapter published in this book has been scrutinized by our experts. Their significance has been extensively debated. The topics covered herein carry significant findings which will fuel the growth of the discipline. They may even be implemented as practical applications or may be referred to as a beginning point for another development.

The contributors of this book come from diverse backgrounds, making this book a truly international effort. This book will bring forth new frontiers with its revolutionizing research information and detailed analysis of the nascent developments around the world.

We would like to thank all the contributing authors for lending their expertise to make the book truly unique. They have played a crucial role in the development of this book. Without their invaluable contributions this book wouldn't have been possible. They have made vital efforts to compile up to date information on the varied aspects of this subject to make this book a valuable addition to the collection of many professionals and students.

This book was conceptualized with the vision of imparting up-to-date information and advanced data in this field. To ensure the same, a matchless editorial board was set up. Every individual on the board went through rigorous rounds of assessment to prove their worth. After which they invested a large part of their time researching and compiling the most relevant data for our readers.

The editorial board has been involved in producing this book since its inception. They have spent rigorous hours researching and exploring the diverse topics which have resulted in the successful publishing of this book. They have passed on their knowledge of decades through this book. To expedite this challenging task, the publisher supported the team at every step. A small team of assistant editors was also appointed to further simplify the editing procedure and attain best results for the readers.

Apart from the editorial board, the designing team has also invested a significant amount of their time in understanding the subject and creating the most relevant covers. They scrutinized every image to scout for the most suitable representation of the subject and create an appropriate cover for the book.

The publishing team has been an ardent support to the editorial, designing and production team. Their endless efforts to recruit the best for this project, has resulted in the accomplishment of this book. They are a veteran in the field of academics and their pool of knowledge is as vast as their experience in printing. Their expertise and guidance has proved useful at every step. Their uncompromising quality standards have made this book an exceptional effort. Their encouragement from time to time has been an inspiration for everyone.

The publisher and the editorial board hope that this book will prove to be a valuable piece of knowledge for researchers, students, practitioners and scholars across the globe.

List of Contributors

Francisco Renan Doth Sales, Georgia Alexsandra Colantonio Dourado, Ana Carolina Montes Ribeiro, Humberto de Holanda Madeira Barros, David Sucupira Cristino, Antonio Augusto Guterres Castro and Francisco José Cabral Mesquita
Department of Urology, Doctor Cesár Cals General Hospital, Fortaleza, Ceará, Brazil

Irene Chua
Department of Paediatric Surgery, Perth Children's Hospital, Western Australia, Australia

Naeem Samnakay
Department of Paediatric Surgery, Perth Children's Hospital, Western Australia, Australia
Division of Surgery, Medical School, The University of Western Australia, Western Australia, Australia

K. G. Fossi, A. S. Salihou, D. E. C. Dikongue, Salihou Fadi and Bienvenu Binwe
Faculty of Medicine and Biomedical Sciences, University of Yaounde I, Cameroon

E. Njuma Tamufor
Yaounde Gyneco-Obstetric and Pediatric Hospital, Cameroon
Faculty of Medicine and Biomedical Sciences, University of Yaounde I, Cameroon

Landry Mbouché and F. F. Mouafo Tambo
Faculty of Medicine and Biomedical Sciences, University of Yaounde I, Cameroon
Yaounde Gynaeco-Obstetric and Paediatric Hospital, Cameroon

Zachary Werner, Ali Hajiran and Osama Al-Omar
Suite 6300, Health Sciences Center, Morgantown, WV 26506, USA

Oumar Gaye, Ngor Mack Thiam, Yaya Sow, Boubacar Fall and Alain Khassim Ndoye
Urology-Andrology Department, Hôpital Aristide Le Dantec, Senegal

Ayun Cassell
Urology-Andrology Department, Hôpital Général Idrissa Pouye, Senegal

Serigne Mourtalla Gueye
Centre National de Transfusion Sanguine, Dakar, Senegal

Sarah Bouri, Jean-Christophe Noël, Xavier Catteau, Nicky D'Haene and Sandrine Rorive
Department of Pathology, Erasme Hospital, Université Libre de Bruxelles, Brussels, Belgium
Department of Pathology, Centre Universitaire Inter Regional d'Expertise en Anatomie Pathologique Hospitalière, Jumet, Belgium

Walid Al Hajj Obeid, Ilyas Svistakov and Thierry Roumeguère
Department of Urology, Erasme Hospital, Université Libre de Bruxelles, Brussels, Belgium

Ethan Vargo and Neel Parekh
Cleveland Clinic Akron General Department of Urology, Akron General Avenue, Akron, OH 44307, USA

Bryson Cook
Northeast Ohio Medical University, 4209 St, OH-44, Rootstown, OH 44272, USA

Jason Lane and Eric Speakman
Cleveland Clinic Akron General Department of Pathology, Akron General Avenue, Akron, OH 44307, USA

Astrid Van Daele, Johan Schurmans and Raf Van Reusel
AZ Turnhout, Rubensstraat 166, 2300 Turnhout, Belgium

Pietro Pepe, Letterio D'Arrigo, Domenico Patane', Ludovica Pepe, Giuseppe Candiano and Michele Pennisi
Urology Unit-Cannizzaro Hospital, via Messina 829, Catania, Italy
Imaging Department-Cannizzaro Hospital, Catania, Italy

L. O.Mbouché, G. Ondobo Andzé, A. L. Amenglé, J. Zé Mikandé and F. F. Angwafo III
Yaounde Gyneco-Obstetric and Pediatric Hospital, Cameroon
Faculty of Medicine and Biomedical Sciences of University of Yaoundé I, Cameroon

A. S. Nwaha Makon and D. Nyanit Bob
Yaounde Gyneco-Obstetric and Pediatric Hospital, Cameroon

P. Y. Mure
University Teaching Hospital of Lyon, France

Maazou Halidou
Department of Urology, Zinder National Hospital, Zinder, Niger
Faculty of Health Sciences, University of Zinder, Zinder, Niger

Ibrahim Amadou Magagi and Harissou Adamou
Faculty of Health Sciences, University of Zinder, Zinder, Niger
Department of General Surgery, Zinder National Hospital, Zinder, Niger

Amadou Roua
Department of Urology, Regional Hospital Center of Maradi, Maradi, Niger

Mohamed Rouga
Department of General Surgery, Regional Hospital Center of Maradi, Maradi, Niger

Ousseini Adakal
Department of General Surgery, Regional Hospital Center of Maradi, Maradi, Niger
Faculty of Health Sciences, Dan Dicko Dankoulodo University, Maradi, Niger

Soumana Amadou and Rachid Sani
Department of Surgery and Surgical Specialties, Faculty of Health Sciences, University of Niamey, Niamey, Niger

Taisuke Ezaki, Tansei Sanjo and Takeshi Masuda
Department of Urology, Saitama City Hospital, Saitama, Japan

Seiya Akatsuka
Division of Pathology, Department of Central Laboratory, Saitama City Hospital, Saitama, Japan

Umesh Jayarajah and Sanjeewa Seneviratne
Department of Surgery, Faculty of Medicine, University of Colombo, Colombo, Sri Lanka

Lalani de Silva and Chandu de Silva
Department of Pathology, Faculty of Medicine, University of Colombo, Colombo, Sri Lanka

Niall P. Kelly, Adrian Fuentes-Bonachera, William P. Shields, Ivor M. Cullen and Padraig J. Daly
Department of Urology, University Hospital Waterford, Waterford, Ireland

Shivika Ahuja, Hannah Sullivan, Mark Noller, Yun Tan and Daniel Daly
Center for Anatomical Science and Education, Department of Surgery, Saint Louis University School of Medicine, Saint Louis, MO 63104, USA
Urological Surgeons of Northern California, San Jose, CA 95124, USA

Raymond Saa-Eru Maalman and Yaw Otchere Donkor
Department of Basic Medical Sciences, School of Medicine, University of Health and Allied Sciences, Ho, Volta Region, Ghana

Ali Mahamudu Ayamba
Department of Basic Medical Sciences, School of Medicine, University of Health and Allied Sciences, Ho, Volta Region, Ghana
Consultant Urologist, Department of Surgery, School of Medicine, University of Health and Allied Sciences, Ho, Volta Region, Ghana

John Noah Anyorigiya
Medical Officer, Margaret Maquart Catholic Hospital, Kpando, Volta Region, Ghana

Ebtehal Althobaiti, Maryam Aloqalaa and Raghdah Alsharif
Faculty of Medicine, Umm Al-Qura University, Makkah, Saudi Arabia

Hattan Badr
Department of Urology, King Abdullah Medical City, Makkah, Saudi Arabia

Naif Alqarni
Pediatric Urology Division, Pediatric Surgery Department, Maternity and Children Hospital, Makkah, Saudi Arabia

Takanori Sekito, Takuya Sadahira, Kohei Edamura, Motoo Araki and Yasutomo Nasu
Department of Urology, Dentistry and Pharmaceutical Sciences, Okayama University Graduate School of Medicine, 2-5-1 Shikatacho, Kita-ku, Okayama 700-8558, Japan

Masahiro Sugihara
Division of Surgery, Nishi Fukuyama Hospital, 340-1 Matsunagacho, Fukuyama City, Hiroshima 729-0104, Japan

Alhareth Baarimah
Department of Urology, International Medical Center (IMC), Jeddah, Saudi Arabia

Saeed Alshahrani and Latif Dar
Department of Pediatric Urology, Abha Maternity and Child Hospital (AMCH), Abha, Saudi Arabia

Rayan Dashnan, Mohammed Beaiti and Khaled ALDhabaan
Department of Pediatric Urology, Khamis Mushayt Maternity and Children Hospital, Khamis Mushayt, Saudi Arabia

Ibrahim Alnadhari, Ausama Abdulmuhsin, Omar Ali, Ahmad Shamsodini, Morshed Salah and Osama Abdeljaleel
Division of Urology, Department of Surgery, AlWakra Hospital, Hamad Medical Corporation, Doha, Qatar

Ahmed Ibrahimi and Idriss Ziani
Department of Urology A, Ibn Sina University Hospital, Rabat, Morocco
Faculty of Medicine and Pharmacy, Mohammed V University in Rabat, Morocco

Yassine Nouini
Department of Urology A, Ibn Sina University Hospital, Rabat, Morocco
Faculty of Medicine and Pharmacy, Mohammed V University in Rabat, Morocco
Faculty of Medicine and Pharmacy of Rabat Morocco, Ibn Sina Hospital, Department of Urology A, Mohammed V University, Morocco

Hachem El Sayegh and Lounis Benslimane
Faculty of Medicine and Pharmacy of Rabat Morocco, Ibn Sina Hospital, Department of Urology A, Mohammed V University, Morocco
Department of Urology A, Ibn Sina University Hospital, Rabat, Morocco
Faculty of Medicine and Pharmacy, Mohammed V University in Rabat, Morocco

Abdelmoughit Hosni, Laila Jroundi and Fatima Zahra Laamrani
Faculty of Medicine and Pharmacy, Mohammed V University in Rabat, Morocco
Emergency Radiology Department, Ibn Sina University Hospital, Rabat, Morocco

M. Hevia Palacios
Member of Urology Department, Ramon y Cajal Hospital, Spain

M. Álvarez-Maestro
Member of Urology Department, La Paz Universitary Hospital, Spain

J. Gómez Rivas
Member of Urology Department, Clinico San Carlos Hospital, Spain

A. Aguilera Bazan
Section Chief, La Paz Universitary Hospital, Spain

L. Martínez-Piñeiro
Chief Urology Department, La Paz Universitary Hospital, Spain

Seiichi Saito
Art Park Urology Hospital & Clinic, Ishiyama-Higashi 3-1-31, Minami-ku, Sapporo 005 0850, Japan

Mark Arthur
Albany Medical College, Department of General Surgery, Division of Urology, Albany, NY, USA

Jonathan Canete
Albany Medical College, Department of General Surgery, Section of Colon and Rectal Surgery, Albany, NY, USA
Albany Stratton Veterans Affairs Medical Center, Albany, NY, USA

Charles Welliver
Albany Medical College, Department of General Surgery, Division of Urology, Albany, NY, USA
Albany Stratton Veterans Affairs Medical Center, Albany, NY, USA

A. M. Omar Mohamed Ozaal, B. Pragalathan and S. Lavanya
General Surgery, University Surgical Unit, Teaching Hospital Jaffna, Sri Lanka

S. T. Sarma
University Surgical Unit, Teaching Hospital Jaffna, Sri Lanka

Ahmad Dahman
West Virginia University School of Medicine, Morgantown, WV 26506, USA

Daniel McClelland
Department of Urology, West Virginia University School of Medicine, Morgantown, WV 26506, USA

Stanley Zaslau and Robert Shapiro
Department of Urology, West Virginia University School of Medicine, Morgantown, WV 26506, USA
Department of Obstetrics & Gynecology, West Virginia University School of Medicine, Morgantown, WV 26506, USA

Valerie Galvan Turner and Omar Duenas
Department of Obstetrics & Gynecology, West Virginia University School of Medicine, Morgantown, WV 26506, USA

Youssef Kadouri
Faculty of Medicine and Pharmacy of Rabat Morocco, Ibn Sina Hospital, Department of Urology A, Mohammed V University, Morocco

Damien Carnicelli
Department of Urology and Andrology, Center Hospitalier Métropole Savoie, Chambery, France

Mathew Yamoah Kyei
Department of Surgery and Urology, University of Ghana Medical School, Accra, Ghana

Robert Djagbletey
Department of Anaesthesia, University of Ghana Medical School, Accra, Ghana

Afua Darkwa Abrahams
Department of Pathology, University of Ghana Medical School, Accra, Ghana

James Edward Mensah
Department of Surgery and Urology, University of Ghana Medical School, Accra, Ghana

Maria Erodotou, Maria Isaia, Georgios Fragkiadakis and Nikolaos Nikolaou
General Surgery Department, Larnaca General Hospital, Larnaca, Cyprus

Theocharis Tontikidis, Kosmas Tyriakidis and Spyridon Palaiologos
Urology Department, Larnaca General Hospital, Larnaca, Cyprus

Amin A. Karadaghy, Matthew T. Bell and Daniel T. Daly
Center for Anatomical Science and Education, Department of Surgery, Saint Louis University School of Medicine, Saint Louis, MO 63104, USA

Félix Campos-Juanatey
Urology Department, Marqu´es de Valdecilla University Hospital, Institute of Investigation Marqu´es de Valdecilla (IDIVAL), Santander, Spain

José Antonio Portillo Martín
Urology Department, Marqués de Valdecilla University Hospital, University of Cantabria, Santander, Spain

Luisana Castillo Carvajal
University Foundation of Health Sciences, San Jose Hospital, Bogotá, Colombia

Ryan Morris
Texas A&M Health Science Center, USA

John Barnard and Chad Morley
West Virginia University Health Science Center, USA

Andris Romašovs
University of Latvia, Riga, Latvia

Aldis Puķītis and Viktorija Mokricka
University of Latvia, Riga, Latvia
Center of Gastroenterology, Pauls Stradins Clinical University Hospital, PilsoHu iela 13, Riga LV-1002, Latvia

Elina Frolova
Medical Faculty, Riga Stradins University, Riga, Latvia

Victor A. Abdullatif, Jacob Novack, Philip J. Shalhoub, Todd G. Campbell and Joel E. Abbott
Urology, Ascension Macomb-Oakland Hospital, Warren, 48093 MI, USA

Antonio Nacchia, Ferdinando di Giacomoa and Giuseppe Disabato
Urology Department, IRCCS CROB, Rionero in Vulture (PZ), Italy

Arcangelo Di Cerbo, Massimo Dante Di Somma, Giuseppe Patitucci and Giulia Vita
Anatomical Pathology Department, IRCCS CROB, Rionero in Vulture (PZ), Italy

Raquel Varea-Malo and Paola Calleja Hermosa
Urology Department, Marqués de Valdecilla University Hospital, Santander, Cantabria, Spain

Daniel Martínez Revuelta
GP Department, Marqués de Valdecilla University Hospital, Santander, Cantabria, Spain

Felix Campos-Juanatey
Urology Department, Marqués de Valdecilla University Hospital, Santander, Cantabria, Spain
Valdecilla Research Institute (IDIVAL), Santander, Cantabria, Spain

Miguel Angel Correas Gómez
Urology Department, Marqués de Valdecilla University Hospital, Santander, Cantabria, Spain
School of Medicine, University of Cantabria, Santander, Cantabria, Spain

Pierre Azzi
Faculty of Medicine, University of Ottawa, Ottawa, Ontario, Canada

Surasak Puvabanditsin, Miry Shim, Jeffrey Suell, Jeffrey Manzano, Kristin Blackledge, Avram Bursky-Tammam and Rajeev Mehta
Department of Pediatrics, Rutgers Robert Wood Johnson Medical School, New Brunswick, New Jersey, USA

Dominique Bossé
Division of Medical Oncology, The Ottawa Hospital Cancer Center, Ottawa, Ontario, Canada

Ilias Cagiannos
Division of Urology, The Ottawa Hospital, Ottawa, Ontario, Canada

Paul Borowy-Borowski
Department of Pathology and Laboratory Medicine, The Ottawa Hospital, Ottawa, Ontario, Canada

David Tiberi
Division of Radiation Oncology, The Ottawa Hospital Cancer Center, Ottawa, Ontario, Canada

Ali Barki and Anouar El Moudane
Department of Urology, Mohammed IV University Medical Center Oujda, Morocco

Siv Venkat, Andre Matteliano and Darrel Drachenberg
Section of Urology, University of Manitoba, Winnipeg, MB, Canada

Orla Cullivan, Silviu David and Syed Jaffry
Department of Urology, Galway University Hospital, Galway, Ireland

Index

T

U

V

Z

www.ingramcontent.com/pod-product-compliance
Lightning Source LLC
LaVergne TN
LVHW082234200926
848484LV00008B/2351